BODY STRUCTURES & FUNCTIONS

SEVENTH EDITION

DELMAR PUBLISHERS INC.®

ELIZABETH FONG • ELVIRA B. FERRIS • ESTHER G. SKELLEY

NOTICE TO THE READER

Cover illustration by Sheri Amsel

Delmar Staff

Executive Editor: Leslie F. Boyer
Associate Editor: Marjorie A. Bruce
Editing Manager: Barbara A. Christie

Project Editor: Ruth East
Design Coordinator: Susan Mathews
Publications Coordinator: Linda Helfrich

For information, address Delmar Publishers Inc.
2 Computer Drive West, Box 15-015
Albany, New York 12212

Printed in the United States of America
Published simultaneously in Canada
by Nelson Canada,
a division of International Thomson Limited

10 9 8 7 6 5 4 3 2 1

Library of Congress Cataloging in Publication Data

Fong, Elizabeth
    Body structures and functions / Elizabeth Fong, Elvira B. Ferris,
Esther G. Skelley.
        p.   cm.
    Ferris's name appears first on the 6th edition.
    Includes index.
    ISBN 0-8273-3481-8 (pbk.). IBSN 0-8273-3482-6
(instructor's guide)
        1. Human physiology. 2. Anatomy, Human. 3. Nursing. I. Ferris,
Elvira B. (Elvira Binello). II. Skelley, Esther G.
III. Title.
QP34.5.F66 1989   88-20411
    612--dc19   CIP

CONTENTS

CHAPTER
1

THE BODY
AS A WHOLE

CHAPTER
2

THE BODY
FRAMEWORK

CHAPTER
5

BREATHING
PROCESSES

CHAPTER
6

DIGESTION
OF FOOD

CHAPTER
7

ELIMINATION
OF WASTE
MATERIALS

CHAPTER 8

HUMAN REPRODUCTION

CHAPTER 9

REGULATORS OF BODY FUNCTIONS

CHAPTER
10

**COORDINATION
OF BODY
FUNCTIONS**

PREFACE

Introduction

The 7th edition of *Body Structures and Functions* has been extensively revised to reflect content areas of increased importance to those preparing for entry into the various health science careers. More than ever before, numerous job opportunities in health care exist for those who have successfully completed an approved course of instruction. It is projected that the changing health care delivery system in the United States will require more and more certified and licensed health professionals well into the twenty-first century.

The intent of the 7th edition of this text is to help learners master the essential concepts of the organization and structure of the body components (anatomy) and the functions (physiology) of each structure and the interrelationships between structures. This base of information is crucial to successfully completing the course and entering a health care career.

Using an easily readable writing style and numerous well-executed line drawings, the text presents an overview of each body system. Explanations are provided of how these systems work together to achieve a balanced state—homeostasis. Clear and concise discussions of common disorders (pathophysiology) introduce the student to the effects of dysfunction.

Special Features of This Edition

- Expanded use of color in the illustrations and tables to highlight key concepts, show changes in state or position, and emphasize details.

- New units include:

  Unit 2   Chemistry of Living Things (introduces biochemistry and the functioning of human cells)

  Unit 6   Tissue Repair (explains the physiology of how tissues begin the process of healing following a trauma)

  Unit 32   Role of Nutrients, Vitamins, and Minerals in Health Care

  Unit 39   Menstrual Cycle and Menopause (describes the stages of the menstrual cycle and the changes in the menopausal female—anatomical, physiological, and psychological)

Unit 40   Genetics and Genetically Linked Diseases (provides the basic theory of the genetic transmission of disease and describes several of the more common genetically linked diseases such as Downs Syndrome and Tay-Sachs Disease)

- Unit 7 (was Unit 32) on the Integumentary System was reorganized and expanded to reflect the importance of the skin as the largest organ of the body, the first line of defense against infectious organisms, and as a temperature regulator, among other functions.

- Greatly expanded number of tables summarizes essential information and provides a means of ready reference; they are listed at the end of the Contents for improved accessibility.

- Key words in the text are printed in boldface for easy recognition.

- Expanded unit on principal skeletal muscles includes 6 new tables of major muscles, effects of sports training and work on muscle strength and efficiency, and the effects of massage on muscles.

- More pathophysiology (study of common disorders) has been added to all body systems sections.

- Expanded coverage of the male and female reproductive systems includes new content and illustration of cell division.

- In the unit on the blood, an added section explains the inflammation process.

- In the unit on the lymphatic system, major sections have been added on natural and acquired immunities, autoimmunity, hypersensitivity, AIDS and ARC.

Features Retained From Previous Editions

In addition to the major changes described previously, the 7th edition of *Body Structures and Functions* retains the following features for an effective teaching/ learning approach to the subject:

- Content is organized by body system in the sequence usually taught.

- Specific and measurable learning objectives are listed at the beginning of each unit.

- A list of key words at the beginning of each unit alerts learners to their use within the text.

- A 16-page insert with 20 full-color anatomical illustrations and a full-color chart show pH color changes for common acids, bases, and human body fluids.

- Topics for further study and discussion appear at the end of each unit to promote learner involvement in the subject and to provide opportunities for further enrichment and application of knowledge.

- Where appropriate, guidelines for laboratory study are presented.

- Well-organized tables summarize important concepts/data for ready reference (expanded for 7th edition).

- Nearly 500 unit review questions test student comprehension of concepts; they are helpful in identifying areas where learners may require further study.

- Self-evaluation tests for each section further reinforce learning and understanding of content.

- Comprehensive glossary of terms with a pronunciation guide is located at the back of the text (expanded for 7th edition).

Supplements

The supplements for the 7th edition include an Instructor's Guide and a slide set. The Instructor's Guide includes answers to all assignment and self-evaluation questions. In addition, transparency masters are provided to help the instructor in the preparation of visuals to augment classroom instruction. The Guide also contains a section of anatomical drawings with instructions for coloring to help students learn the components of the human body.

The augmented slide set contains slides of anatomical illustrations designed to facilitate and reinforce classroom instruction.

About The Authors

Previous editions of *Body Structures and Functions* were written by the late Esther G. Skelley and Elvira Ferris. Both authors were actively involved in education and had several books published. Esther Skelley was the author of *Medications and Mathematics for the Nurse;* and Elvira Ferris wrote *Microbiology for Health Careers,* with Elizabeth Fong as her co-author for the most recent edition. Elizabeth Fong, as assistant chairperson of the Biology Department at Brooklyn Technical High School, New York, pioneered a new and innovative biomedical program. In addition to *Body Structures and Functions,* she is also co-author of the successful second edition of *Microbiology for Health Careers.*

Acknowledgments

The author and staff of Delmar Publishers wish to thank Professor Loretta Chiarenza for her contributions to the 7th edition of *Body Structures and Functions.*

Professor Chiarenza teaches anatomy and physiology at the State University of New York at Farmingdale, New York. Units 32 and 40 were technically edited and expanded by Professor Chiarenza. In addition, she served as a technical consultant for the revised manuscript. Her efforts on behalf of the new edition are very much appreciated.

Appreciation is also expressed to the instructors who provided recommendations for the revision and who reviewed the manuscript for the new edition at various stages:

Grace Turner, RN, Connersville Area Vocational School,
 Connersville, IN
Dorethea Y. Carter, Harding Business College, Maple Heights, OH
Roy A. Schreck, Jordan College, Fremont, MI
Joanne Brickley, Thompson School for Practical Nurses,
 Brattleboro, VT
Joan M. Wolf, RN, MS, Buckeye Joint Vocational School,
 New Philadelphia, OH
Linda Niosi, Brookhaven Occupational Center, Belport, NY
Michael L. Decker, BS, MA, Omaha College of Health Careers,
 Omaha, NB
Barbara Simon, Missouri School for Doctor's Assistants,
 St. Louis, MO
Jan Blake, Sawyer College, Dayton, OH
Katherine Kucinkas, RN, Mansfield Business College, San Antonio, TX
Lisa Staples, Draughons Junior College, Memphis, TN
Alice M. Pfeninger, Greater New Bedford Vocational-Technical
 High School, New Bedford, MA

Reviewers

Daniel M. Greenfield, DC, Empire Technical Schools, New York, NY
Teri Sword, RN, Huntington Junior College of Business, Huntington, WV
Mary E. Arnold, BSN, RN, CMA, Western Career College, Sacramento, CA
Clyde Victoria Staples, Draughons Junior College, Memphis, TN
Linda Cox, American Careers, San Antonio, TX
Maureen Sparks, Lawton School, San Jose, CA
Ollie Eldridge, RN, Mansfield Business College, Charleston, SC
Virginia Sasser, RN, Mansfield Business College, Charleston, SC
Loretta Chiarenza, MA, MS, State University of New York at Farmingdale,
 Farmingdale, NY

COLOR PLATES AND TABLES

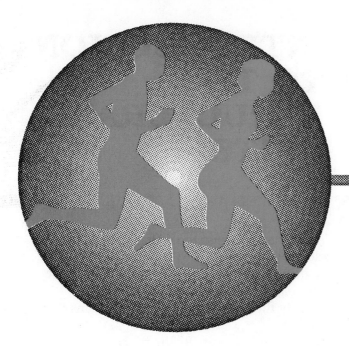

CHAPTER 1

THE BODY AS A WHOLE

UNIT
1

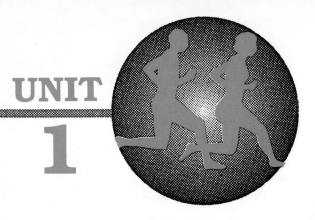

INTRODUCTION TO THE STRUCTURAL UNITS

KEY WORDS

abdominal cavity
abdominopelvic
   cavity
anabolism
anatomical
   position
anatomy
angiology
anterior
arthrology
biology
catabolism
caudal
comparative
   anatomy
coronal
   (frontal)
cranial
cytology
deep
dermatology
developmental
   anatomy
diaphragm

distal
dorsal
embryology
endocrinology
external
gametes
gross anatomy
histology
homeostasis
inferior
internal
lateral
life function
medial
mediastinum
metabolism
microscopic
   anatomy
morphology
myology
nasal cavity
neurology
oral (buccal)
   cavity

orbital cavity
organ system
osteology
pelvic cavity
physiology
pleura
posterior
proximal
regional
   (topographic)
   anatomy
sagittal
splanchnology
spinal cavity
sternum
superficial
superior
systematic anatomy
thoracic cavity
transpyloric plane
transtubercular
   plane
transverse
ventral

OBJECTIVES

- Identify and discuss the different branches of anatomy
- Identify the terms referring to location, direction, planes, and sections of the body
- Identify the body cavities and the organs they contain
- Identify and discuss the life functions
- Define the Key Words that relate to this unit of study

ANATOMY AND PHYSIOLOGY

Both anatomy and physiology are branches of a much larger science called **biology.** Biology, itself, is the study of all forms of life. Biology studies microscopic one-celled organisms, multicelled organisms, plants, animals, and humans.

Anatomy studies the shape and structure of an organism's body and the relationship of one body part to another. The word anatomy comes from the Greek, *ana,* meaning apart, and *temuein,* to cut; thus, the acquisition of knowledge on human anatomy comes basically from dissection. However, one cannot fully appreciate and understand anatomy without the study of its sister science, **physiology.** Physiology studies the function of each body part and how the functions of the various body parts coordinate to form a complete living organism.

Branches of Anatomy

Anatomy, itself, is subdivided into many branches based on the investigative techniques used, the type of knowledge sought after, or the parts of the body under study.

1. **Gross Anatomy.** Gross anatomy is the study of large and easily observable structures on an organism. This is done through dissection and visible inspection with the naked eye. In it the different body parts and regions are studied with regard to their general shape, external features, and main divisions. The study of shape is called **morphology.** The study of the different regions of the body by dissection and by way of sections taken through the body at different angles is known as **regional** or **topographic anatomy.**

2. **Microscopic Anatomy.** With the invention and perfection of the microscope, the knowledge of gross anatomy can be extended down to the microscopic level. Microscopic anatomy is subdivided into two branches. One is called **cytology,** which is the study of the structure, function, and development of cells that make up the different body parts. For example, cytology can study the heart cells or the nerve cells comprising the brain. The other subdivision is **histology,** which studies the tissues and organs making up the entire body of an organism.

3. **Developmental Anatomy.** This part of anatomy studies the growth and development of an organism during its lifetime. More specifically, **embryology** studies the formation of an organism from the fertilized egg to birth.

4. **Comparative Anatomy.** Man is one of many animals found in the Animal Kingdom. As such, the different body parts and organs of man can be studied with regard to similarities and differences to other animals in the Animal Kingdom.

5. **Systematic Anatomy.** Systematic anatomy is the study of the structure and function of various organs or parts making up a particular organ system. Depending upon the particular organ system under study, a specific term is applied:

    a. **angiology**—the study of the circulatory system

    b. **arthrology**—the study of joints

    c. **dermatology**—the study of the integumentary system (skin, hair, and nails)

    d. **endocrinology**—the study of the endocrine or hormonal system

    e. **myology**—the study of the muscular system

    f. **neurology**—the study of the nervous system

    g. **osteology**—the study of the skeletal system

    h. **splanchnology**—the collective study of the digestive, respiratory, reproductive, and urinary systems.

ANATOMIC TERMINOLOGY

In the study of anatomy and physiology, special words are used to describe the specific location of a structure or organ, or the relative position of one body part to another. Refer to figure 1-1 frequently while studying the following terms.

The following terms are used to describe the human body as it is standing in the **anatomical position.** A human being in such a position is standing erect, with face forward, arms at the side, and palms forward.

Terms Referring to Location or Position and Direction

- **anterior** or **ventral** means "front" or "in front of." For example, the knees are located on the anterior surface of the human body. A ventral hernia may protrude from the front or belly of the abdomen.

- **posterior** or **dorsal** means "back" or "in back of." For example, human shoulder blades are found on the posterior surface of the body. The dorsal aspect of the foot is the back or sole of the foot.

- **cranial** and **caudal** refer to direction; cranial means the head end of the body, caudal means the tail end. For example, cranial pressure causes headache. Caudal anesthesia is injected in the lower spine.

- **superior** and **inferior**—superior means "upper" or "above another," inferior refers to "lower" or "below another." For example, the heart and lungs are situated superior to the diaphragm, while the intestines are inferior to it.

- **medial** and **lateral**—medial (sometimes called mesial) signifies "toward the midline or median plane of the body," while lateral means "away, or toward the side of the body."

- **proximal** and **distal**—proximal means "toward the point of attachment to the body, or toward the trunk of the body," distal means "away from the point of attachment or origin, or farthest from the trunk." For example, the hand is proximal to the wrist; the elbow is distal to the shoulder. Note: these two words are used primarily to describe the appendages or extremities.

- **superficial** or **external** and **deep** or **internal**—superficial implies on or near the surface of the body. For instance, a superficial wound just involves an injury to the outer skin. A deep injury involves damage to an internal organ such as the stomach. The terms external and internal are specifically used to refer to body cavities and hollow organs.

Terms Referring to Body Planes and Sections

- **sagittal, coronal,** and **transverse planes** — a sagittal or median plane is a lengthwise cut that divides the body into right and left halves. It starts from the middle of the skull, bisecting the breastbone (sternum) and the vertebral column, figure 1-1. The word **sagittal** is derived from the sagittal suture along the skull, which coincides with the midline of the body.

A coronal (frontal) plane is a vertical cut at right angles to the sagittal plane, dividing the body into anterior and posterior portions. The term **coronal** comes from the coronal suture which runs perpendicular (at a right angle) to the sagittal suture. A **transverse** or cross section is a horizontal cut that divides the body into upper and lower parts.

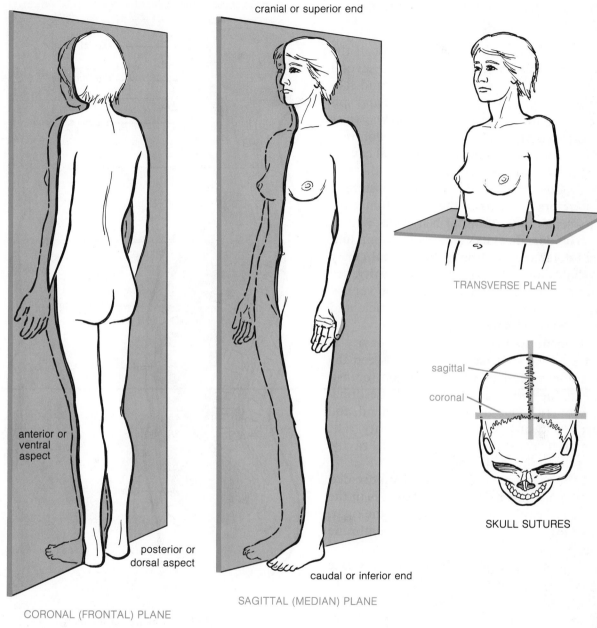

Figure 1-1   **Anatomical terms are used to describe body divisions into parts.**

Terms Referring to Cavities of the Body

The organs which comprise most of the nine body systems are organized into several cavities: cranial, spinal, thoracic, and abdominopelvic, figure 1-2. The cranial and spinal cavities are within a larger region known as the dorsal cavity. The thoracic and abdominopelvic cavities are found in the ventral cavity. The dorsal and ventral cavities are the two major body cavities. The **dorsal** (posterior) cavity refers to the back; the **ventral** (anterior) cavity refers to the front or belly side.

The dorsal cavity contains the brain and spinal cord: the brain is in the **cranial cavity** and the spinal cord is in the **spinal cavity**, see figure 1-2. The **diaphragm** divides the ventral cavity into two parts: the upper thoracic and lower abdominopelvic.

The midpoint of the thoracic cavity is known as the **mediastinum.** It is between the lungs and extends from the **sternum** (breastbone) to the vertebrae of the back. The esophagus, bronchi, lungs, trachea, thymus gland, and heart are located in the thoracic cavity. The heart itself is contained within a smaller cavity, called the pericardial cavity.

The **thoracic cavity** is further subdivided into two pleural cavities: the left lung is in the left pleural cavity, the right lung is in the right. Each lung is covered with a thin membrane which we call the **pleura.**

The **abdominopelvic cavity** is really one large cavity with no separation between the abdomen and pelvis. In order to avoid confusion, this cavity is usually referred to separately – as the abdominal cavity and the pelvic cavity. The **abdominal cavity** contains the stomach, liver, gallbladder, pancreas, spleen, kidneys, small intestine, appendix, and part of the large intestine, see color plate 1. The kidneys are in the back under the lining of the abdominal cavity.

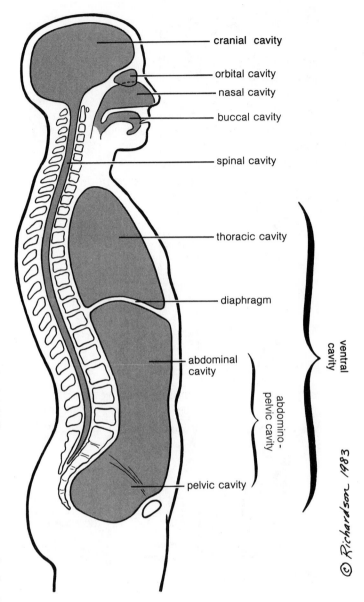

Figure 1-2 Cavities of the body

The urinary bladder, the reproductive organs, the rectum, the remainder of the large intestine, and the appendix are in the **pelvic cavity.**

Terms Referring to Regions in the Abdominopelvic Cavity _____

In order to locate the abdominal and pelvic organs more easily, anatomists have subdivided the abdominopelvic cavity into nine regions and four imaginary planes. The four planes are: two horizontal planes called the **transpyloric** and the **transtubercular** and two sagittal planes called the right lateral and the left lateral planes, see figure 1-3.

The nine regions are located in the upper, middle, and lower parts of the abdomen:

- Upper — The right hypochondriac, epigastric, and left hypochondriac regions lie above the upper line (transpyloric plane). Note that the plane crosses the abdomen at the tip of the ninth rib cartilage.

- Middle — The left lumbar, umbilical, and right lumbar regions are located below the transpyloric plane and above an imaginary line (transtubercular plane) that crosses the abdomen at the top of the hip bones.

- Lower — The left iliac, hypogastric, and right iliac regions lie below the transtubercular plane.

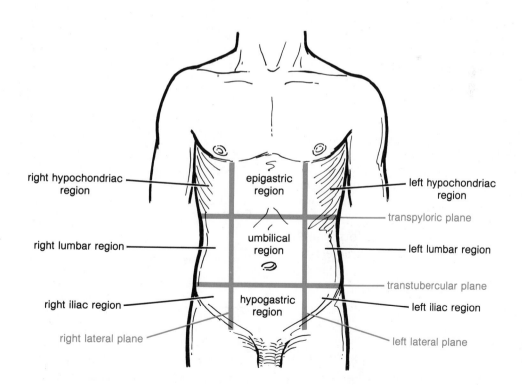

right hypochondriac region

epigastric region

left hypochondriac region

transpyloric plane

right lumbar region

umbilical region

left lumbar region

transtubercular plane

right iliac region

hypogastric region

left iliac region

right lateral plane

left lateral plane

© Richardson 1983

Figure 1-3   Diagram showing the nine regions of the abdominal area

Smaller Cavities

In addition to the **cranial cavity,** the skull also contains several smaller cavities. The eyes, eyeball muscles, optic nerves, and lacrimal (tear) ducts are within the **orbital cavity.** The **nasal cavity** contains the parts that form the nose. The **oral** or **buccal cavity** encloses the teeth and tongue.

LIFE FUNCTIONS

When we examine humans, plants, one-celled organisms, or multicelled organisms, we recognize that all of them have one thing in common: that of being alive.

All living organisms are capable of carrying on life functions. **Life functions** are a series of highly organized and related activities which help living organisms to live, grow, and maintain themselves.

These vital life functions include movement, ingestion, digestion, transport, respiration, synthesis, assimilation, growth, secretion, excretion, regulation (sensitivity) and reproduction, see table 1-1.

HUMAN DEVELOPMENT

A person is born, grows into maturity, and eventually dies. In the intervening years between birth and death, the body carries on a number of life functions which keep us alive and active. As is true of all living things, each one of us inherits a range of size, form, and a lifespan. We inherit these many characteristics through the gametes from our parents. **Gametes** are the sperm and egg cells.

Living depends upon the constant release of energy in every cell of the body. Powered by the energy that is released from food, the cells are able to maintain their own living condition and thus, the life of human beings.

Table 1-1 Review of the Life Functions

LIFE FUNCTIONS	DEFINITION
Movement	The ability of the whole organism — or a part of it — to move
Ingestion	The process by which an organism takes in food
Digestion	The breakdown of complex food molecules into simpler food molecules
Transport	The movement of necessary substances to, into, and around cells, and of cellular products and wastes out and away from cells
Respiration	The burning or oxidation of food molecules in a cell to release energy, water and carbon dioxide
Synthesis	The combination of simple molecules into more complex molecules to help an organism build new tissue
Assimilation	The transformation of digested food molecules into living tissue for growth and self-repair
Growth	The enlargment of an organism due to synthesis and assimilation, resulting in an increase in the number and size of its cells
Secretion	The formation and release of substances from a cell or structure
Excretion	The removal of metabolic waste products from an organism
Regulation (sensitivity)	The ability of an organism to respond to its environment so as to maintain a balanced state (homeostasis)
Reproduction	The ability of an organism to produce offspring with similar characteristics. This is *essential* for species survival as opposed to individual survival

A complex life form like a human being consists of over fifty thousand billion cells. Early in human development, certain groups of cells become highly specialized for specific functions, like motion or response.

Special cells, grouped according to function, shape, size, and structure are called tissues. Tissues, in turn, form larger functional and structural units known as organs. For example, human skin is an organ made up of epithelial, connective, muscular, and nervous tissue. In much the same way, our kidneys are composed of highly specialized connective and epithelial tissue.

The functional activities of cells that result in growth, repair, energy release, use of food, and secretions are combined under the heading of metabolism. Metabolism consists of two processes which are opposite to each other: anabolism and catabolism. **Anabolism** means the building up of complex materials from simpler ones. **Catabolism** is the breaking down and changing of complex substances into simpler ones, with a release of energy. The sum of all the chemical reactions within a cell is, therefore, called **metabolism.**

The proper function and maintenance of the human body depends upon a number of activities. The body must constantly respond to changes in the environment by exchanging substances between its surroundings and its cells. Maintaining the body's cellular environment and function helps to insure regular body functions. Thus optimum cell functioning requires a stable cellular environment (within very narrow limits of acidity, nutrients, oxygen, and temperature).

The maintenance of such (optimal) internal environmental conditions is known as **homeostasis.** Human survival ultimately depends on maintenance or restoration of homeostasis.

The organs of the human body do not operate independently. They function interdependently with one another to form a whole, live, functioning organism. Furthermore, some organs are grouped together because they perform a related function. Such a grouping is called an **organ system.** One example is the digestive system, which is composed of all the organs involved in digestion. The circulatory system includes all the organs related to circulation.

The functioning of complex organisms like human beings includes the combined activities of cells, tissues, organs, and systems. The remainder of this section will cover the structure and functions of cells, specialized groups of cells which are called tissues, and the organs which make up the various systems. In other units of the text, each of the body systems will be discussed in more detail.

Assignment

A. Associate each term in column I with its correct description in column II.

Column I	Column II
_____ 1. catabolism	a. the sum of all the chemical reactions within the cell
_____ 2. pelvic cavity	b. constructive chemical processes which use food to build complex materials of the body
_____ 3. cranial cavity	
_____ 4. anabolism	
_____ 5. abdominal cavity	c. useful breakdown of food materials resulting in the release of energy
_____ 6. dorsal cavity	d. contained within the thoracic cavity
_____ 7. metabolism	e. cavity in which the reproductive organs, urinary bladder, and lower part of large intestine are located
_____ 8. tissue	
_____ 9. kidneys, ureters, and adrenal glands	f. cavity in which the stomach, liver, gallbladder, pancreas, spleen, appendix, cecum, and colon are located
_____ 10. heart and lungs	
_____ 11. life function	g. the cavity containing both the cranial and spinal cavities
_____ 12. organ system	h. a group of cells which together perform a particular job
	i. portion of the dorsal cavity containing the brain
	j. divides the ventral cavity into two regions
	k. structures located behind the abdominal cavity and under its lining
	l. located in the abdominopelvic cavity
	m. organs grouped together because they have a related function
	n. an activity that a living thing performs to help it live and grow

B. Briefly answer the following questions.

1. Define the terms anatomy and physiology.

2.   Describe what is studied in each of the following branches of anatomy.
     a. Gross anatomy

     b. Developmental anatomy

     c. Comparative anatomy

     d. Systematic anatomy

3.   Define the terms coronal section and sagittal section.

4.   Name the body cavities and list the organs in each cavity.

5.   List four life functions and describe how they help to maintain homeo-
     stasis in the body.

UNIT 2

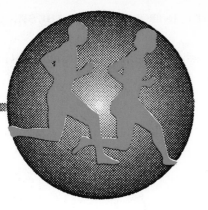

CHEMISTRY OF LIVING THINGS

KEY WORDS

acid
alkali
amino acid
apoenzyme
base
biochemistry
buffer
carbohydrate
coenzyme
compound
dehydration
   synthesis
disaccharide
element

enzyme
formula
hydrolysis
hydronium ion
hydroxide
ionize
lustrous
messenger RNA
   (m = RNA)
molecule
monosaccharide
multicellular
neutralization
nucleotide

organic catalysts
organic compound
oxidation
pH scale
phase
polymer
polysaccharide
property
salt
trace elements
transfer RNA
   (t = RNA)
unicellular
yield

OBJECTIVES

- Relate the importance of chemistry and bio-chemistry to health care
- Explain the value of a formula and give at least four examples
- Describe the difference between a dilute solution and a concentrated solution
- Describe the difference between an inorganic compound and an organic compound, and list some examples of each
- Differentiate between the messenger RNA molecule and the transfer RNA molecule
- Explain the process of neutralization and list the products it forms
- Explain indicators and give some examples
- Describe a pH scale and tell what it attempts to measure
- Explain why the maintenance of a specific pH is crucial to all living organisms
- Define the key words that relate to this unit of study

In order for an individual to be an effective health care professional, an understanding of the normal and abnormal functioning of the human body is essential. To this end, a knowledge of basic chemistry and biochemistry is needed.

Chemistry is the study of the structure of matter, the composition of substances, their properties, their chemical reactions, and synthesis. There are many chemical reactions that occur in the human body. These reactions can range from the digestion of a piece of meat in the stomach and formation of urine in the kidneys to the manufacture of proteins in a microscopic human cell. Ultimately, the chemical reactions necessary to sustain life occur in the cells. Thus, the study of the chemical reactions of living things is called **biochemistry.**

BASIC CHEMISTRY

Despite the small size of microorganisms, their ability to live and thrive has affected many areas of our daily life. Health care professionals must have knowledge of the behavior of microbes in order to control them. The behavior and function of all microorganisms is dependent upon many biochemical processes and reactions which occur inside of them. In the study of microbes at the molecular level, scientists have gained an insight into the chemical basis of life. In order to reach some understanding of microbiology at the molecular level, it is wise to have some knowledge of basic chemistry.

The basic chemistry in this chapter will serve as background or reference information for many microbiological ideas mentioned throughout the book. Students with a prior knowledge of chemistry will find it to be a helpful review, while others will encounter it for the first time.

ELEMENTS

All matter can exist in one of three states or **phases** — solid, liquid, or gas. Nonliving matter under a given temperature and pressure exists in only one phase. Although living matter appears somewhat solid, it usually contains more than one phase. For instance, in humans we find bone (basically solid), body fluid (basically liquid), and the contents of the lungs (basically gaseous).

If matter (whether living or nonliving) was broken down into its smallest basic particles, we would discover that all of these particles are the same. These basic building blocks of all matter are called **elements.** An element is a substance in its simplest form that cannot be broken down any further by ordinary means. There are 92 elements that are found naturally in nature. Besides the natural elements, there are at least 13 additional elements that have been made by humans. Some of these human-made elements are curium, neptonium, and plutonium. All of the elements are represented by a chemical symbol or an abbreviation. Generally, the symbol comes from the first letter or first two letters of the element. Other symbols come from the Latin term for the element, such as aurum (Au) for gold and argentum (Ag) for silver. Table 2–1 shows a sampling of some elements and their chemical symbols.

Of the 105 elements, there are about 20 elements that are generally found in all living things. Among these 20 elements, there are 4 elements that make up 97 percent of all living matter. These are carbon (C), oxygen (O), hydrogen (H), and nitrogen (N) in varying combinations. The other 16 elements are: sodium

Table 2–1 Some Sample Elements and Their Symbols

ELEMENT	SYMBOL
Aluminum	Al
Calcium	Ca
Carbon	C
Gold	Au
Hydrogen	H
Iodine	I
Iron	Fe
Mercury	Hg
Nitrogen	N
Oxygen	O
Phosphorus	P
Silicon	Si
Silver	Ag

(Na), chlorine (Cl), magnesium (Mg), phosphorus (P), sulfur (S), calcium (Ca), potassium (K), iron (Fe), copper (Cu), manganese (Mn), zinc (Zn), boron (B), tin (Sn), vanadium (V), cobalt (Co), and molybdenum (Mo). The last nine are called trace elements because they are present in such small quantities in the body.

COMPOUNDS

Various elements can combine together, in a definite proportion by weight, to form **compounds.** A compound has different characteristics or **properties** from the elements that make them up. For example, the compound water (H_2O) is made of two parts of hydrogen and one part of oxygen. Separately hydrogen and oxygen are gaseous elements, but when combined together to form water, the resulting compound is a liquid. Common table salt is a compound made from the two elements sodium (Na) and chlorine (Cl), and it is chemically called sodium chloride (NaCl). Separately, sodium is a metallic element. It is light, silver-white, and **lustrous** (shiny) when freshly cut, but rapidly becomes dull and gray when exposed to air. Chlorine, on the other hand, is an irritating, greenish-yellow poisonous gas with a very suffocating odor. However, the chemical combination of both sodium and chlorine results in sodium chloride, which is a crystalline powder that can be dissolved in water.

Just as elements are represented by symbols, compounds are represented by something called a **formula.** A formula shows the types of elements present and the proportion of each element present by weight. Some common formulas are H_2O (water), NaCl (common table salt), HCl (hydrogen chloride or hydrochloric acid), $NaHCO_3$ (sodium bicarbonate or baking powder), NaOH (sodium hydroxide or lye), $C_6H_{12}O_6$ (glucose or grape sugar), $C_{12}H_{22}O_{11}$ (sucrose or common table sugar), CO_2 (carbon dioxide), and CO (carbon monoxide).

A living organism, whether it is a **unicellular** (one-celled) microbe or a **multicellular** animal or plant, can be compared to a chemical factory. Most living organisms will take the 20 essential elements and change them into needed compounds for the maintenance of the organism. In many living organisms, the elements carbon, hydrogen, and oxygen are united to form **organic compounds** (compounds found in living things containing the element carbon). One group of organic compounds manufactured are **carbohydrates,** such as sugars and starches.

MOLECULES

The smallest unit of a compound that still has the properties of the compound and has the capability to lead its own stable and independent existence is called a **molecule.** For example, the common compound water can be broken down into smaller and smaller droplets. Finally, when the absolutely smallest unit is reached, one has a molecule of water, H_2O.

TYPES OF COMPOUNDS

The various elements can combine to form a great number of compounds. All known compounds, whether natural or synthetic, can be classified into two groups—inorganic compounds and organic compounds.

Inorganic Compounds

Inorganic compounds are compounds that do not contain the element carbon. A few exceptions are carbon dioxide (CO_2) and calcium carbonate ($CaCO_3$). Many inorganic compounds are found in living organisms. Table 2-2 shows a sampling of some inorganic compounds.

Organic Compounds

Organic compounds are compounds found in living things and the products they make. These compounds always contain the element carbon combined with hydrogen and other elements. Carbon has the ability to combine with other carbons and other elements to form a large number of organic compounds. There are more than a million known organic compounds. Their molecules are comparatively large and very complex. By comparison, inorganic molecules are much smaller. There are four main groups of organic compounds: carbohydrates, lipids, proteins, and nucleic acids.

CARBOHYDRATES

All **carbohydrates** are compounds composed of the elements carbon (C), hydrogen

Table 2–2 Different Types of Inorganic Compounds

INORGANIC COMPOUND	CHEMICAL FORMULA
Calcium carbonate	$CaCO_3$
Calcium phosphate	$Ca(PO_4)_2$
Hydrochloric acid	HCl
Phosphoric acid	H_3PO_4
Potassium chloride	KCl
Sulfuric acid	H_2SO_4
Sodium bicarbonate	$NaHCO_3$
Sodium chloride	NaCl
Water	H_2O

(H), and oxygen (O). These elements have twice as many hydrogen as oxygen atoms. Carbohydrates are divided into three groups. They are the monosaccharides, disaccharides, and polysaccharides.

Monosaccharides

Monosaccharides (Gr. **mono,** meaning one, and **sakcharon,** meaning sugar) are sugars that cannot be broken down any further. Hence, they are also called single or simple sugars. There are three types of monosaccharide sugars—glucose, fructose, and galactose.

Glucose (dextrose or grape sugar) is a very important sugar. It is the main source of energy in cells. Glucose is carried by the bloodstream to individual cells. This is why it is also called blood sugar. In the cell, glucose combines with oxygen in a chemical reaction called **oxidation** that produces energy for a cell.

Fructose is a sugar found in fruits and honey, and is the sweetest monosaccharide.

Galactose is found in small amounts in agar and flaxseed.

Disaccharides

A **disaccharide** is known as a double sugar because it is formed from two monosaccharide molecules by a chemical reaction called **dehydration synthesis.** Dehydration synthesis involves the synthesis of a large molecule from small ones by the loss of a molecule of water. Table 2-3 illustrates the process of dehydration synthesis.

Table 2–3 The Monosaccharide Composition of Sucrose, Maltose, and Lactose

MONOSACCHARIDE + MONOSACCHARIDE − H_2O (DEHYDRATION SYNTHESIS)	FORMS	DISACCHARIDE
Glucose + Fructose − H_2O	→	Sucrose
Glucose + Glucose − H_2O	→	Maltose
Glucose + Galactose − H_2O	→	Lactose

The opposite reaction to dehydration synthesis is **hydrolysis.** In this reaction, a large molecule is broken down into smaller molecules by the addition of water. Examples of disaccharides are sucrose (table sugar), maltose (malt sugar), and lactose (milk sugar).

Polysaccharides

A large number of carbohydrates found in or made by living organisms and microbes are polysaccharides. **Polysaccharides** are large, complex molecules made up of hundreds to thousands of glucose molecules bonded together in one long chainlike molecule. Such a collection of many similar, repeating molecules forming a large molecule is called a **polymer** (meaning "many parts"). Examples of polysaccharide polymers are starch, cellulose, and glycogen. Under the proper conditions, polysaccharides can be broken down into disaccharides and then finally into monosaccharides.

Starch is made in plant cells where it serves as the storage form of glucose. Cellulose is a "tough" molecule that gives support to plant cells. It is the main carbohydrate found in cotton, paper, cellophane, and wood. Glycogen or "animal starch" is the storage form of glucose that is found in the liver and muscles of vertebrates.

LIPIDS

Lipids are molecules containing the elements carbon, hydrogen, and oxygen. Lipids are different from carbohydrates because there is proportionately much less oxygen in relation to hydrogen. For instance, the formula for castor oil is $C_{18}H_{34}O_3$. Examples of lipids are fats, oils, and waxes.

Characteristics of Lipids

At room temperature, fats are solid and oils are liquid even though they have the same molecular structure. Lipids are much better sources of energy than carbohydrates. This simply means that for a given quantity of fat which is oxidized, it will **yield** (give up) more energy than does the same quantity of carbohydrate. However, more glucose molecules are oxidized in a cell for energy than lipids because lipids are harder to oxidize.

Lipids are found in many living organisms, and they are categorized into three groups: simple lipids, compound lipids, and derived lipids.

Simple lipids contain the elements carbon, hydrogen, and oxygen. Examples are fats and oils such as butter, margarine, and corn, olive, peanut, and safflower oils. Other simple lipids are waxes such as beeswax and lanolin.

Compound lipids are composed of carbon, hydrogen, oxygen, nitrogen, and phosphorus. They include the phospholids, which are found in cell membranes, and the glycolipids in brain and nerve cells.

Finally, there are the derived lipids containing only carbon, hydrogen, and oxygen. These include the steroids found in the male and female sex hormones and cholesterol and the fat-soluble vitamins A, D, E, and K.

PROTEINS

Proteins are organic compounds containing the elements carbon, hydrogen, oxygen, and nitrogen and, most times, phosphorus and sulfur. Proteins are among the most diverse and essential organic compounds found in all living organisms. Proteins are found in every part of a living cell. They are found in the nucleus, the cellular organelles, and in the cell membrane. (A more detailed discussion of cellular structures and their functions is found in Unit 3.) Proteins are also an important part of the outer protein coat of all viruses. Proteins also serve as binding and structural components of all living things. For example, large amounts of protein are found in fingernails, hair, cartilage, ligaments, tendons, and muscle.

The small molecular units that make up the very large protein molecules are called **amino acids.** Proteins are large polymers of amino acids. There are 22 different amino acids that can be combined in any number and sequence to make up the various kinds of proteins.

Table 2-4 gives a listing of the 20 naturally occurring amino acids along with their 3-letter symbol. Note that most of the amino acids tend to end in -*ine.*

Table 2–4 The 20 Naturally Occurring Amino Acids

AMINO ACID	SYMBOL
Alanine	Ala
Arginine	Arg
Asparagine	Asn
Aspartic acid	Asp
Cysteine	Cys
Glutamic acid	Glu
Glutamine	Gln
Glycine	Gly
Histidine	His
Isoleucine	Ileu
Leucine	Leu
Lysine	Lys
Methionine	Met
Phenylalanine	Phe
Proline	Pro
Serine	Ser
Threonine	Thr
Tryptophan	Trp
Tyrosine	Tyr
Valine	Val

Table 2–5 The 9 Essential Amino Acids

ESSENTIAL AMINO ACIDS	SYMBOL
Histidine	His
Isoleucine	Ileu
Leucine	Leu
Lysine	Lys
Methionine	Met
Phenylalanine	Phe
Threonine	Trp
Tryptophan	Try
Valine	Val

Table 2-5 gives a list of the nine essential amino acids. Essential amino acids must be ingested because they cannot be made by the body.

Large protein molecules are constructed from any number and sequence of these amino acids. The number of amino acids in any given protein molecule can number from 300 to several thousand. Therefore, the structure of proteins is quite complicated.

ENZYMES

Enzymes are specialized protein molecules that are found in all living cells. They help to finely control the various chemical reactions occurring in a cell, so each reaction occurs at just the right moment and at the right speed. Enzymes help provide energy for the cell, assist in the making of new cell parts, and control almost every process in a cell. Because enzymes are capable of such activity, they are known as **organic catalysts.** An enzyme or organic catalyst affects the rate or speed of a chemical reaction without itself being changed. Enzymes can also be used over and over again. An enzyme molecule is highly specific in its action.

Composition of Enzymes

Enzyme molecules are very large and complex protein molecules. Enzymes are made up of either all protein or part protein attached to a nonprotein part. The protein part of an enzyme molecule is known as an **apoenzyme,** while the nonprotein component is called the **coenzyme.** Minerals such as calcium (Ca), iron (Fe), magnesium (Mg), and copper (Cu) and vitamins like C and B-complex serve as coenzymes.

The name of an enzyme usually ends in -*ase.* The -*ase* ending is added to the stem word taken from the substrate.

Table 2-6 shows some examples of enzyme names.

NUCLEIC ACIDS

Nucleic acids are very important organic compounds containing the elements carbon, oxygen, hydrogen, nitrogen, and phosphorus. There are two types of nucleic acids: one is deoxyribonucleic acid (DNA) and the other is ribonucleic acid (RNA). DNA is involved in the process of heredity. Specific genetic information is carried in the DNA molecule that is found in the nuclear chromosomes and genes of all cells. This genetic information tells a cell what structures it will possess and what functions and behavior it will have. The DNA molecule passes on this genetic information from cell to cell and eventually from one generation to the next. DNA can also be found in the plasma membrane, mitochondria, centrioles, and chloroplasts. (For a more detailed discussion of the cell and its cellular parts and function, see Unit 3.) RNA is essential in helping a cell to synthesize proteins. Proteins are needed to help a cell grow and repair damaged or worn-out parts. Large amounts of RNA can be found in the nucleoli, cytoplasm, and ribosomes of cells.

Structure of Nucleic Acids

Nucleic acids are the largest known organic molecules. They are very high molecular-weight polymers made from thousands of smaller, repeating subunits called **nucleotides.** A nucleotide, itself, is a very complex molecule. It is composed of three different molecular groups. Figure 2–1 shows a typical nucleotide. Group 1 is a phosphate or phosphoric acid group, H_3PO_4, while group 2 represents a five-carbon sugar. Depending upon the nucleotide, the sugar could be either a ribose or a deoxyribose sugar. Finally, group 3 represents a nitrogenous base. There are two groups of nitrogenous bases—one is the purines and the other is the pyrimidines. The purines are either adenine (A) or guanine (G), while the pyrimidines are cytosine (C), thymine (T), or uracil (U).

DNA Structure

The nucleotide structure of a DNA molecule consists of a phosphate group, the deoxyribose* sugar, and any one of the four nitrogenous bases: adenine, thymine, cytosine, and guanine.

Table 2–6 Examples of Some Enzymes and Their Substrates

ENZYME	SUBSTRATE
Amylase	Starch
Lactase	Lactose
Lipase	Lipids
Maltase	Maltose
Protease	Proteins
Sucrase	Sucrose

---

*A deoxyribose sugar is a sugar that has one less oxygen atom than the ribose sugar.

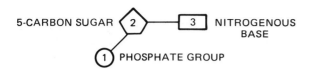

Figure 2-1   Structure of a typical nucleotide

RNA Structure

The RNA nucleotide consists of a phosphate group, the ribose sugar, and any one of the following nitrogenous bases: adenine, cytosine, guanine, and uracil instead of thymine. The RNA molecule is a single-stranded molecule, while the DNA molecule is a double-stranded molecule.

There are three different types of RNA in a cell, the **messenger RNA (m-RNA)**, the **transfer RNA (t-RNA)**, and the **ribosomal RNA (r-RNA).** Messenger RNA carries the instructions for protein synthesis from the DNA molecule located in the nucleus of a cell into the cytoplasm. The m-RNA molecule carries the code for protein synthesis from the DNA in the nucleus to the ribosomes in the cytoplasm. The transfer RNA molecule picks up amino acid molecules in the cytoplasm and transfers them to the ribosomes where they are put together to form proteins. The ribosomal RNA helps in the attachment of the M-RNA to the ribosome. Table 2–7 shows the basic differ-ences between the DNA molecule and the RNA molecule.

ACIDS, BASES, AND SALTS

Before ending the discussion of basic chemistry and biochemistry, a brief discussion of acids, bases, salts, and pH is essential.

Many inorganic and organic compounds found in living organisms are ones that we use in our daily lives. They can be classified into one of three groups—acids, bases, and salts. We are familiar with the sour taste of citrus fruits (grapefruits, lemons, and limes) and vinegar. The sour taste is due to the presence of compounds called acids. What characteristics do acids have to set them apart from the bases and salts?

Acids

An **acid** is a substance that, when dissolved in water, will **ionize*** into positively charged **hydronium ions** (H_3O^+) or **hydrogen ions** (H^+) and negatively charged ions of some other element. (Basically, an acid is a substance that yields hydronium ions (H_3O^+) in solution.) For example, hydrogen chloride

---

*Ionize means the ability of a substance to separate into either positively or negatively charged particles when in solution.

Table 2–7 Differences Between the DNA and RNA Molecules

TYPE OF NUCLEIC ACID	TYPE OF SUGAR PRESENT	TYPE OF BASES PRESENT	PHOSPHATE GROUP	LOCATION	NUMBER OF STRANDS PRESENT
DNA	Deoxyribose	A, T, G, C	Same as RNA	Plasma membrane, mitochondria, chromosomes, chloroplasts, centrioles	2
RNA	Ribose	A, U, G, C	Same as DNA	Cytoplasm, nucleoli, ribosomes	1

(HCl) in pure form is a gas, but when bubbled into water, it becomes hydrochloric acid. How does this happen? Simply, in a water solution hydrogen chloride ionizes into one hydronium ion and one negatively charged chloride ion.

$$HCl + H_2O \longrightarrow H_3O^+ + Cl^-$$
Hydrogen chloride in solution $\longrightarrow$ Hydronium ion + Chloride ion

It is the presence of the hydronium ions that gives hydrochloric acid its acidity and sour taste. (However, one should **not** taste any inorganic acid to identify it as an acid. There are other more reliable and safer methods for the identification of an acid.) A substance can be tested for its acidity through the use of special dyes called litmus paper. In the presence of an acid, blue litmus paper turns red. Table 2–8 gives the names of some

common acids, their formulas, and where they are found.

Bases _____

A **base** or **alkali** is a substance that, when dissolved in water, ionizes into negatively charged **hydroxide** (OH^-) ions and positively charged ions of a metal. For example, sodium hydroxide (NaOH) ionizes into one sodium ion (Na^+) and one hydroxide ion (OH^-). The reaction can be shown as follows:

$$NaOH \longrightarrow Na^+ + OH^-$$
Sodium hydroxide in solution $\longrightarrow$ Sodium ion + Hydroxide ion

Bases have a bitter taste and feel slippery between the fingers. They turn red litmus paper blue. Table 2–9 gives the names of some common bases, their formulas, and location or use.

Table 2–8 Names, Formulas, Location or Use of Some Common Acids

NAME OF ACID	FORMULA	WHERE FOUND OR USAGE
Acetic acid	CH_3COOH	Found in vinegar
Boric acid	H_3BO_3	Weak eyewash
Carbonic acid	H_2CO_3	Found in carbonated beverages
Hydrochloric acid	HCl	Found in stomach
Nitric acid	HNO_3	Industrial oxidizing acid
Sulfuric acid	H_2SO_4	Found in batteries and industrial mineral acid

Table 2–9 Names, Formulas, Location or Use of Some Common Bases

NAME OF BASE	FORMULA	WHERE FOUND OR USAGE
Ammonium hydroxide	NH_4OH	Household liquid cleaners
Magnesium hydroxide	$Mg(OH)_2$	Milk of magnesia
Potassium hydroxide	KOH	Caustic potash
Sodium hydroxide	NaOH	Lye

Neutralization and Salts

When an acid and a base are combined, they form a salt and water. This type of reaction is called a **neutralization.** In a neutralization reaction, hydrogen ions (H^+) from the acid and hydroxide ions (OH^-) from the base join to form water. At the same time, the negative ions of the acid combine with the positive ions of the base to form a compound called a **salt.** For example, hydrochloric acid and sodium hydroxide combine to form sodium chloride and water. The hydrogen ions from the acid unite with the hydroxide ions from the base to form water. The sodium ions (Na^+) combine with the chloride ions (Cl) to form sodium chloride (NaCl). When the water evaporates, solid salt remains. The neutralization reaction is written as shown in figure 2–2.

INDICATORS

Indicators are special chemicals used to test the hydrogen ion concentration present in a particular solution. They are able to do this by changing color according to the hydrogen ion concentration present in a solution. Some of these indicators are litmus paper, bromthymol blue, and phenolphthalein. We have already discussed the value of blue and red litmus paper. Bromthymol blue will turn yellow in the presence of an acid but remains blue in the presence of a base. Phenolphthalein is colorless in an acid solution but changes to pink in a basic solution.

pH

Often it is necessary to determine the pH of a solution. pH is a measure of the acidity or alkalinity (basicity) of a solution. As previously mentioned, special indicators can be used for this purpose, along with special pH meters, to determine the hydrogen or hydroxide ion concentration of a solution on a scale called the *pH scale.* The pH scale, which is used to measure the acidity or alkalinity of a solution, ranges from 0 to 14. A pH of 7 indicates that a particular solution has the same number of hydrogen ions as hydroxide ions. This is a neutral pH, and pure water is neutral with a pH value of 7.0. A pH value of 8 is 10 times as alkaline as a pH of 7; a pH of 9 is 10 times that of 8, etc. Any pH value between zero and 6.9 indicates an acidic solution. The lower the pH number, the stronger the acid or higher hydrogen ion concentration. Any pH value between 7.1 and 14.0 means a solution is basic or alkaline. Thus, the greater the number above 7.0, the stronger the base or greater hydroxide ion concentration. Figure 2-3 shows the pH values of some common acids, bases, and human body fluids. Plate 2 illustrates the color changes that occur on a pH strip when used to test body fluids.

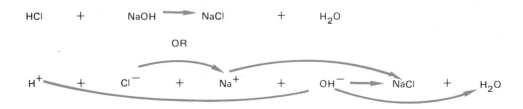

Figure 2-2 The neutralization reaction

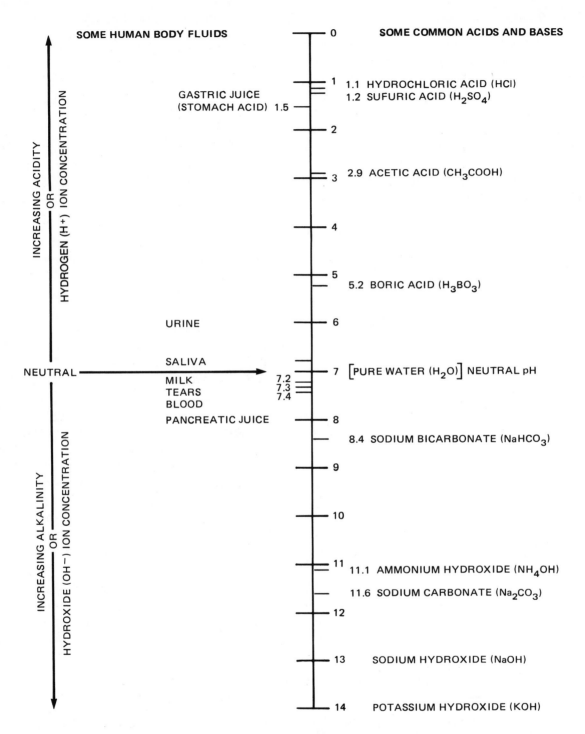

Figure 2-3 pH values of some common acids, bases, and human body fluids

pH of Living Things

As shown in Figure 2-3, living cells and the fluids they produce are usually neither strongly acidic nor strongly alkaline. (The one notable exception is gastric juice, containing hydrochloric acid, that is found in the human stomach.) These fluids, in fact, are nearly neutral. For instance, human tears have a pH of 7.3 and human blood has a pH of 7.4

In order for living cells to function optimally, their biochemical reactions must occur at a given pH. Any marked deviation in the pH causes disruption in the sensitive biochemical processes, illness, or even death of the organism. In humans and other living organisms, the maintenance of a balanced pH, where the fluids are neither too acidic nor too basic, is achieved through a compound called a **buffer.** Sodium bicarbonate ($NaHCO_3$) acts as a buffer in many living organisms. Thus buffers help a living organism to maintain a constant pH value which contributes to the homeostasis or balanced state within all living things.

Further Study and Discussion

- Individually, prepare a brief report on at least 30 of the 105 elements discussing how the name of each element originated.

- Lipids and oils play an important role in our daily lives. Make a list of the various lipids and oils you use every day. Divide the list into the following categories:

FOODS	COOKING OILS	COSMETICS AND DRUGS	HOUSEHOLD USE

- There is much news and controversy over a substance called cholesterol. Prepare a report using library references and contribute your information via a class discussion that should include the following items on cholesterol:
  1. What is cholesterol?
  2. What part of the human body can cholesterol build up in?
  3. How can cholesterol be a health hazard to humans?
  4. What foods should be eliminated or minimized that are very rich in cholesterol?

5. What type of activity and diet would you recommend to an individual who has a cholesterol problem?

• Vitamins are essential in our daily diet. Discuss why this is so. Make a list of at least six vitamins and include the following information:

VITAMIN	FOODS FOUND IN	USES IN THE HUMAN BODY

Assignment

A. Select the letter of the choice which best completes the statement.

1. Organic catalysts are called
   a. enzymes.
   b. indicators.
   c. acids.
   d. ions.

2. Although carbon dioxide contains carbon, it is considered to be an inorganic compound because it lacks the element
   a. sulfur.
   b. hydrogen.
   c. phosphorus.
   d. nitrogen.

3. When an acid and a base are combined, the reaction between the hydrogen ions (H^+) and the hydroxide ions (OH^-) is called
   a. neutralization.
   b. ionization.
   c. dehydration synthesis.
   d. hydrolysis.

4. If blue litmus paper is dipped into gastric juice, it will turn
   a. blue.
   b. colorless.
   c. red.
   d. yellow.

5. Of the following acids, the weakest is
   a. sulfuric.
   b. acetic.
   c. hydrochloric.
   d. nitric.

6. Salt that dissolves in water is called a
   a. solute.
   b. solvent.
   c. mixture.
   d. gas.

7. When proper amounts of an acid and a base are combined, the products formed are a salt and
   a. a gas.
   b. water.
   c. another base.
   d. another acid.

8. An example of an element is
   a. sugar.
   b. starch.
   c. water.
   d. sodium.

9. A solution with a pH of 12 is
   a. neutral.
   b. a base.
   c. organic
   d. an acid.

10. A pH of 5 compared to a pH of 1 represents a hydrogen ion concentration that is
    a. ½ as large.
    b. four times as large.
    c. greater.
    d. less.

11. Compounds that are added to a solution to prevent sudden deviations in pH are known as
    a. ionic.
    b. precipitate.
    c. indicators.
    d. buffers

12. Another name for glucose is
    a. grape sugar.
    b. table sugar.
    c. cane sugar.
    d. milk sugar.

13. A sugar that is used by most cells as a primary source of energy is
    a. deoxyribose.
    b. glucose.
    c. lactose.
    d. maltose.

14. Compounds that are carried to a cell's ribosomes via the t-RNA molecules are
    a. amino acids.
    b. fatty acids.
    c. sugars.
    d. lipids.

15. The formula that represents a carbohydrate compound is
    a. $C_3H_4O_3$.
    b. $CaHPO_4$.
    c. $C_{12}H_{22}O_{11}$.
    d. C_2H_5OH.

16. In cells, the molecule that can release the most energy is
    a. ATP.   c. DNA.
    b. ADP.   d. RNA.

17. Chemical processes that occur within most cells generally occur at a pH that is closest to
    a. 9.1   c. 12.8
    b. 1.1   d. 7.1

18. Vitamins are necessary for the maintenance of living things because vitamins function as
    a. nucleotides.   c. nucleic acids.
    b. coenzymes.   d. apoenzymes.

19. A nucleotide consists of a phosphate group, a sugar group, and a (an)
    a. hydroxide group.   c. amino group.
    b. nitrogenous base.   d. carboxyl group.

20. The pH scale ranges from
    a. 0–13.   c. 1–12.
    b. 1–14.   d. 0–14.

B. Complete each statement with the appropriate word or words to make the statement correct.

1. The sugars glucose, galactose, and fructose are examples of compounds called _____ .

2. The smallest part of an element that still possesses the original properties of the element is called a (an) _____ .

3. Elements that are present in very minute quantities in living things are called _____ elements.

4. The smallest part of a compound that still has the original properties of the compound is called a (an) _____ .

5. Most inorganic compounds separate into ions when the compounds are dissolved in _____ .

6. Compounds that are basic have a (an) _____ taste.

7. A water solution of a substance containing an excess of hydroxide ions is called a (an) _____ .

8. Pure water has a pH of _____ .

9. Compounds that are acidic have a (an) _____ taste.

10. Starch and cellulose molecules are the same in that both consist of many linked molecules of _____ .

11. All organic compounds contain the elements carbon, hydrogen, and _____ .

12. In liver and muscle cells, glucose molecules may be united into large storage molecules called _____ .

13. The building blocks of large protein molecules are called _____ .

14. The type of sugar present in an RNA molecule is called _____ .

15. Guanine and adenine are _____ .

UNIT 3 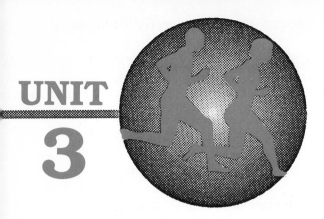 CELLS

KEY WORDS

absolute zero
active transport
anaphase
astral rays
ATP (adenosine
  triphosphate)
carrier-molecule
  complex
cell
cell membrane
cellular
  respiration
centriole
centromere
centrosome
chondrion
chromatid
chromatin
chromosome
cristae
cyclosis
cytokinesis
cytoplasm
deoxyribonucleic
  acid (DNA)
diffusion
diploid number of
  chromosomes
  (2n)

ectoplasm
endoplasm
endoplasmic
  reticulum
  (smooth
  and rough)
enzyme
equatorial plane
equilibrium
filtration
Golgi apparatus
hypertonic
  solution
hypotonic
  solution
interphase
isotonic solution
karyokinesis
karyolymph
lipid
lysosome
metaphase
microtubule
mitochondria
mitosis
multicellular
nuclear
  membrane
nuclear sap

nucleolus
nucleoplasm
nucleus
organelle
osmolality
osmosis
osmotic pressure
phagocytosis
phase
pinocytic vesicle
pinocytosis
pores
polyribosomes
prophase
replication
ribosome
selective
  permeable
  membrane
solutes
solvent
somatic cell
spindle-fiber
  apparatus
telophase
unicellular
vacuole

OBJECTIVES

- Identify the structure of a typical cell
- Define the function of each component of a typical cell
- Relate the function of cells to the function of the body
- Describe the processes that will transport materials in and out of a cell
- Define the Key Words relating to this unit of study

When a field of grass is seen from a distance it looks just like a solid green carpet. Closer observation, however, shows that it is not a solid mass but is made up of countless separate blades of grass. So it is with the body of a plant or animal; it seems to be a single entity, but when any portion is examined under a microscope it is found to be made up of many small discrete parts. These tiny parts, or units, are called **cells.** All living things, whether plant or animal, unicellular or multicellular, large or small, are composed of cells. A cell is microscopic in size. *The cell is the basic unit of structure and function of all living things.*

Since cells are microscopic, a special unit of measurement is employed to determine their size. This is the micrometer (μm), or micron (μ). It is used to describe both the size of cells and their cellular components, table 3-1.

To better understand the structure of a cell, let us compare a living entity—such as a human being—to a house. The many individual cells of this living organism are comparable to the many rooms of a house. Just as each room is bounded by four walls, floor and ceiling, a cell is bounded by a cell membrane. Cells, like rooms, come in a variety of shapes and sizes. Every kind of room or cell has its own unique function. A house can be made up of a single room or many. In much the same fashion, a living thing can be made up of only one cell (**unicellular**), or many cells (**multicellular**).

"Basic" and "typical" are terms used to identify structures common to most living cells.

THE CELL MEMBRANE

Every *cell* is surrounded by a cell membrane. It is sometimes called a plasma membrane. The **cell membrane** separates the cell's *cytoplasm* from its external environment and from the neighboring cells. It also regulates the passage or transport of certain molecules into and out of the cell, while preventing the passage of others. This is why the cell membrane is often called a "selective semi-permeable membrane." The cell membrane is made of protein and **lipid** (fatty substance) molecules arranged in a double layer. This arrangement is rather like a sandwich: the lipid molecules are the filling, and the two layers of protein molecules are the slices of bread.

THE CYTOPLASM

The **cytoplasm** is a sticky semi-fluid material found between the nucleus and the cell membrane. Cytoplasm may be divided into two layers: an outer layer known as the **ectoplasm** and an inner layer called the **endoplasm.** Chemical analysis of the cytoplasm shows that it consists of proteins, lipids, carbohydrates, minerals, salts, and a great deal of water (70%–90%). Each of these substances varies greatly from one cell to the next and from one organism to the next. The cytoplasm is the background for all the chemical reactions which take place in a cell, such as protein synthesis and cellular respiration. Molecules are transported about the cell by the circular motion of the cytoplasm, (**cyclosis**). Embedded in the cytoplasm are **organelles,** or cell structures that help a cell to function. These are the nucleus, mitochondria, ribosomes, Golgi apparatus, endoplasmic reticulum, and the lysosomes. Table 3-2 summarizes the organelles and their functions.

THE NUCLEUS

The **nucleus** is the most important organelle within the cell. It has two vital functions: to control the activities of the cell and to facilitate cell division. This spherical organelle is usually located in or near the center of the cell. Various dyes or stains, like iodine, can be used to make the nucleus stand out. The nucleus

Table 3–1 Units of Length in the Metric System

1 meter	= 39.37 inches
1 centimeter (cm)	= 1/100 or 0.01 meters
1 millimeter (mm)	= 1/1000 or 0.001 meters
1 micrometer (μm) or micron (μ)	= 1/1,000,000 or 0.000001
1 nanometer (nm)	= 1/1,000,000,000 or 0.000000001 meters
1 angstrom (Å)	= 1/10,000,000,000 or 0.0000000001 meters

Table 3–2 Summary Table of Cell Organelles

ORGANELLE	FUNCTION
Cell membrane	Regulates transport of substances into and out of the cell.
Cytoplasm	Provides an organized watery environment in which life functions take place by the activities of the organelles contained in the cytoplasm.
Nucleus	Serves as the "brain" for the control of the cell's metabolic activities and cell division.
Nuclear membrane	Regulates transport of substances into and out of the nucleus.
Nucleoplasm	A clear, semifluid medium that fills the spaces around the chromatin and the nucleoli.
Nucleolus	Functions as a reservoir for RNA.
Ribosomes	Serve as sites for protein synthesis.
Endoplasmic reticulum	Provides passages through which transport of substances occurs in cytoplasm.
Mitochondria	Serve as sites of cellular respiration and energy production.
Golgi apparatus	Manufactures carbohydrates and packages secretions for discharge from the cell.
Lysosomes	Serve as centers of cellular digestion
Pinocytic vesicles	Transport of large particles into a cell.
Centrosome and centrioles	Contains two centrioles that are functional during animal cell division.

stains vividly because it contains **DNA (deoxyribonucleic acid)** and protein. Both readily absorb stains. Surrounding the nucleus is a membrane called the **nuclear membrane.**

The DNA and protein are arranged in a loose and diffuse state called **chromatin.** When the cell is ready to divide, the chromatin condenses to form short, rodlike structures called **chromosomes.** There is a specific number of chromosomes in the nucleus for each species. The number of chromosomes for the human being is 46, or 23 pairs.

When a cell reaches a certain size, it may divide to form two new cells. When this occurs, the nucleus divides first by a process called **mitosis.** During this process, the nuclear material is distributed to each of the two new nuclei. This is followed by division of the cytoplasm into two approximately equal parts through the formation of a new membrane between the two nuclei. It is only during the process of nuclear division that the chromosomes can be seen.

Chromosomes are important because they store the hereditary material—deoxyribonucleic acid (DNA)—which is passed on from one generation of cells to the next.

THE NUCLEAR MEMBRANE

The **nuclear membrane** is a double-layered membrane that has openings at regular intervals. Through these **pores** materials can pass from either the nucleus to the cytoplasm or from the cytoplasm to the nucleus. The outer layer of the nuclear membrane is continuous with the endoplasmic reticulum of the cytoplasm and may have small round projections on them called ribosomes. (A discussion of the ribosomes and endoplasmic reticulum follows shortly.)

THE NUCLEOPLASM

The **nucleoplasm** is also called by two other names. One is **nuclear sap** and the other is **karyolymph.** The nucleoplasm is a clear, semifluid medium that fills the spaces around the chromatin and the nucleoli.

THE NUCLEOLUS AND THE RIBOSOMES

Within the nucleus are one or more **nucleoli.** Each nucleolus is a small, round body, see figure 3-1. It contains **ribosomes** made up of ribonucleic acid and protein. The ribosomes can pass from the nucleus through the nuclear pores into the cytoplasm. There the ribosomes aid in protein synthesis. They may exist freely in the cytoplasm, be in clusters called **polyribosomes,** or be attached to the walls of the endoplasmic reticulum.

THE CENTROSOME AND CENTRIOLES

The **centrioles** are two cylindrical organelles found near the nucleus in a tiny round body called the **centrosome.** The centrioles are perpendicular to each other. Figure 3-1 shows two centrioles near the nucleus. Each centriole is made up of nine groups of three microtubules. During eukaryotic mitosis, or cell division, the two centrioles separate from each other. In the process of separation, thin cytoplasmic spindle fibers form between the two centrioles. This structure is called a **spindle-fiber apparatus.** The spindle fibers attach themselves to individual chromosomes to help in the even and equal distribution of these chromosomes to two daughter cells.

THE ENDOPLASMIC RETICULUM

Crisscrossing the cellular cytoplasm is a fine network of tubular structures called the **endoplasmic reticulum** (reticulum means "network"). Some of this endoplasmic reticulum connects the nuclear membrane to the cell membrane. Thus it serves as a channel for the transport of materials in and out of the nucleus. Sometimes the endoplasmic reticulum will accumulate large masses of proteins and act as a storage area.

There are two types of endoplasmic reticulum: **rough endoplasmic reticulum** and **smooth endoplasmic reticulum.** Rough endoplasmic reticulum has ribosomes studding the outer membrane. This gives it a coarse appearance. Smooth endoplasmic reticulum has no ribosomes on the outer membrane.

THE MITOCHONDRIA

All of a cell's energy comes from spherical or rod-shaped organelles called **mitochondria** (singular, mitochondrion; *mito* means thread, **chondrion** means granule). These mitochondria vary in shape and number. There can be as few as a single one in each cell or as many as a thousand or more. Cells that need the most energy have the greatest number of mitochondria. Because they supply the cell's energy mitochondria are also known as the "powerhouses" of the cell.

The electron microscope identifies the mitochondrion as a double-membraned structure: it has an outer membrane and an inner membrane. The inner membrane is folded inward to form shelflike ridges called **cristae. Enzymes** are chemicals found in the cristae. These enzymes help the mitochondrion to undergo cellular respiration. **Cellular respiration** is a chemical reaction that breaks down carbohydrate, lipid, and protein molecules to release energy, carbon dioxide, and water.

THE GOLGI APPARATUS

The **Golgi apparatus** was discovered in 1898 by the Italian scientist, Camillo Golgi. It is also called Golgi bodies or the Golgi complex. It is an arrangement of layers of membranes resembling a "stack of pancakes." Scientists believe that this organelle synthesizes

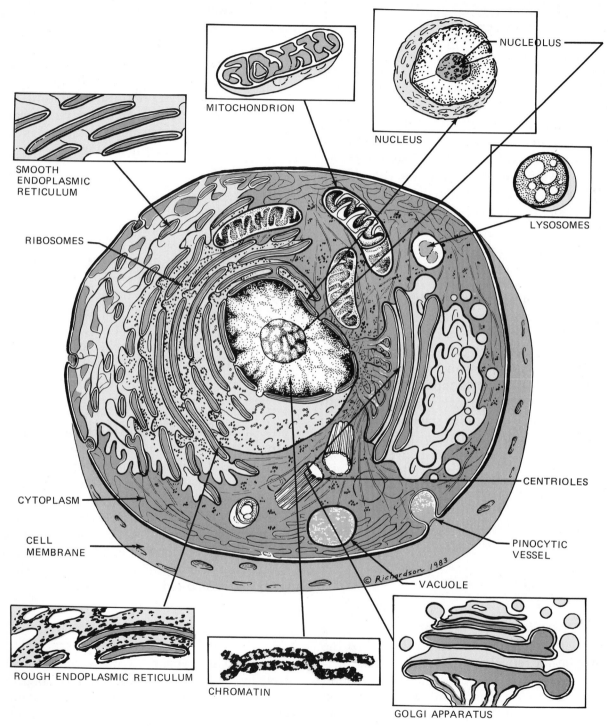

SMOOTH
ENDOPLASMIC
RETICULUM

MITOCHONDRION

NUCLEOLUS

NUCLEUS

LYSOSOMES

RIBOSOMES

CYTOPLASM

CELL
MEMBRANE

CENTRIOLES

PINOCYTIC
VESSEL

© Richardson 1983

VACUOLE

ROUGH ENDOPLASMIC RETICULUM

CHROMATIN

GOLGI APPARATUS

Figure 3-1   Fine structure of a typical animal cell

carbohydrates and combines them with protein molecules as they pass through the Golgi apparatus. In this way the Golgi apparatus stores and packages secretions for discharge from the cell. It follows logically that these organelles are abundant in the cells of gastric glands, salivary glands and pancreatic glands.

LYSOSOMES

Lysosomes are oval or spherical bodies found in the cellular cytoplasm. They contain powerful digestive enzymes that digest protein molecules. The lysosome thus helps to digest old, wornout cells, bacteria and foreign matter. If a lysosome should rupture, as sometimes happens, the lysosome will start digesting the cell's proteins, causing it to die. For this reason lysosomes are also known as "suicide bags."

PINOCYTIC VESICLES

Large molecules like protein and lipids, which cannot pass through the cell membrane, will enter a cell by way of the pinocytic vesicles. The **pinocytic vesicles** form by having the cell membrane fold inward to form a pocket. Some of the fluid surrounding the cell flows into this pocket. The fluid contains large molecules in solution. The edges of the pocket then close and pinch away from the cell membrane, forming a bubble or **vacuole** in the cytoplasm. The contents of the vacuole are separated from the cytoplasm by a cell membrane. This process by which a cell forms pinocytic vesicles to take in large molecules is called **pinocytosis** or "cell drinking."

MICROTUBULES AND MICROFILAMENTS

Microtubules, as the name implies, are an array of long, thin microscopic tubules. They play a role in cytoplasmic membrane function and cell shape as well as helping to form the spindle fibers in the mitotic spindle-fiber apparatus. In addition, microtubules help to move various substances and organelles within the cell.

CELL DIVISION

Both the growth and the maintenance of all the cells in the human body are achieved through cell division. Some human body cells (**somatic cells**) live only a short time, while others are subjected to continual "wear and tear" and are destroyed. The cells that are destroyed must be replaced. The process of cell division or **mitosis** will produce new cells. Many different types of cells in the human body will undergo mitosis. However, the neurons do not. How often a cell undergoes mitosis depends upon its particular cell type and species of organism it belongs to.

Mitosis

Cell division or mitosis is divided into two distinct processes:

1. **Mitosis.** The exact duplication of the nucleus to form two identical nuclei. This involves a doubling of the DNA hereditary material followed by the division of the nucleus, which is called **karyokinesis.**

2. **Cytoplasmic division.** The division of the cytoplasm into two approximately equal parts following nuclear division is called **cytokinesis.**

Mitosis essentially is an orderly series of steps by which the DNA in the nucleus of a cell is precisely and equally distributed to two daughter nuclei.

Mitosis in a Typical Animal Cell _____

Mitosis is a smoothly continuing process. However, for ease and convenience of study, five stages or **phases** have been identified by the cell biologist. These five phases are discussed subsequently with accompanying diagrams. The normal human somatic cell contains 46 chromosomes in the nucleus, which is equal to 23 pairs of chromosomes. This particular chromosome number (46) is called the **diploid number of chromosomes.** There is a characteristic diploid number of chromosomes for different organismal species. The diploid number is symbolized by *2n.* So, the 2n number for the human species is 46. The illustration of a cell in interphase that follows is a representative animal cell with a diploid number of 6 chromosomes. This cell will help to illustrate the process of mitosis.

Phase 1—Interphase (Resting Stage). In the **interphase** or "resting" stage, an animal cell undergoes **all** metabolic cellular activities to help in the maintenance of cell homeostasis. The term "resting" **only** refers to the fact that the cell isn't undergoing the visible steps of mitosis yet. Interphase occurs between nuclear divisions. During early interphase, an exact duplicate of each nuclear chromosome is made. This process is called **replication.** Replication is the duplication of the molecules of DNA within a chromosome.

At the start of mitosis, each chromosome has already replicated. Each strand of the replicated chromosome is called a **chromatid.** The two chromatid strands are joined together by a small structure called the **centromere,** see figure 3–2. During interphase, two centrioles located near the periphery of the nucleus are quite visible. The two centrioles are found in an area called the **centrosome,** see figure 3–3. They also replicate during interphase in preparation for the next cell division.

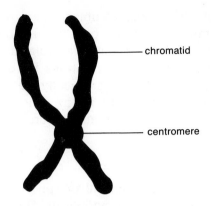

Figure 3-2   A replicated chromosome with two chromatids joined together by a centromere

Phase 2—Prophase. During prophase (see figure 3–3), the two pairs of centrioles start to separate towards the opposite ends or poles of the cell. As the two pairs of centrioles migrate, an array of cytoplasmic microtubules forms between them. These microtubules are called **spindle fibers.** Some short cytoplasmic fibers called **astral rays** radiate out of the centrioles. This whole structure consisting of the astral rays, centrioles, and the spindle fibers is called the **spindle-fiber apparatus** (SFA).

There are changes in the nucleus as well. The nuclear membrane starts to dissolve and the nucleolus disappears. The DNA in the chromosomes becomes more highly coiled or condensed and forms very deeply-staining, rod-like structures.

Phase 3—Metaphase. During **metaphase** (see figure 3–3), the nuclear membrane has dissolved completely. The chromatid pairs arrange themselves in a single file, one chromatid pair per spindle fiber between the two centrioles. The area that the chromatid pairs line up along is called the equatorial plate.

Phase 4—Anaphase. During **anaphase** (see figure 3–3), the chromatid pairs separate and are

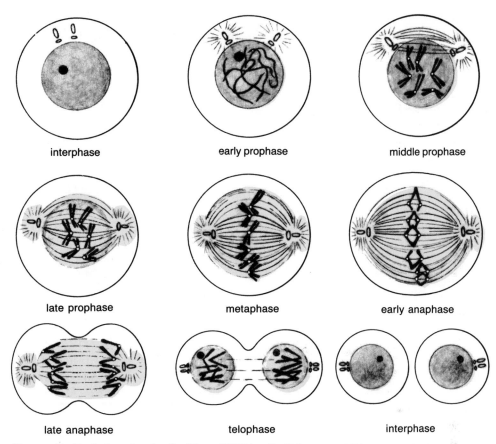

interphase   early prophase   middle prophase

late prophase   metaphase   early anaphase

late anaphase   telophase   interphase

Figure 3-3   Stages of mitosis in animal cells (From William D. Schraer and Herbert J. Stoltze, *Biology: The Study of Life,* 2nd edition. Copyright © 1987 by Allyn and Bacon, Inc.)

pulled by the shortening spindle fibers towards the centrioles. The two chromatids of each replicated chromosome are now fully separated.

Phase 5—Telophase. During **telophase** (see figure 3–3), the chromosomes migrate to the opposite poles of the cell. There they start to uncoil or decondense to become loosely arranged chromatin granules. The nuclear membrane and the nucleolus reappear to help reestablish the nucleus as a definite organelle again.

The astral rays and the spindle fibers of the SFA dissolve back into the cytoplasm.

When cytoplasmic division is finished, two new daughter cells are formed.

Cytokinesis

The actual process of dividing one cell into two new approximately equal-sized daughter cells is called **cytokinesis.** In the animal cell, this division is accompanied by a pinching in of the cell membrane.

MOVEMENT OF MATERIALS ACROSS CELL MEMBRANES

The cell membrane, aside from housing the cellular organelles, also controls passage of substances into and out of the cell. This is important because a cell must be able to acquire materials from its surrounding medium, after which it either secretes synthesized substances or excretes wastes. The physical processes which control the passage of materials through the cell membrane are: **diffusion, osmosis, filtration, active transport, phagocytosis,** and **pinocytosis.** Diffusion, osmosis, and filtration are passive processes, which means they do not need energy in order to function. Active transport, phagocytosis, and pinocytosis are active processes which do require an energy source.

Diffusion

Diffusion is a physical process whereby molecules of gases, liquids, or solid particles spread or scatter themselves evenly through a medium. When solid particles are dissolved within a fluid, they are known as **solutes.** Diffusion also applies to a slightly different process, where solutes and water pass across a membrane to distribute themselves evenly throughout the two fluids, which remain separated by the membrane. Generally, *molecules move from an area where they are greatly concentrated to an area where they are less concentrated.* The molecules will, eventually, distribute themselves evenly within the space available; when this happens, the molecules are said to be in a state of **equilibrium,** see figure 3–4.

The three common states of matter are gases, liquids, and solids. Molecules will diffuse more quickly in gases and more slowly in solids. Diffusion occurs due to the heat energy of molecules. As a result of this, molecules are always in constant motion, except at **absolute zero** ($-273°C$). In all cases, the movement of molecules increases with an increase in temperature.

A few familiar examples of the rates of diffusion may be helpful. For instance, if one thoroughly saturates a wad of cotton with ammonia and places it in a far corner of a room, the entire room will soon smell of ammonia. Air currents quickly carry the ammonia fumes throughout the room. Another test for diffu-

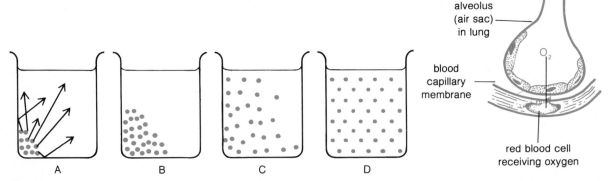

Diffusion:
(A) A small lump of sugar is placed into a beaker of water, its molecules dissolve and begin to diffuse outward. (B&C) The sugar molecules continue to diffuse through the water from an area of greater concentration to an area of lesser concentration. (D) Over a long period of time, the sugar molecules are evenly distributed throughout the water, reaching a state of equilibrium.

Example of diffusion in the human body: Oxygen diffuses from an alveolus in a lung where it is in greater concentration, across the blood capillary membrane, into a red blood cell where it is in lesser concentration.

Figure 3-4 The process of diffusion

sion is to place a pair of dye crystals on the bottom of a water-filled beaker. Eventually, they will uniformly permeate and color the water. This diffusion process will take quite a while, especially if no one stirs, shakes or heats the beaker. In still another test, a dye crystal placed on an ice cube moves even more slowly through the ice. Diffusion of the dye can be accelerated by melting the ice.

The diffusion rate of molecules in the various media (gas, liquid, and solid) depends upon the distances between each molecule and how freely they can move. In a gas, molecules can move more freely and quickly; within a liquid, molecules are more tightly held together. In a solid substance, molecular movement is highly restricted and thus very slow.

Diffusion plays a vital role in permitting molecules to enter and leave a cell. Oxygen diffuses from the bloodstream, where it dwells in greater concentration. From the bloodstream, the oxygen enters the fluid surrounding a cell, then into the cell itself, where it is far less concentrated. In this manner, the flow of blood through the lungs and bloodstream provides a continuous supply of oxygen to the cells. Once

oxygen has entered a cell, it is utilized in metabolic activities.

Osmosis

Osmosis is the diffusion of water or any other *solvent* molecule through a selective permeable membrane (like the cell membrane). A **selective permeable membrane** is any membrane through which some solutes can diffuse, but others cannot.

Sausage casing is a selective permeable membrane which can be used to substitute for a cell membrane. A solution of salt, sucrose (table sugar), and gelatin is placed into the sausage casing. This mixture is then suspended into a beaker filled with distilled water, figure 3–5. The sausage casing is permeable to water and salt, but not to gelatin and sucrose. Thus only the water and salt molecules can pass through the casing. Eventually more salt molecules will move out because we began with a greater concentration of these molecules inside. At the same time, more water molecules move into the casing, since there were more outside when we began.

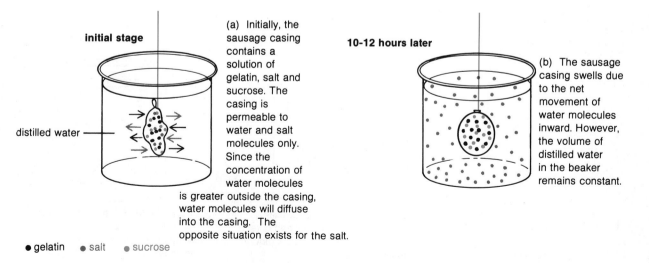

Figure 3-5 Osmosis: the diffusion of water through a selective permeable membrane is illustrated here. (A sausage casing is an example of a selective permeable membrane.)

This is yet another example of diffusion whereby molecules move from a region of higher concentration to a region of lower concentration. The volume of water increases inside the casing, causing it to expand because of the entry of water molecules. When the number of water molecules entering the casing are equal to the number exiting, an equilibrium has been achieved; the casing will expand no further.

The pressure exerted by the water molecules within the casing at equilibrium is called the **osmotic pressure,** which is expressed as millimeters of mercury (mm Hg). It is important to remember that every solution has a potential osmotic pressure.

The osmotic pressure of a solution is dependent upon the number of molecules of solute dissolved in a solution. The higher the osmotic pressure (**osmolality**) of a solution, the greater the number of molecules in that solution. And the greater the concentration of molecules, the stronger the "pull" or attraction for water molecules. Simply stated, *water molecules move toward the area of greater osmolality.*

In physiology, the osmotic characteristics of various solutions are determined by the manner in which they affect red blood cells. In other words, the osmolality of a given solution is compared to that of blood serum. For instance, if a human red blood cell is placed into a solution with the same osmotic pressure as human blood serum, the red blood cell will remain unchanged. This type of solution is known as an **isotonic solution.** In a **hypotonic solution,** the osmolality is lower than that of blood serum, and the red blood cell will swell and burst. This is caused by the water molecules moving into the cell. However, a red blood cell placed inside a **hypertonic solution,** such as seawater (with a higher osmolality than that of blood serum), will shrink and wrinkle up because of the water moving out of the cell, figure 3–6.

Filtration

Filtration is the movement of solutes and water across a semi-permeable membrane. This results from some mechanical force, such as blood pressure or gravity. The solutes and water move from an area of higher pressure to

hypertonic solution

hypotonic solution

isotonic solution

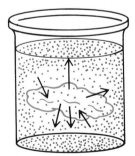 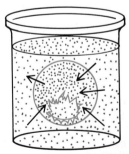 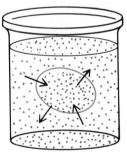

Hypertonic solution (seawater)
a red blood cell will shrink and wrinkle up because water molecules are moving out of the cell.

• water molecules

Hypotonic solution (freshwater)
a red blood cell will swell and burst because water molecules are moving into the cell.

Isotonic solution (human blood serum)
a red blood cell remains unchanged, because the movement of water molecules into and out of the cell are the same.

Figure 3-6   Movement of water molecules in solutions of different osmolalities

an area of lower pressure. The size of the membrane pores determines which molecules are to be filtered. Thus filtration allows for the separation of large and small molecules. Such filtration takes place in the kidneys. The process allows larger protein molecules to remain within the body and smaller molecules to be excreted as waste, figure 3–7.

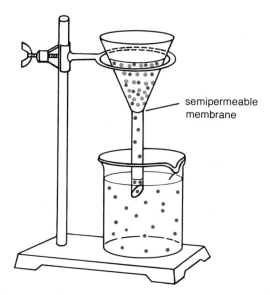

Filtration: Small molecules are filtered through the semipermeable membrane, while the large molecules remain in the funnel.

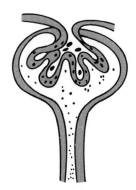

Example of filtration in the human body: Glomerulus of kidney, large particles like red blood cells and proteins remain in the blood, and small molecules like urea and water are excreted as a metabolic excretory product—urine.

Figure 3-7   Filtration: a passive transport process

Active Transport

Active transport is a process whereby molecules move across the cell membrane from an area of lower concentration, against a concentration gradient, to an area of higher concentration. This process requires the high energy chemical compound called **ATP (adenosine-triphosphate).** The ATP is supplied by the cell membrane.

How does active transport work? One theory suggests that a molecule is picked up from the outside of the cell membrane and brought inside by a carrier molecule. Both molecule and carrier are bound together, forming a temporary **carrier-molecule complex.** This carrier molecule complex shuttles across the cell membrane; the molecule is released at the inner surface of the membrane, from where it enters the cytoplasm. At this point, the carrier acquires energy at the inner surface of the cell membrane. Then it returns to the outer surface of the cell membrane to pick up another molecule for transport. Accordingly, the carrier can also convey molecules in the opposite direction, from the inside to the outside, figure 3–8.

Phagocytosis

Phagocytosis, or "cell eating," is quite similar to pinocytosis, with an important difference: in pinocytosis, the substances engulfed by the cell membrane are in solution; however, in phagocytosis, the substances engulfed are within particles. Human white blood cells undergo phagocytosis. They will phagocytize bacteria, cell fragments, or even a damaged cell. The particulate substance will be engulfed by an enfolding of the cell membrane to form a vacuole enclosing the material. When the material is completely enclosed within the vacuole, digestive enzymes pour into the vacuole from the cytoplasm to destroy the entrapped substance.

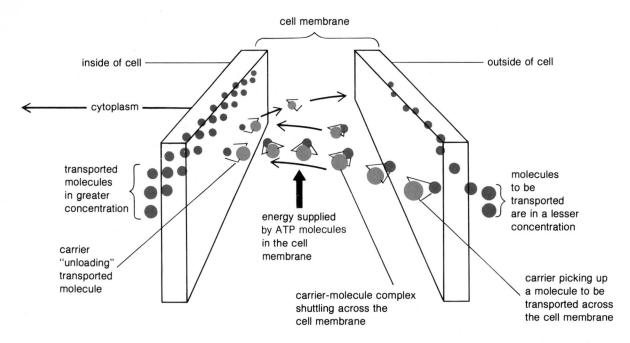

Figure 3-8 Diagram showing the active transport of molecules from an area of lesser concentration to an area of greater concentration, according to one theoretical model

Pinocytosis

As stated earlier, pinocytosis or "cell drinking" involves the formation of pinocytic vesicles which engulf large molecules in solution. The cell then ingests the nutrient for its own use.

SPECIALIZATION

There are many kinds of cells of different shapes and sizes. Most of them have the characteristics shown in figure 3-1, which is a generalized diagram of a basic cell. Some of the more specialized types, such as nerve cells and red blood cells, look very different, figure 3–9.

Human beings are composed entirely of cells and the nonliving substances which cells build up around themselves. The interaction of the various parts of the cell within the cellu-lar structure constitutes the life of the cell. These interactions result in the life activities, life processes, or life functions that were discussed in unit 1. However, in complex organisms, groups of cells become specialists in a particular function. Nerve cells, for example, have become specialized in response; red blood cells, in oxygen transport.

Specialized cells may lose the ability to perform some of the other functions, such as reproduction (cell division). Normally, when nerve cells are destroyed or damaged, others cannot be formed to replace them. Specialization also has resulted in an interdependence among cells — certain cells depend on other kinds of cells to aid them in carrying on the total life activities of the organism. In humans, this specialization and interdependence extends to the organs.

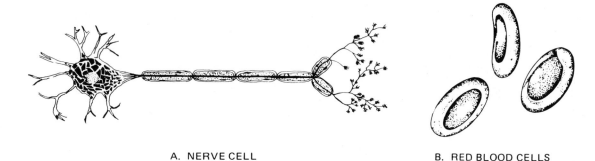

A. NERVE CELL

B. RED BLOOD CELLS

Figure 3-9 Specialized cells

Further Study and Discussion

Complete each of the laboratory exercises under the supervision of your instructor.

Laboratory Lesson 1

A. **Objective:** To make a slide so as to observe and study the typical cell structure of a cheek cell

B. **Equipment and materials**

- One box of flat-ended toothpicks
- One compound light microscope
- One microscope slide
- One bottle of Lugol's iodine solution
- One cover slip
- Paper towels
- Lens paper
- An eye dropper

C. **Procedure**

1. If necessary, clean the microscope slide and coverslip carefully with the lens paper.
2. Insert the wide, flat end of a toothpick into your mouth. *Gently* scrape the inside of your cheek. (If you have a cold, use your laboratory partner's cheek cells)!
3. Place the wide, flat end of the toothpick against the surface of the microscope slide. Slide the toothpick horizontally across it to make a smear of the cheek cells.
4. Place one or two small drops of Lugol's iodine (solution) on the smear.
5. *Gently* lower the cover slip over a portion of the stained smear.
6. Place your prepared cheek cell slide on the microscope stage. Gently place the stage clips over the slide to secure it.

7. First use the low power objective to focus in on your cells. (Do *not* focus on clumps of cells: only on the separate yellowish cheek cells).

8. Now rotate the low power objective out of its position. Rotate and click the high power objective to focus in on your cells.

D. **Observations**

1. On a separate sheet of paper, draw a cheek cell (as you see it) under low power.
   — Label the structures on the cell.

2. Observing the slide under high power, focus in on the nucleus.
   a. What structure is found within the nucleus?

   b. How many of these are in the nucleus?

3. What is the name of the structure surrounding the entire cheek cell?

4. State what happens to a cheek cell if you move the slide:
   a. to the right?

   b. to the left?

   c. towards you?

   d. away from you?

E. **Conclusions**
    1. Why are some cheek cells clumped together and others separate?

    2. Describe the general shape of a cheek cell.

    3. Explain why Lugol's iodine solution was added to the cheek cell smear.

    4. What is the function of the cell membrane: (a) on the cheek cell, (b) on the nucleus in the cheek cell?

Laboratory Lesson 2

A. **Objective:** To prepare a slide for observation and study of a human red blood cell

B. **Equipment and Materials**
    - One compound microscope
    - Four microscope slides
    - Two cover slips
    - Two sterile disposable lancets
    - Sterile absorbent cotton
    - 70%-90% alcohol
    - One watch glass
    - Wright's stain
    - Distilled water
    - One pipette
    - One beaker
    - Tap water
    - Paper towels

C. **Procedure**

1. Dampen a small wad of sterile absorbent cotton with the alcohol. Swab the tip of the little finger of your left hand.

2. Using a single-wrapped sterile disposable lancet, quickly prick the cleaned area.

3. Immediately squeeze the puncture; a drop of blood should appear.

4. Carefully place the drop of blood half an inch from the edge of a clean glass slide. (Swab the skin puncture with another wad of sterile cotton dampended with alcohol).

5. Use the edge of a second glass slide as a spreader. Hold the spreader slide, with its edge just touching the drop of blood, at a 45 degree angle to the first slide.

6. Allow a few seconds for the drop of blood to spread along the edge of the spreader slide, then push it toward the opposite end of the first slide, figure 3–10.

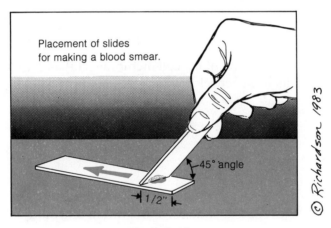

Figure 3-10

7. Cover the blood smear with a cover slip; examine the slide under the low power lens, then with the high power lens.

Second part of procedure: Perform the same exercise, using Wright's stain.

1-6. Repeat steps of preceding exercise in this lesson.

7. Allow two minutes for the blood smear to dry.

8. Rest the slide on top of a watch glass, then add 10 drops of Wright's stain to the slide. Let the excess stain drip into the watch glass.

9. After one minute, add 10 drops of distilled water. Allow 5 minutes for the stain to act.

10. Gently dip the slide in a beaker of tap water to remove any excess stain.

11. Wipe *only* the *lower* surface of the blood smear with paper towels.

12. Cover the blood smear with a cover slip; examine the slide under the low power lens, then with the high power lens.

D. **Observations**

1. How many different types of blood cells did you see?

2. Name the most abundant cell found in blood.

3. Describe the color and shape of these cells.

4. Do these cells contain a nucleus?

5. Did you see a blood cell containing a nucleus?

6. What is the name of this blood cell?

7. Describe the appearance of these cells.

8. Name the smallest blood cell; describe its appearance.

9. How do the red blood cells and the white blood cells compare in number?

E. **Conclusions**
   1. What is the function of the red blood cell?

   2. What is the function of the white blood cell?

   3. What is the function of the platelets?

Assignment

A. Study the diagram of a typical cell, figure 3–11. Enter the names of the structures after the proper numbered callouts, as listed below.

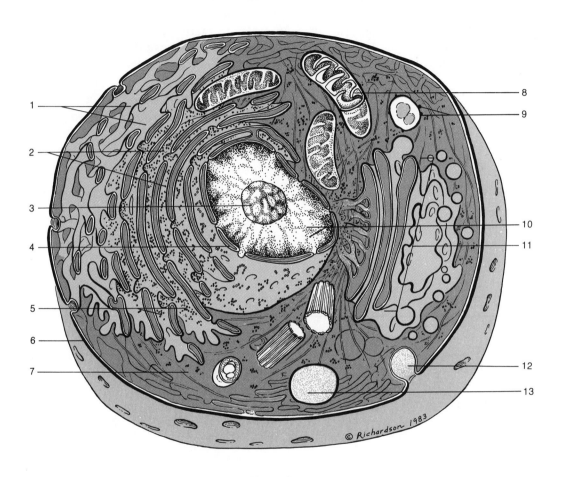

Figure 3-11

1 _____	8 _____	
2 _____	9 _____	
3 _____	10 _____	
4 _____	11 _____	
5 _____	12 _____	
6 _____	13 _____	
7 _____		

B. Associate each of the terms in column I with its correct description in column II.

Column I	Column II
_____ 1. nucleus	a. small units of which all plants and animals are made
_____ 2. chromatin material	
_____ 3. DNA	b. the exposed outer edge of the cell
_____ 4. cytoplasm	c. the process by which cells divide
_____ 5. nerve	d. an example of a specialized cell
_____ 6. reproduction	e. the dense inner portion of the cell
_____ 7. cells	f. the cell powerhouse from which energy is released
_____ 8. mitosis	
_____ 9. mitochondrion	g. the light outer portion of the cell
_____ 10. cell membrane	h. an ability lost by some specialized cells
	i. the hereditary material within the chromosome
	j. cell structure where chromosomes are located
	k. hereditary chemical which transmits traits from one generation to the next.

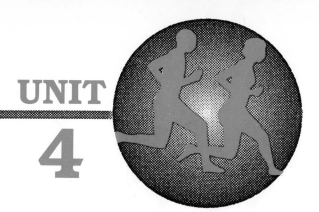

UNIT 4

TISSUES

OBJECTIVES

- Describe how cells are organized into tissues
- List the four main types of tissues
- Define the function and location of tissues
- Define the Key Words relating to this unit of study

Multicellular organisms are composed of many different types of cells. Although they are not randomly arranged, each of these cells performs a special function. These millions of cells are grouped according to their similarity in shape, size, structure, and function. Cells so grouped are called **tissues.**

Specialization of cells can be seen in a study of the epithelial cells which make up epithelial tissue. Epithelial cells that cover the body's external and internal surfaces have a typical shape, either columnar, cubical, or platelike. This variation is necessary so the epithelial cells can fit together smoothly in order to line and protect the bodily surface. Also,

muscle cells making up muscle tissue are long and spindle-like so they can contract. Nerve cells (**neurons**) that make up nerve tissue are specialized to carry electrical messages.

Some tissues are comprised of both living cells and various nonliving substances which the cells build up around themselves. This is especially true of the supporting tissues, such as bones and cartilage, figures 4–1 and 4–2.

There are four main types of tissue: (1) epithelial, (2) connective, (3) muscle, and (4) nervous. Each has a specialized structure to perform a particular function. The variations, functions, and locations of each type are described in table 4–1.

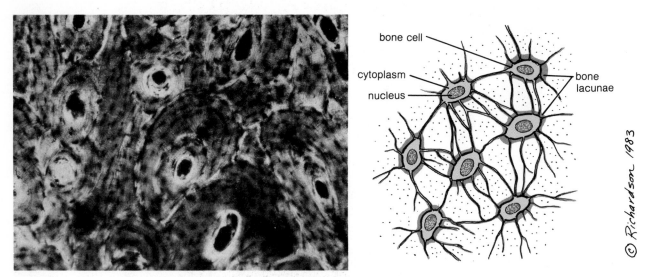

Figure 4-1 **Bone tissue (Photograph reprinted, by permission, from Joan G. Creager, *Human Anatomy and Physiology, 95)***

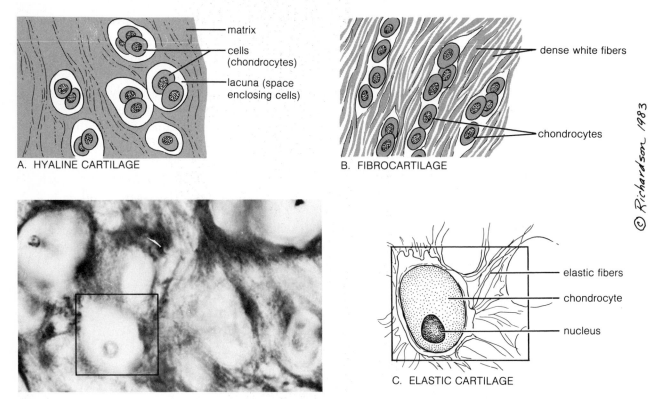

Figure 4-2 **Cartilage tissues (Photograph courtesy of Armed Forces Institute of Pathology, negative 71-9216)**

Table 4–1 Different Kinds of Human Tissue

TYPE OF TISSUE	FUNCTION	CHARACTERISTICS AND LOCATION	MORPHOLOGY
I. **EPITHELIAL**	Cells form a continuous layer covering internal and external body surfaces, provide protection, produce secretions (digestive juices, hormones, perspiration) and regulate the passage of materials across themselves.		
	A. Covering and lining tissue These cells can be stratified (layered), ciliated or keratinized.	**1. Squamous epithelial cells** These are flat, irregularly-shaped cells. They line the heart, blood and lymphatic vessels, body cavities, and alveoli (air sacs) of lungs. The outer layer of the skin is composed of stratified and keratinized squamous epithelial cells. The stratified squamous epithelial cells on the outer skin layer protect the body against microbial invasion.	I-A-1
		2. Cuboidal epithelial cells These are the cube-shaped cells that line the kidney tubules, and which cover the ovaries and secretory parts of certain glands.	I-A-2
		3. Columnar epithelial cells Elongated, with the nucleus generally near the bottom and often ciliated on the outer surface. They line the ducts, digestive tract (especially the intestinal and stomach lining), parts of the respiratory tract, and glands.	I-A-3

© Richardson 1983

Table 4–1 Different Kinds of Human Tissue (continued)

TYPE OF TISSUE	FUNCTION	CHARACTERISTICS AND LOCATION	MORPHOLOGY
I. EPITHELIAL (continued)	B. **Glandular or secretory tissue** These cells are specialized to secrete materials like digestive juices, hormones, milk, perspiration and wax. They are columnar or cuboidal shaped.	**Endocrine gland cells** These cells form ductless glands which secrete their substances (hormones) directly into the bloodstream. For instance, the thyroid gland secretes thyroxin, while adrenal glands secrete adrenalin. Exocrine glands secrete their substnaces into ducts. The mammary glands, sweat glands, and salivary glands are examples.	duct (where secretions leave) secretory cells exocrine (duct) gland cell e.g. sweat and mammary glands I-B
II. **CONNECTIVE**	Cells whose intercellular secretions (matrix) support and connect the many organs and tissues of the body.	Connective tissue is found almost everywhere within the body: bones, cartilage, mucous membranes, muscles, nerves, skin, and all internal organs.	
	A. **Adipose tissue** Stores lipid (fat); acts as filler tissue; cushions, supports, and insulates the body.	A type of loose, connective tissue composed of sac-like adipose cells; they are specialized for the storage of fat. Adipose cells are found throughout the body: in the subcutaneous skin layer, around the kidneys, within padding around joints and in the marrow of long bones.	cytoplasm collagen fibers nucleus vacuole (for fat storage) II-A © Richardson 1983
	B. **Areolar (loose) connective** Surrounds various organs, supports both nerve cells and blood vessels which transport nutrient materials (to cells) and wastes (away from) cells. Areolar tissue also (temporarily) stores glucose, salts and water.	It is composed of a large, semifluid matrix, with many different types of cells and fibers embedded in it. These include fibroblasts (fibrocytes), plasma cells, macrophages, mast cells and various white blood cells. The fibers are bundles of a strong, flexible white fibrous protein called *collagen,* and elastic single fibers of *elastin.* It is found in the epidermis of the skin and in the subcutaneous layer with adipose (fat) cells.	matrix reticular fibers mast cell collagen fibers plasma cell elastic fiber fibroblast cell macrophage cell II-B

Table 4–1 Different Kinds of Human Tissue (continued)

TYPE OF TISSUE	FUNCTION	CHARACTERISTICS AND LOCATION	MORPHOLOGY
II. CONNECTIVE (continued)	**C. Dense fibrous** This tissue forms ligaments, tendons and aponeuroses. *Ligaments* are strong, flexible bands (or cords) which hold bones firmly together at the joints. *Tendons* are white, glistening bands attaching skeletal muscles to the bones. *Aponeuroses* are flat, wide bands of tissue holding one muscle to another or to the periosteum (bone covering). *Fasciae* are fibrous connective tissue sheets that wrap around muscle bundles to hold them in place.	Dense fibrous tissue is also called white fibrous tissue, since it is made from closely packed white collagen fibers. Fibrous tissue is flexible, but not elastic. It is found in aponeuroses, fasciae, ligaments and tendons.	closely packed collagen fibers / fibroblast cell **II-C**
	D. Supportive **1. Bone (osseous) tissue —** Comprises the skeleton of the body, which supports and protects underlying soft tissue parts and organs, and also serves as attachments for skeletal muscles.	Connective tissue whose intercellular matrix is *calcified* by the deposition of mineral salts (like calcium carbonate and calcium phosphate). Calcification of bone imparts great strength. The entire skeleton is composed of bone tissue.	bone cell / cytoplasm / nucleus / bone lacunae **II-D-1**
	2. Cartilage — Provides firm but flexible support for the embryonic skeleton and part of the adult skeleton. **a. Hyaline —** appears as a bluish white, glossy mass.	Hyaline cartilage is found upon articular bone surfaces, and also at the nose tip, bronchi and bronchial tubes. Ribs are joined to the *sternum* (breastbone) by the *costal cartilage*. It is also found in the larynx and the rings in the trachea.	matrix / cells (chondrocytes) / lacuna (space enclosing cells) **II-D-2a**
	b. Fibrocartilage — a strong, flexible, supportive substance; found between bones and wherever great strength (and a degree of rigidity) is needed.	Fibrocartilage is located within *intervertebral discs* and *pubic symphysis* between the *pubic bones*.	dense white fibers / chondrocytes **II-D-2b**

© Richardson 1983

Table 4–1 Different Kinds of Human Tissue (continued)

TYPE OF TISSUE	FUNCTION	CHARACTERISTICS AND LOCATION	MORPHOLOGY
II. CONNECTIVE (continued)	D. **Supportive (continued)** c. **Elastic cartilage** — the intercellular matrix is embedded with a network of elastic fibers.	Elastic cartilage is located inside the auditory ear tube, external ear, epiglottis, and larynx.	
	E. **Vascular (liquid blood tissue)** 1. **Blood** — Transports nutrient and oxygen molecules to cells, and metabolic wastes away from cells (can be considered as a liquid tissue). Contains cells that function in the body's defense and in blood clotting.	Blood is composed of two major parts: a liquid called plasma, and a solid cellular portion known as blood cells (or corpuscles). The plasma suspends corpuscles, of which there are two major types: *red* blood cells (erythrocytes) and *white* blood cells (leucocytes). A third cellular component (really a cell fragment) is called platelets (thrombocytes). Blood circulates within the blood vessels (arteries, veins and capillaries) and through the heart.	
	2. **Lymph** — Transports tissue fluid, proteins, fats and other materials from the tissues to the circulatory system. This occurs through a series of tubes called the lymphatic vessels.	Lymph is a fluid made up of water, glucose, protein, fats and salt. The cellular components are lymphocytes and granulocytes. They flow in tubes called lymphatic vessels, which closely parallel the veins and bathe the tissue spaces between cells.	

Table 4–1 Different Kinds of Human Tissue (continued)

TYPE OF TISSUE	FUNCTION	CHARACTERISTICS AND LOCATION	MORPHOLOGY
III. MUSCLE	A. **Cardiac** These cells help the heart contract in order to pump blood through and out of the heart.	Cardiac muscle is a striated (having a cross-banding pattern), involuntary (not under conscious control) muscle. It makes up the walls of the heart.	 centrally located nucleus striations branching of cell intercalated disc III-A
	B. **Skeletal (striated voluntary)** These muscles are attached to the movable parts of the skeleton. They are capable of rapid, powerful contractions and long states of partially sustained contractions, allowing for voluntary movement.	Skeletal muscle is: *striated* (having transverse bands that run down the length of muscle fiber); *voluntary,* because the muscle is under conscious control; and *skeletal,* since these muscles are attached to the skeleton (bones, tendons and other muscles).	 nucleus myofibrils III-B
	C. **Smooth (nonstriated involuntary)** These provide for involuntary movement. Examples include the movement of materials along the digestive tract, controlling the diameter of blood vessels and the pupil of the eyes.	Smooth muscle is *nonstriated* because it lacks the striations (bands) of skeletal muscles; its movement is *involuntary.* It makes up the walls of the digestive, genitourinary, respiratory tracts, blood vessels and lymphatic vessels.	spindle-shaped cell nucleus cells separated from each other III-C
IV. NERVE	**Neuronal** Cells have the ability to react to stimuli. *Irritability —* ability of nerve tissue to respond to environmental changes. *Conductivity —* ability to carry a nerve impulse (message).	Nerve tissue is composed of neurons (nerve cells). Neurons have branches through which various parts of the body are connected and their activities coordinated. They are found in the brain, spinal cord, and nerves.	dendrites cell body nucleus axon myelin sheath terminal end branch IV

© Richardson 1983

Further Study and Discussion

- Observe prepared microscope slides of the following tissues: muscle, nerve, epithelial, blood, bone, cartilage, fat, white fibrous, and yellow elastic.

Assignment

Match each term in column I with its correct description in column II.

Column I	Column II
_____ 1. heart	a. provides protection to the body and produces secretion
_____ 2. vascular tissue	
_____ 3. epithelial tissue	b. hardest body tissue providing support
_____ 4. cartilage tissue	c. slightly flexible tissue found in the intervertebral disks and the ribs
_____ 5. differentiation	
_____ 6. tissue interspaces	d. primarily transports nutrients and wastes
_____ 7. smooth muscle	
_____ 8. bone tissue	e. provides for involuntary movements
_____ 9. nervous tissue	f. provides for voluntary movement
_____ 10. skeletal muscle	g. carries impulses and messages throughout the body
	h. location of cardiac muscle
	i. result of cell specialization
	j. location of most loose fibrous connective tissue
	k. fluid in tissue interspaces
	l. cell digestion

UNIT 5

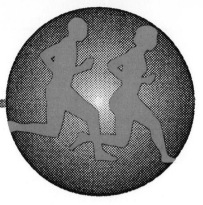

ORGANS AND SYSTEMS

KEY WORDS

digestive system   circulatory   organ
division of labor   system   organ system

OBJECTIVES

- Define an organ
- Define an organ system
- Relate various organs to their respective systems
- Define Key Words relating to this unit of study

An **organ** is a structure made up of several tissues grouped together to perform a single function. For instance, the stomach is an organ composed of highly specialized vascular, connective, epithelial, muscular, and nerve tissues. All of these tissues function together so as to enable the stomach to undergo digestion and absorption.

The skin which covers our bodies is no mere simple tissue, but a complex organ composed of connective, epithelial, muscular and nervous tissue. These tissues enable the skin to protect the body and remove its wastes (water and inorganic salts), making us sensitive to our environment.

The various organs of the human body do not function separately. Instead, they coordinate their activities to form a complete, functional organism. A group of organs which act together to perform a specific, related function is called an **organ system,** see figure 5–1.

The **digestive system** has the special function of processing solid food into liquid for absorption into the bloodstream. This organ system includes the mouth, salivary glands, esophagus, stomach, small intestine, liver, pancreas, gallbladder and large intestine. The **circulatory system** transports materials to and from cells. It is comprised of the heart, arteries, veins, capillaries, lymphatic vessels and spleen.

Each of the nine organ systems is highly specialized to perform a specific function; together they coordinate their functions to form a whole, live, functioning organism. This type of specialization is known as **division of labor** a process which occurs in multicellular organisms.

The systems of the body are the skeletal, muscular, digestive, respiratory, circulatory, reproductive, excretory, endocrine nervous, and integumentary systems. The functions and organs of each system are shown in table 5–1.

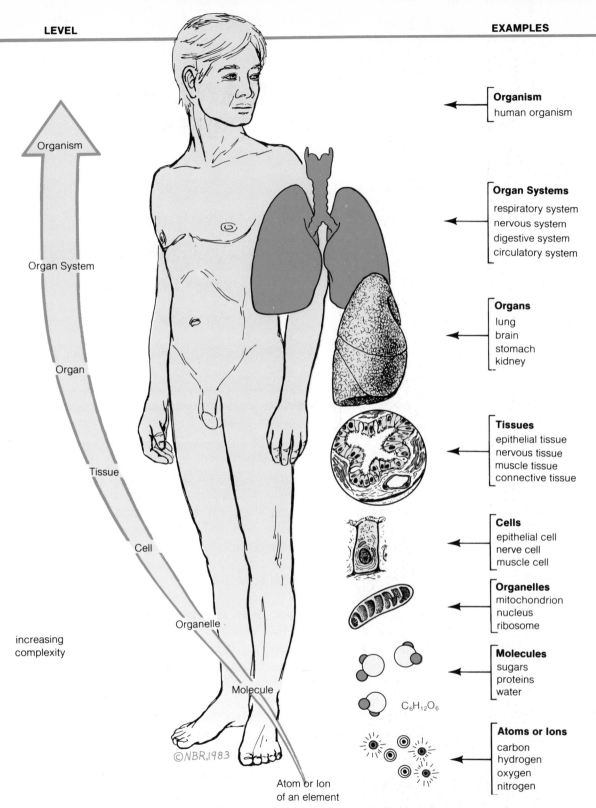

LEVEL

Organism

Organ System

Organ

Tissue

Cell

Organelle

Molecule

Atom or Ion
of an element

increasing
complexity

©NBR,1983

EXAMPLES

Organism
human organism

Organ Systems
respiratory system
nervous system
digestive system
circulatory system

Organs
lung
brain
stomach
kidney

Tissues
epithelial tissue
nervous tissue
muscle tissue
connective tissue

Cells
epithelial cell
nerve cell
muscle cell

Organelles
mitochondrion
nucleus
ribosome

Molecules
sugars
proteins
water

$C_6H_{12}O_6$

Atoms or Ions
carbon
hydrogen
oxygen
nitrogen

Figure 5-1 Formation of the human organism progresses from different levels of complexity.

Table 5–1 The Ten Body Systems

SYSTEM	SYSTEM FUNCTIONS	ORGANS
Skeletal	Gives shape to body; protects delicate parts of body; provides space for attaching muscles; is instrumental in forming blood; stores minerals.	Skull, Spinal Column, Ribs and Sternum, Shoulder Girdle, Upper and Lower Extremities, Pelvic Girdle.
Muscular	Determines posture; produces body heat; provides for movement.	Voluntary Muscles (Skeletal) Involuntary Muscles Cardiac Muscle
Digestive	Prepares food for absorption and use by body cells through modification of chemical and physical states.	Mouth (salivary glands, teeth, tongue), Pharynx, Esophagus, Stomach, Intestines, Liver, Gallbladder, Pancreas.
Respiratory	Acquires oxygen; rids body of carbon dioxide.	Nose, Pharynx, Larynx, Trachea, Bronchi, Lungs.
Circulatory	Carries oxygen and nourishment to cells of body; carries waste from cells; body defense.	Heart, Arteries, Veins, Capillaries, Lymphatic Vessels, Lymph Nodes, Spleen.
Excretory	Removes waste products of metabolism from body.	Skin, Lungs, Kidneys, Bladder, Ureters, Urethra.
Nervous	Communicates; controls body activity, coordinates body activity.	Brain, nerves, Spinal Cord, Ganglia.
Endocrine	Manufactures hormones to regulate organ activity.	Glands (ductless): Pituitary, Thyroid, Parathyroid, Pancreas, Adrenal, Gonads (ovaries, testes)
Reproductive	Reproduces human beings.	*Male* — Testes, Scrotum, Epididymis, Vas deferens, Seminal vesicles, Ejaculatory duct, Prostate gland, Cowper's gland, Penis, Urethra *Female* — Ovaries, Fallopian tubes, Uterus, Vagina, Bartholin glands, External genitals (vulva), Breasts (mammary glands)
Integumentary	Helps regulate body temperature, establishes a barrier between the body and the environment; eliminates waste; synthesizes Vitamin D; contains receptors for temperature, pressure, and pain.	Epidermis, dermis, sweat glands, oil glands.

Further Study and Discussion

- Identify all the types of tissue present in the arm.
- Discuss how each system is involved in the functioning of the arm.

Assignment

A. Briefly answer the questions.

   1. Explain the relationship of cells to tissues, organs and systems.

2. Briefly define an organ and an organ system.

3. State the functions of the skeletal system.

4. What is meant by the division of labor between organ systems?

5. List the different types of tissue present in the stomach.

B. Name three organs found in each of the ten body systems.

Skeletal	Excretory
Muscular	Nervous
Digestive	Endocrine
Respiratory	Reproductive
Circulatory	Integumentary

UNIT 6

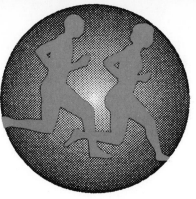

TISSUE REPAIR

KEY WORDS

bactericidal
clean wound
cicatrix
coagulum
endothelium

fibroblast
graft
granulation
intravenously
primary repair

scab
secondary repair
serous fluid
sutures

OBJECTIVES

■ Identify the two main types of tissue repair
■ Describe the processes involved in the two types of tissue repair
■ Describe the process of granulation
■ Discuss measures of minimizing disfigurement in patients with extensive tissue damage
■ Identify the types of vitamins needed in tissue repair
■ Discuss the functions of tissue repair vitamins
■ Define the Key Words related to this unit of study

DEGREE OF TISSUE REPAIR

Repair of damaged tissues occurs continually under the everyday activities of living. For example, skin tissue would undergo tissue repair more often because it is subjected to lots of "wear and tear."

Depending upon the type of damage or injury and the location of the tissue, some tissues will be easily and quickly repaired. These include surface epithelium, connective tissue, and liver cells. Bone tissue repairs slowly because broken bone ends must be kept aligned and immobilized until the repair is done. Damaged muscle tissue repairs itself minimally, and neurons destroyed by infection or injury do *not* grow back.

PROCESS OF EPITHELIAL TISSUE REPAIR

There are two types of epithelial tissue repair. One is called **primary repair** and the other one is called **secondary repair.**

Primary Repair

Primary repair takes place in "clean" wounds. A **clean wound** is a cut or incision on the skin where infection is not present. In a simple skin injury, the deep layer of stratified squamous epithelium divides. The new stratified squamous epithelial cells "push" themselves upward toward the surface of the skin.

The damage or wound is quickly and completely restored to normal. However, if the damage is over a larger area, then the underlying connective tissue cells and **fibroblasts*** are also involved.

Primary Repair Over A Larger Skin Area

If a larger area of skin is damaged, fluid will escape from the broken capillaries. This capillary fluid dries and seals the wound, and the typical "scab" forms. Epithelial cells multiply at the edges of the scab and continue to grow over the damaged area until it is covered. If even a much larger area of skin is destroyed, skin **grafts** are needed to help in wound healing.

Primary Repair Of Deeper Tissues

When there is damage to deeper tissues, the edges of the wound must be brought together with **sutures.** For example, in operative incisions or wounds, there is a tremendous amount of **serous fluid** that leaks out onto the wound. This helps to form a **coagulation** (clot) that seals the wound. The coagulum contains tissue fragments and white blood cells. In 24 to 36 hours, the epithelial cells lining the capillaries (**endothelium**) and fibroblasts of connective tissue are rapidly regenerating. The newly formed cells remain along the edges of the wound. On the third day, new vascular tissue starts to form. These multiply across the wound along with connective tissue formation.

On the fourth or fifth day, fibroblast cells start to be very active. They will help to make new collagen fibers. In addition, capillaries grow and "reach" across the wound, holding the edges firmly together. Towards the end of the healing process, the collagenous fibers shorten, and scar tissue is reduced to a minimum.

Secondary Repair

A process called **granulation** occurs in a large open wound with small or large tissue loss. The granulation process will form new vertically upstanding blood vessels. These new blood vessels are surrounded by young connective tissue and wandering cells of different types. Granulation causes the surface area to have a pebbly texture. Fibroblasts will be quite active in their production of new collagenous fibers. With all this activity going on, the large open wound eventually heals up. It also should be mentioned that as granulation occurs, a fluid is secreted. This fluid has very strong **bactericidal** (bacterial destruction) properties. This is important to help reduce the risk of infection during wound healing.

As in any type of tissue repair, there is always some amount of scar tissue that will be formed. The amount of scar (**cicatrix**) tissue formed depends upon the extent of tissue damage. Much careful attention must be given to patients whose body or body parts are undergoing massive tissue repair. These include burn victims with burned areas involving the neck and chest, the chest after breast removal, etc. These areas *must* be kept in alignment and immobile at the beginning. However, later on active movement should be encouraged so as new tissue forms, pulling from scar tissue will not occur. It is the role of the health care professional to help prevent or minimize excessive scar tissue formation that can lead to disfigurement.

---

*Fibroblast is a large, flat branching cell. It helps to form the flexible skin collagen fibers.

A health care professional should be doubly aware that burn victims lose a large amount of blood plasma. A large amount of electrolytes and blood proteins are also lost in the blood plasma. This causes an imbalance to the body's fluid balance. So, it is very important that the health care professional give lots of fluids either orally or **intravenously** to their patient. This must be done regularly until the tissues heal properly and completely.

A health care professional should also be mindful that proper nutrition plays an important part in the healing act. Newly growing tissues require lots of protein for repair, thus the need for protein-rich foods is important.

Vitamins also play an essential role in wound repair. They help the patient develop resistance to and help prevent infections. Table 6–1 gives a listing of some vitamins that are needed in tissue repair.

Table 6–1 Vitamins Favorable To Tissue Repair

VITAMIN	FUNCTION
Vitamin A	Repairs epithelial tissue, especially the epithelial cells lining the respiratory tract.
Vitamin B (Thiamine, nicotinic acid, and riboflavin)	Helps to promote the general well-being of the individual. Specifically helps to promote appetite, metabolism, vigor, and pain relief in some cases.
Vitamin C	Helps in the normal production of and maintenance of collagen fibers and other connective tissue substances.
Vitamin D	Needed for the normal absorption of calcium from the intestine; possibly helps in the repair of bone fractures.
Vitamin K	Helps in the process of blood coagulation.
Vitamin E	Helps healing of tissues by acting as an antioxidant protector. It prevents important molecules and structures in the cell from reacting with oxygen. (When delicate components of living protoplasm are attacked by oxygen, they are literally "burnt.")

Further Study and Discussion

First conduct your own individual research using library reference materials, science magazines, etc., on tissue and organ transplants. Include the following information in your report:

- What are tissue and organ transplants?
- What types of tissues and organs have been transplanted successfully?
- Why is it easier to transplant tissues from one part of the same body to another part on the same body and between identical twins.?
- What are the problems encountered in tissue and organ transplants between two different individuals?

After you have completed your own library research, share your findings in a group discussion with class members.

Assignment

Briefly answer the following questions:

1. Explain the relationship between wound healing and nutrition.

2. Define the term primary repair.

3. What is a "scab"?

4. What is "coagulum" and what does it contain?

5. What is granulation?

6. Name three vitamins important to tissue repair and their role in tissue repair.

UNIT 7

INTEGUMENTARY SYSTEM

KEY WORDS

acne vulgaris
albinism
arector pili
   muscle
athlete's foot
   (dermato-
   phytosis)
callus
carbuncle
corn
cortex
dermis (corium
   or cutis vera)
dermatitis
   actinica
dermatitis
   medica-
   mentosa
eczema
end organs of
   Krause
end organs of
   Ruffini

epidermis
   (cuticle)
friction ridges
fungi
furuncles
gangrene
hair follicle
impetigo
   contagiosa
integument
   (integumentary
   system)
inunction
keratin
matrix (nail bed)
medulla
Meissner's
   corpuscles
melanin
melanocyte
necrosis
Pacinian
   corpuscles

papillae
pili
pruritus
psoriasis
ringworm
root
sarcoptes scabies
scabies
sebaceous gland
sebum
shaft
shingles (herpes
   zoster)
stratum corneum
   (horny layer)
stratum
   germinativum
sudoriferous
   gland
ungues
urticaria (hives or
   nettle rash)
yeast

OBJECTIVES

- Describe the functions of the skin
- Describe the structures found in the two skin layers
- Explain how the skin serves as a channel of excretion
- Describe the action of the sweat glands
- Recognize some common skin disorders
- Define the Key Words related to this unit of study

The skin is our protective covering and is called the **integument** or **integumentary system.** It is tough, pliable, and multi-functional. Skin is first thought of as a covering for the underlying, deeper tissues, protecting them from dehydration, injury, and germ invasion. The skin also helps regulate body temperature by controlling the amount of heat loss. Evaporation of water from the skin, in the form of perspiration, helps rid the body of excess heat. Only a very small amount of waste is eliminated through the skin.

Since the skin is well supplied with nerves, it is sensitive to changes in its surrounding environment. These include changes in temperature (heat or cold), pain, pressure, and touch sensations.

The skin has tissues for the temporary storage of fat, glucose, water, and salts like sodium chloride. Most of these substances are later absorbed by the blood and transported to other parts of the body.

The skin is designed to screen out any harmful ultraviolet radiation contained in sunlight. It also absorbs certain drugs, and other chemical substances. The administration of drugs through the skin is called **inunction.** This absorptive quality can be harmful if insecticides, gas, or lead salts enter the body through the skin.

STRUCTURE OF THE SKIN

The skin consists of two basic layers: (1) The **epidermis** or **cuticle** and (2) The **dermis corium** or **cutis vera** (true skin).

Epidermis

The two most functionally important cellular layers of the epidermis are the **stratum corneum** and the **stratum germinativum.** The cytoplasm of the cells making up the stratum corneum is replaced by a hard, nonliving protein substance called **keratin.** This keratin layer acts as a waterproof covering. Cells making up the stratum corneum are flattened and scalelike. They flake off from the constant friction of clothing, rubbing, and washing. For this reason the stratum corneum is sometimes called the **horny layer.** As the cells of the horny layer are flaked off, they are replaced by new cells from the lower stratum germinativum.

The stratum corneum forms the body's first line of defense against invading bacteria. Because it is slightly acidic, many kinds of organisms which come in contact with the stratum corneum are destroyed. The thickness of the horny layer varies in different parts of the body. It is thickest on the palms of the hands and on the soles of the feet due to constant friction. Sometimes the thickening develops outwardly in a concentrated area forming a **callus.** If the thickening grows inward, a **corn** may form.

The stratum germinativum is a very important epidermal layer. The replacement of cells in the epidermis depends upon the division of cells in this layer. As new germinativum cells form, they push their way upward towards the epidermis. Eventually they become keratinized like the other epidermal cells within the horny layer.

Skin pigmentation is found in germinativum cells called **melanocytes.** Melanocytes contain a skin pigment called **melanin.** Melanin can be black, brown, or have a yellow tint, depending upon racial origin. The amount of melanin (and other skin pigments like carotene and hemoglobin) in the melanocytes determines the various shades of human skin color. Members of the Caucasian (white) race have a reduced amount of melanin in their melanocytes. Other races, on the other hand, possess a higher amount of melanin. Absence of pigments (other than hemoglobin) causes **albinism.** The skin of an albino has a pinkish tint. Basic skin coloring is inherited from our parents.

Environment is another factor which can modify skin coloring. For example, exposure to sunlight may result in a temporary increase in melanin within the melanocytes. This is the darkened, or tanned effect with which we are all familiar. Tanning is produced by the ultraviolet (UV) rays of sunlight. It should be noted that prolonged exposure to sunlight is unwise because it may lead to the development of skin cancers.

As seen in figure 7–1, the lower edge of the stratum germinativum is thrown into ridges. These ridges are known as the **papillae** of the skin. In the skin of the fingers, soles of the feet, and the palms of the hands, these papillae are quite pronounced. So much so, in fact, that they raise the skin into permanent ridges. These ridges are so arranged that they provide maximum resistance to slipping when grasping and holding objects. Thus they are also referred to as **friction ridges.** The ridges on the inner surfaces of the fingers create individual and characteristic fingerprint patterns

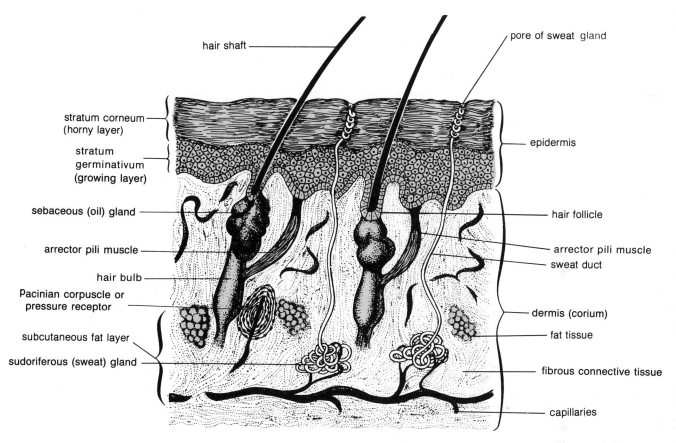

hair shaft

pore of sweat gland

stratum corneum (horny layer)

stratum germinativum (growing layer)

epidermis

sebaceous (oil) gland

hair follicle

arrector pili muscle

arrector pili muscle

sweat duct

hair bulb

Pacinian corpuscle or pressure receptor

dermis (corium)

subcutaneous fat layer

fat tissue

sudoriferous (sweat) gland

fibrous connective tissue

capillaries

Figure 7-1 Cross section of the skin (Adapted from W. Schraer and R. Noelle, *A Learning Program for Biology,* Fairfield, New Jersey: Cebco Publishing Co.)

used in identification. Newborn infants are also footprinted for means of identity.

Dermis

The dermis, or **corium,** is the thicker, inner layer of the skin. It contains matted masses of connective tissue, strong fibrous tissue bands, elastic fibers (through which pass numerous blood vessels), lymphatics, nerve endings, muscles, hair follicles; oil and sweat glands, and fat cells. The thickness of the dermis varies over different parts of the body. It is, for instance, thicker over the soles of the feet and the palms of the hand. The skin cover-

ing the shoulders and back is thinner than that over the palms, but thicker than the skin over the abdomen and thorax.

There are many nerve receptors of different types in the dermal layer. The sensory nerves end in receptors which are sensitive to heat. They are called the **end organs of Ruffini.** Those sensitive to cold are the **end organs of Krause. Meissner's corpuscles** detect the sensation of touch, while the deeper lying **Pacinian corpuscles** detect pressure. There are also nerve endings to sense pain located under the epidermis and around the hair follicles. These pain receptors are especially numerous on the lower arm, breast, and forehead.

APPENDAGES OF THE SKIN

The appendages of the skin include the hair, nails, the sudoriferous (sweat) glands, the sebaceous (oil) glands, and their ducts.

Hair

Hairs (**pili**) are distributed over most of the surface area of the body. They are missing from the palms of hands, soles of feet, the glans penis, and the inner surfaces of the vaginal labia.

The length, thickness, type, and color of hair varies with the different body parts and different races. The hairs of the eyelids, for example, are extremely short, while hair from the scalp can grow to a considerable length. Facial and pubic hair are quite thick. The hair of Asian people is straight; that of Africans is very curly.

Microscopic examination reveals that a hair is composed of three layers: the outer **cuticle** layer, the **cortex,** and the inner **medulla.** The cuticle consists of a single layer of flat, scalelike, keratinized cells that overlap each other. The cortex is comprised of elongated, keratinized, nonliving cells. Hair pigment is located in the cortex, or in the medulla if one is present. In dark hair the cortex contains pigment granules; white hair indicates the presence of air.

A hair consists of a **root** and a **shaft.** The root is the part of the hair that is implanted in the skin. The shaft is that part which projects from the skin surface. The root is embedded in an inpocketing of the epidermis called the **hair follicle.** Toward the lower end of the hair follicle is a tuft of tissue called the **papilla,** which extends upward into the hair root. The papilla contains capillaries which nourish the hair follicle cells. This is important because the division of cells in the hair follicle gives rise to a new hair.

Attached to each hair follicle on the side toward which it slopes is a smooth muscle called the **arrector pili muscle.** When the pili muscle is stimulated, as by a sudden chill, it contracts and causes the skin to pucker around the hair. This occasions the so-called "goosebumps" or "gooseflesh" condition. When this occurs, a small amount of oil is produced, due to pressure on the sebaceous glands.

Nails

The nails (**onyz, onych**) are hard structures covering the dorsal surfaces of the last phalanges of the fingers and toes. They are slightly convex on their upper surfaces and concave on their lower surfaces. A nail is formed in the **nail bed,** or **matrix.** Here the epidermal cells first appear as elongated cells. These then fuse together to form hard, keratinized plates. As long as a nail bed remains intact, a nail will always be formed. Occasionally, a nail is lost due to an injury or disease. However, if the nail bed is not damaged, a new nail will be produced.

Sweat Glands

Actual excretion is a minor function of the skin; certain wastes dissolved in perspiration are removed. Perspiration is 99 percent water with only small quantities of salt and organic materials (waste products). Sweat, or **sudoriferous,** glands are distributed over the entire skin surface. They are present in large numbers under the arms, on the palms of the hands, soles of the feet, and forehead.

Sweat glands are tubular, with a coiled base and a tubelike duct which extends to form a pore in the skin, figure 7-1. Perspiration is excreted through the pores. Under the control of the nervous system, these glands may be activated by several factors including heat, pain, fever, and nervousness.

The amount of water lost through the skin is almost 500 milliliters a day. However, this varies according to the type of exercise and the environmental temperature. In profuse sweating a great deal of water may be lost; it is vital to replace the loss of water as soon as possible.

Sebaceous Glands

The skin is protected by a thick, oily substance known as **sebum** secreted by the **sebaceous glands.** Sebum lubricates the skin, keeping it soft and pliable.

THE INTEGUMENT AND ITS RELATIONSHIP TO MICROORGANISMS

Most of the surface of the skin is not a favorable place for microbial growth because it is too dry. Microbes live only on moist skin areas where they adhere to and grow on the surfaces of dead cells that compose the outer epidermal layer. The type of microbes found are of the Staphylococcus or Corynebacterium bacterial species type. The other types are **fungi*** and **yeasts***.

Most skin bacteria are associated with the hair follicles or sweat glands where nutrients are present and the moisture content is high. "Underarm perspiration odor" is caused by the interaction of bacteria on perspiration. This odor can be minimized or prevented either by decreasing perspiration with antiperspirants or killing the bacteria with deodorant soaps. Each hair follicle is associated with a sebaceous gland that secretes a lubricant. This lubricant fluid contains amino acids, lactic acid, lipids, salts and urea. These are substances that can support microbial growth.

A health care professional must exercise proper handwashing in order to minimize or remove skin microbes. Depending upon skin conditions and number of microbes present, it takes seven to eight minutes of scrubbing to remove most of the temporary skin bacteria. However, more permanent, resident bacteria are removed less easily. Sometimes, washing may increase the number of microbes on the skin surface because it draws out bacteria embedded in the hair follicles.

REPRESENTATIVE DISORDERS OF THE SKIN

Acne vulgaris is a common and chronic disorder of the sebaceous glands. Its exact cause is presently unknown. Somehow the sebaceous glands secrete excessive oil, or sebum, which is deposited at the openings of the glands. Eventually this oily deposit becomes hard, or keratinized, plugging up the opening. This prevents the escape of the oily secretions, and the area becomes filled with leukocytes. The leukocytes cause the accumulation of pus. Acne occurs most often during adolescence and is marked by blackheads, cysts, pimples, and scarring. While there is no definite evidence to support the theory, it is believed that acne may be associated with the oversecretion of sex hormones.

Athlete's foot (dermatophytosis) is a contagious fungal infection. The fungus, or dermatophyte, infects the superficial skin layer and leads to skin eruptions. These eruptions are characterized by the formation of small blisters between the fingers and most often, the toes. Accompanied by cracking and scaling, this condition is usually contracted in public baths or showers. Treatment involves thorough cleansing and drying of the affected area. In addition, special antifungal antibiotics

*Fungi are low form of microscopic plant life lacking chlorophyll; may be filamentous (mold) or unicellular (yeast).
*Yeast is a microscopic, single-celled member of the fungi division.

(such as Amphotericin B) are administered and antifungal powders are applied liberally.

Eczema is an acute, or chronic, noncontagious inflammatory skin disease. The skin becomes dry, red, itchy, and scaly. Various factors can lead to eczema. These may include diet, tight clothing, cosmetics, creams, medications, or soaps. Eczema caused by ingested drugs is known as **dermatitis medicamentosa.** That caused by sunlight or artificial ultraviolet radiation is called **dermatitis actinica.** Treatment consists of removal or avoidance of the causative agent, as well as application of topical medications containing hydrocortisone. The medication, however, only helps to alleviate the symptoms.

Gangrene is the necrosis, or death, of tissue cells resulting from the blockage of blood supply to an area, or from disease or direct injury. The prompt surgical removal of the gangrenous area is required in order to prevent the spread of necrosis to healthy neighboring tissues.

Impetigo contagiosa is an acute, inflammatory and contagious skin disease seen in babies and young children. It is caused by the staphylococcus or streptococcus organism. This disorder is characterized by the appearance of vesicles which rupture and develop distinct yellow crusts.

Pruritus, an intense itching stimulated by irritation of a peripheral sensory nerve, is a symptom rather than a disease. Diabetes mellitus, liver ailments, and thyroid disorders may cause pruritus. Thus treatment of the respective disease alleviates the pruritis.

Psoriasis is a chronic inflammatory skin disease characterized by the development of reddish patches which are covered with silvery-white scales. It affects the hands, feet and scalp (but not the face). The application of creams or lotions containing a specially re-

fined coal tar compound may alleviate the discomfort and help control the disease.

Ringworm is a highly contagious fungal infection marked by raised, itchy, circular patches with crusts. It may occur upon the skin, scalp, and underneath the nails. Ringworm can be effectively treated with a drug called griseofulvin.

Scabies also known as "seven-year itch," is a contagious skin disorder caused by a tiny insect parasite, **Sarcoptes scabies.** This affliction is characterized by multiple skin lesions, along with intense itching which occurs chiefly during the night. The itching is caused by the female insect burrowing beneath the epidermis to lay her eggs. Specific ointments, frequent baths, and change of clean clothing are prescribed.

Urticaria, hives, or **nettle rash** is a skin condition recognized by the appearance of intensely itching wheals or welts. These welts have an elevated usually white, center with a surrounding pink area. They appear in clusters distributed over the entire body surface. The welts last about a day or two. Urticaria is generally a response to an allergen, such as an ingested drug or foods like citrus fruits, chocolate, fish, eggs, shellfish, strawberries, and tomatoes. Complete avoidance and elimination of the causative factor(s) alleviate the problem.

Furuncles are boils which are usually the result of staphylococcus infections in the hair follicles.

Carbuncles are hard, round, deeply-embedded and painful abscesses of the subcutaneous skin tissue. A carbuncle is much larger than a boil; its flat surface oozes pus from multiple points on its surface. Fever usually accompanies the appearance of carbuncles. When they eventually slough away, they leave a scarred cavity behind. Treatment may require incision, drainage of pus, and use of anti-biotics.

Shingles (herpes zoster) is a skin eruption thought to be due to a virus infection of the nerve endings. It is commonly seen on the chest or abdomen, accompanied by severe pain known as herpetic neuralgia. The condition is especially serious in elderly or debilitated persons. The affected area must be treated by protecting it from air and from the irritation of clothing.

They say that the eyes may be the mirror of the soul, but the skin often shows the condition of the "internal milieu" (environment). The health care professional should be familiar with the different types of skin disorders or lesions. This can indicate to the health professional the presence of a specific type of internal disease or disorder in the patient they are caring for. Sometimes the skin lesions indicates only an outer skin disorder. Table 7–1 describes the different types of skin lesions, their characteristics, and their dimensions.

Table 7–1 Different Types of Skin Lesions, Their Characteristics, Size, and Examples

TYPE OF SKIN LESION	CHARACTERISTICS	SIZE	EXAMPLE(S)
Bulla (blister)	Fluid-filled area	Greater than 5 mm across	A large blister
Macule	A round, flat area usually distinguished from its surrounding skin by its change in color	Smaller than 1 cm	• Freckle • Petechia
Nodule	Elevated solid area, deeper and firmer than a papule	Greater than 5 mm across	Wart
Papule	Elevated solid area	5 mm or less across	Elevated nevus
Pustule	Discrete, pus-filled raised area	Varying size	Acne
Ulcer	A deep loss of skin surface that may extend into the dermis that can bleed periodically and scar	Varies in sizes	Venous stasis ulcer
Tumor	Solid abnormal mass of cells that may extend deep through cutaneous tissue	Larger than 1-2 cm	• Benign (harmless) epidermal tumor • Basal cell carcinoma (rarely metastasizing)
Vesicle	Fluid-filled raised area	5 mm or less across	• Chickenpox • Herpes simplex
Wheal	Itchy, temporarily elevated area with an irregular shape formed as a result of localized skin edema	Varies in size	• Hives • Insect bites

Further Study and Discussion

- Pour an equal amount of cold water in two beakers. Cover the water in one beaker with olive oil to prevent evaporation of water. Place them in a container of boiling water.

  a. In which beaker did the temperature rise more rapidly? Why?

  b. What conclusion may be drawn from this experiment in discussing heat loss and the regulation of body temperature in human beings?

- Take your temperature and record the result.

  a. By mouth

  b. By axilla

  c. By mouth, immediately after a cold drink

  d. By mouth, immediately after a hot drink

  Compare the various temperatures. Discuss the reasons for the differences.

- Inspect the skin on various areas of the body. Look for the skin pores, skin irritations, pimples, scaliness, and dryness. Discuss methods of proper cleansing of the skin; nutrition to improve the skin; the effect of sunshine on the skin; and sensitivity of skin to cosmetics.

Assignment

1. In what way does the skin act as an organ of excretion?

2. What factors stimulate the sweat glands into activity?

3. Under normal circumstances, approximately how much water is lost daily through the skin?

4. What is perspiration?

5. What are the sudoriferous glands?

6. What are the three different types of microorganisms that can be found on the outer epidermal layer?

7. What causes "underarm perspiration odor," and what measures can minimize this perspiration odor?

8. Why is it very important for a health care professional to practice proper handwashing?

THE BODY AS A WHOLE

A. Complete the following statements.

1. A group of similar cells which performs one special function is _____ _____ .

2. Three types of muscle tissue are _____ , _____ , and _____ .

3. Tissue which is found on the surface of the body or lining the body cavities is called _____ .

4. A group of tissues performing one special function is _____ .

5. The part of a cell which directs its activites is _____ .

6. The tissue which provides transportation of materials within the body is _____ .

7. A group of organs which together perform a special function is called _____ .

8. The hardest of the connective tissue adapted to give support and protection is _____ .

9. The tissue which provides for contraction is _____ .

10. Four different kinds of connective tissue are _____ , _____ , _____ , and _____ .

B. Classify each of the following according to its main tissue type.

1. Skin _____   6. Skeleton _____

2. Blood _____   7. Spinal cord _____

3. Adipose _____   8. Walls of the stomach _____

4. Heart _____   9. Lining of the nose _____

5. Brain _____   10. Tendon _____

C. Name the body system to which each of the following organs belongs.

1. Brain_____
2. Adrenal glands _____
3. Spinal column _____
4. Voluntary muscles _____
5. Lungs _____

6. Heart _____
7. Kidneys _____
8. Uterus _____
9. Stomach _____

D. Label the parts indicated in Figure SE1-A.

1 _____
2 _____
3 _____
4 _____
5 _____
6 _____
7 _____

8 _____
9 _____
10 _____
11 _____
12 _____
13 _____

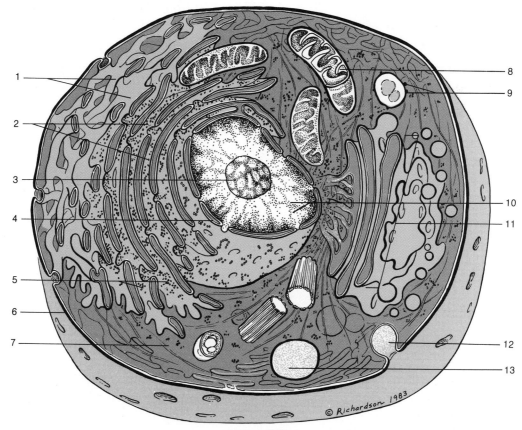

Figure SE1-A

E. Why is the cell called the basic unit of body structure and function?

F. Match each term in column I with its correct definition or description in column II.

Column I	Column II
_____ 1. abdominal cavity	a. location of brain
_____ 2. abdominopelvic cavity	b. another name for chest
_____ 3. dorsal cavity	c. location of diaphragm
_____ 4. thoracic cavity	d. location of liver
_____ 5. ventral cavity	e. location of urinary bladder
_____ 6. spinal cavity	f. sum total of all life functions
_____ 7. diaphragm	g. location of the spinal cord
_____ 8. anabolism	h. synthesis of complex materials from simpler ones
_____ 9. catabolism	i. tissue separating the thorax from the abdominopelvic cavity
_____ 10. metabolism	j. the breakdown of complex materials into simpler ones

G. Briefly answer the following questions.

1. What does embryology study?

2. What is a carbohydrate? Give three examples of a carbohydrate.

3. What is the function of the nuclear membrane?

4. What causes "underarm perspiration odor"?

5. List three vitamins needed in tissue repair and what are their functions?

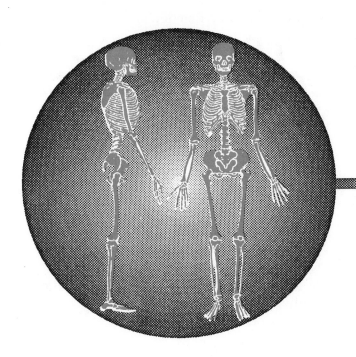

CHAPTER 2

THE BODY FRAMEWORK

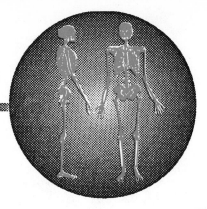

UNIT 8

INTRODUCTION TO THE SKELETAL SYSTEM

KEY WORDS

abduction
adduction
atlas
amphiarthroses
articular
articular
  cartilage
axis
ball and socket
  joint
bursa
diarthroses
extension

fibrous disc
flexion
gliding joint
herniated
  (slipped)
  disc
hinge joint
homeostasis
joint
ligament
pivot joint
pronation
rotation

skeletal system
skeleton
supination
suture
symphysis
  pubis
synarthroses
synovial cavity
synovial fluid
synovial
  membrane
tendon
torso

OBJECTIVES

- List the main function of bones in the body
- Identify and locate four types of bones
- Name and define the main types of joints
- Name the main types of joint motion
- Define the Key Words relating to this unit of study

If you have ever visited a beach, you may have seen a jellyfish floating lightly near the surface. The organs of the jellyfish are buoyed up by the water. But, if a wave should chance to deposit the jellyfish upon the beach, it would collapse into a disorganized mass of tissue. This is because the jellyfish does not possess a supportive framework or **skeleton.** Fortunately, we humans do not suffer such a fate because we have a solid, bony skeleton to support our organs.

The **skeletal system** comprises the bony framework of the body. It is composed of 206 individual bones in the adult; some bones are hinged, while others are fused to one another.

FUNCTIONS

The skeletal system has five specific functions:

1. **Supports** body structures and provides shape to the body.

2. **Protects** the soft and delicate internal organs. For example, the cranium protects the brain, the inner ear, and parts of the eye. The ribs and breastbone protect the heart and lungs; the vertebral column encases and protects the spinal cord.

3. **Movement** and **anchorage** of muscles. Muscles which are attached to the skeleton are called skeletal muscles. Upon contraction, these muscles exert a pull upon a bone and so move it. In this manner, bones play a vital part in body movement, serving as passively operated levers.

4. **Mineral storage.** Bones are a storage depot for minerals like calcium and

phosphorus. In case of inadequate nutrition, the body is able to draw upon these reserves. For example, if the blood calcium dips below normal, the bone releases the necessary amount of stored calcium into the bloodstream. When calcium levels exceed normal, calcium release from the skeletal system is inhibited. In this way the skeletal system helps to maintain blood calcium homeostasis.

5. **Hemopoiesis.** The red marrow of the bone is the site of blood cell formation.

BONE TYPES

Bones are classified as one of four types on the basis of their form, figure 8–1. *Long* bones are found in both upper and lower arms and legs. The bones of the skull are examples of *flat* bones, as are the ribs. *Irregular* bones are represented by bones of the spinal column. The wrist and ankle bones are examples of *short* bones, which appear cube-like in shape.

The bones in the hand are short, making flexible movement possible. The same is true

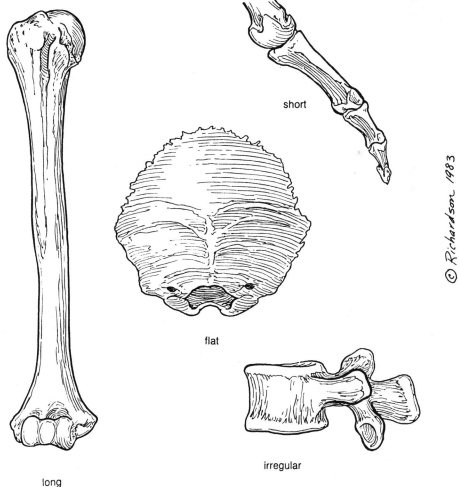

short

© Richardson 1983

flat

irregular

long

Figure 8-1 Bone shapes

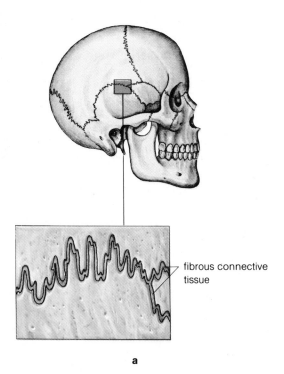

fibrous connective
tissue

a

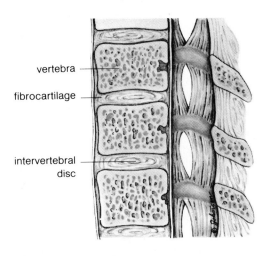

vertebra

fibrocartilage

intervertebral
disc

b

of the irregular bones of the spinal column.
The thigh bone is a long bone, needed for support of the strong leg muscles and the weight
of the body. The degree of movement at a
joint is determined by bone shape and joint
structure.

JOINTS AND RELATED STRUCTURES

Joints are points of contact between two
bones. They are classified into three main
types according to their degree of movement:
diarthroses (movable) joints, **amphiarthroses**
(partially movable) joints, and **synarthroses**
(immovable) joints, figure 8–2.

Most of the joints in our body are diarthroses. They tend to have the same structure.
These movable joints consist of three main
parts: **articular cartilage,** a **bursa** (joint capsule)
and a **synovial** (joint) **cavity.**

When two movable bones meet at a joint,
their surfaces do not touch one another. The
two **articular** (joint) surfaces are covered with a
smooth, slippery cap of cartilage known as **articular cartilage.** This articular cartilage helps
to absorb jolts.

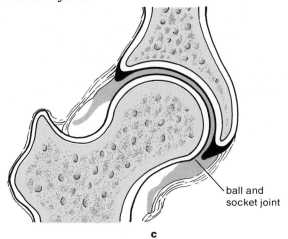

ball and
socket joint

c

**Figure 8-2   Types of joints: (a) a synarthrosis, an immovable fibrous joint (cranial bones); (b) an amphiarthrosis, a
slightly movable cartilaginous joint (ribs or vertebra); (c) a diarthrosis, a freely movable hinge or ball-and-socket joint
(elbow and hip).**

Enclosing two articular surfaces of the bone is a tough, fibrous connective tissue capsule called an **articular capsule.** Lining the **articular capsule** is a synovial membrane which secretes **synovial fluid** (a lubricating substance) into the synovial cavity (an area between the two articular cartilages). The synovial fluid reduces the friction of joint movement.

The clefts in connective tissue between muscles, tendons, ligaments, and bones contain synovial bursae. They are made into closed sacs by synovial lining, similar to that of a true joint. They allow muscles or tendons to glide over bony prominences.

As we advance in age, the joints undergo degenerative changes. The synovial fluid is not secreted as quickly, and the articular cartilaginous surfaces of the two bone ends become ossified. This results in excess bone outgrowths along the joint edges, which tend to stiffen joints, causing inflammation, pain and a decrease in mobility.

There are several types of diarthroses joints: ball-and-socket, hinge, pivot, and gliding joints:

- **Ball and Socket joints** allow the greatest freedom of movement. Here, one bone has a ball-shaped head which nestles into a concave socket of the second bone. Our shoulders and hips have ball-and-socket joints.

- **Hinge joints** move in one direction or plane, as in the knees, elbows and outer joints of the fingers.

- **Pivot joints** are those with an extension rotating in a second, arch-shaped bone. The radius and ulna (long bones of the forearm), wrist and ankle are pivot joints. Another example is the joint between the *atlas* (first cervical vertebra in the neck) which supports the head, and the *axis* (second cervical vertebra) which allows the head to rotate.

- **Gliding joints** are those in which nearly flat surfaces glide across each other, as in the vertebrae of the spine. These joints enable the **torso** to bend forward, backward and sideways, as well as rotate.

Between each body of the vertebrae are found **fibrous disks.** At the center of each fibrous disk is a pulpy, elastic material which loses its resiliency with increased usage and/or age. Disks can be compressed by sudden and forceful jolts to the spine. This may cause a disk to protrude from the vertebrae and impinge upon the spinal nerves resulting in extreme pain. Such a condition is known as a **herniated** or **slipped disk.**

Amphiarthroses are partially movable joints. These joints have cartilage between their articular surfaces. Two examples are: (1) the attachment of the ribs to the spine and **symphysis pubis,** and (2) the joint between the two pubic bones.

Synarthroses are immovable joints connected by tough, fibrous connective tissue. These joints are found in the adult cranium. The bones are fused together in a joint which forms a heavy protective cover for the brain. Such cranial joints are commonly called **sutures.**

Ligaments are fibrous bands which connect bones and cartilages and serve as support for muscles. Joints are also bound together by ligaments. **Tendons** are fibrous cords which connect muscles to bones.

TYPES OF MOTION

Joints can move in many directions, figure 8–3. **Flexion** is the act of bending forward as when the forearm or fingers are bent or

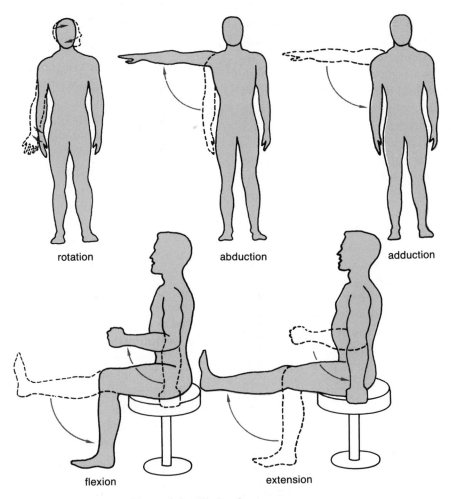

Figure 8-3   Kinds of movements

A **rotation** movement allows a bone to move around one central axis. Two rotation movements are pronation and supination. In **pronation,** the forearm turns the hand so the palm is downward or backward. In **supination,** the palm is forward or upward.

flexed. **Extension** means straightening the forearm or fingers. **Abduction** is the movement of an extremity away from the midline (an imaginary line which divides the body from head to foot). **Adduction** is movement toward the midline.

Further Study and Discussion

- On a human skeleton model, point out the various joints which are movable, partially movable, and those which are immovable.

- Obtain the legs and wings of a turkey or chicken. Identify the bones, muscles, tendons and ligaments. Note the toughness of the tendons and ligaments. Observe the action of the joints, tendons, and ligaments as the leg is bent and straightened or the wing is spread.

- Discuss the differences in the structure of the male and female skeletons.

- Explain why tendons and ligaments are made of very tough tissue.

- Discuss the functions of the skeletal system.

Assignment

Select the letter before the word or phrase which most correctly completes the statement.

1. Supination is one type of
    a. extension   c. adduction
    b. abduction   d. rotation

2. The bones found in the skull are
    a. irregular bones   c. short bones
    b. flat bones   d. long bones

3. The cranium protects the
    a. lungs   c. heart
    b. brain   d. stomach

4. Pivot joints may be found in the
    a. vertebral column   c. wrist
    b. skull   d. shoulder

5. Irregular bones may be found in the
    a. leg   c. arm
    b. vertebral column   d. skull

6. Short bones are found in the
    a. leg   c. vertebral column
    b. arm   d. hand

7. Immovable joints are found in the
    a. infant's skull   c. adult spinal column
    b. adult cranium   d. child's spinal column

8. Flexion means
    a. bending   c. extending
    b. rotating   d. abduction

9. The degree of motion at a joint is determined by
    a. the amount of synovial fluid
    b. the number of bursa
    c. the unusual amount of exercise
    d. bone shape and joint structure

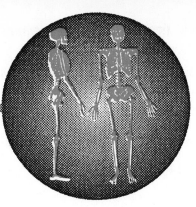

UNIT 9

STRUCTURE AND FORMATION OF BONE

KEY WORDS

articular cartilage
bone collagen
compact bone
diaphysis
endosteum
epiphyseal
  cartilage
epiphysis

erythrocyte
fibroblast
fontanel
growth zone
haversian
  canals
leukocytes
marrow cavity

medullary
  (marrow) canal
ossification
osteoblast
osteoclast
osteocyte
periosteum
spongy bone

OBJECTIVES

- Explain the formation of bones
- Describe bones with regard to composition and construction
- Relate bone changes to body growth
- Define the Key Words relating to this unit of study

Bones are composed of microscopic cells called **osteocytes** (*osteon* — bone; Greek). An **osteocyte** is a mature bone cell. Bone is made up of 35% organic material and 65% inorganic mineral salts.

The organic part derives from a protein called **bone collagen,** a fibrous material. Between these collagenous fibers is a jelly-like material. The organic substances of bone gives it a certain degree of flexibility. The inorganic portion of bone is made from mineral salts like calcium phosphate, calcium carbonate, calcium fluoride, magnesium phosphate, sodium oxide and sodium chloride. These minerals give bone its hardness and durability.

A bony skeleton can be compared to steel-reinforced concrete. The collagenous fibers may be compared to flexible steel supports, and minerals salts to concrete. When tension is applied to a bone, the flexible, organic material prevents bone damage, while the mineral elements resist crushing under pressure.

BONE FORMATION

The embryonic skeleton is initially composed of collagenous protein fibers secreted by the **fibroblasts** (primitive embryonic cells). Later on, during embryonic development, cartilage is deposited between the fibers. At this stage, the embryo's skeleton consists of collagenous protein fibers and hyaline (clear) cartilage. During the eighth week of embryonic development, **ossification** begins. That is, mineral matter starts to replace previously formed cartilage, creating bone. Infant bones are very soft and pliable because of incomplete ossification at birth. A familiar example is the soft spot on a baby's head, the **fontanel,** see color plate 3. The bone has not yet been formed there, although it will become hardened later.

Ossification due to mineral deposits continues through childhood. As bones ossify, they become hard and more capable of bearing weight.

STRUCTURE

A typical long bone is composed of a shaft, or **diaphysis.** This is a hollow cylinder of hard, compact bone. It is what makes a long bone strong and hard yet light enough for movement. At the ends (extremes) of the diaphysis are the **epiphyses,** figure 9–1.

In the center of the shaft is the broad **medullary canal.** This is filled with yellow bone marrow, mostly made of fat cells. The marrow also contains many blood vessels and some cells which form white blood cells, called **leukocytes.** The yellow marrow functions as a fat

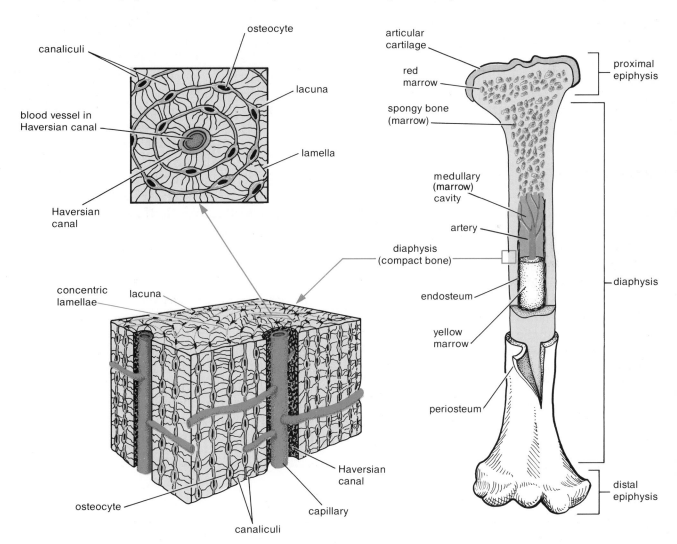

Figure 9-1   A typical long bone

storage center. The marrow canal is lined and the cavity kept intact by the **endosteum.**

The medullary canal is surrounded by **compact** or **hard bone. Haversian canals** branch into the compact bone. They carry blood vessels which nourish the **osteocytes,** or bone cells. Where less strength is needed in the bone, some of the hard bone is dissolved away leaving *spongy* bone.

The ends of the long bones contain the red marrow where some red blood cells called **erythrocytes** and some white blood cells are made. The outside of the bone is covered with the **periosteum,** a tough fibrous tissue which contains blood vessels, lymph vessels and nerves. The periosteum is necessary for bone growth, repair and nutrition.

Covering the epiphysis is a thin layer of cartilage known as the **articular cartilage.** This cartilage acts as a shock absorber between two bones that meet to form a joint.

GROWTH

Bones grow in length and ossify from the center of the diaphysis toward the epiphyseal extremities. Using a long bone by way of example, it will grow lengthwise in an area called the **growth zone.** Ossification occurs here, causing the bone to lengthen; this causes the epiphyses to grow away from the middle of the diaphysis. It is a sensible growth process, since it doesn't interfere with the articulation between two bones.

A bone increases its circumference by the addition of more bone to the outer surface of the diaphysis by osteoblasts. **Osteoblasts** are bone cells that deposit the new bone. As girth increases, bone material is being dissolved from the central part of the diaphysis. This forms an internal cavity called the **marrow cavity,** or **medullary canal.** The medullary canal gets larger as the diameter of the bone increases.

The dissolution of bone from the medullary canal results from the action of cells called osteoclasts. **Osteoclasts** are very large bone cells which secrete enzymes. These enzymes digest the bony material, splitting the bone minerals and enabling them to be absorbed by the surrounding fluid. The medullary canal eventually fills with yellow marrow and cells that will produce white blood cells.

The length of a bone shaft continues to grow until all the epiphyseal cartilage is ossified. At this point, bone growth stops. This fact is helpful in determining further growth in a child. First, an X ray of the child's wrist is taken. If some epiphyseal cartilage remains, there will be further growth. If there is no epiphyseal cartilage left, the child has reached his or her full stature (height).

The average growth in females continues to about 18 years, in males to approximately 20 or 21 years. However, new bone growth can occur in a broken bone at any time. Bone cells near the site of a fracture become active, secreting large amounts of new bone within a relatively short time. Bone healing proceeds quickly and efficiently in youth. The process can be helped along when the fractured ends are properly aligned and immobilized by a cast, splint or by the insertion of a bone pin.

Further Study and Discussion

- Obtain a beef bone from the butcher shop. Have it sawed through the center — lengthwise so that the inner portion of the bone is visible. Identify each part of the bone.

- Discuss how the periosteum is involved in the growth of a bone.

Assignment

A. Briefly answer the following questions.

1. Describe the composition of bone.

2. Explain the function of the red marrow of the bone.

3. Explain the function of the yellow marrow of the bone and what it is made from.

4. Describe the function of the Haversian canals.

5. Why do infant bones tend to be soft and pliable?

6. How may it be determined whether or not a child will have further bone growth?

7. Discuss the pattern of bone growth.

8. How can the process of bone healing be helped along?

B. Match each term in column I with its correct description in column II.

Column I	Column II
_____ 1. mineral matter	a. dietary elements which furnish cells with necessary matérials to manufacture mineral matter
_____ 2. ossification	b. center of the bone shaft
_____ 3. fontanel	c. part of bone containing yellow marrow, blood vessels, and some cells which form white blood cells
_____ 4. endosteum	d. stage of development when bones begin to form
_____ 5. calcium and phosphorus	e. the process of mineral deposition and bone cell growth
_____ 6. epiphysis	f. another term for sodium chloride
_____ 7. periosteum	g. area in infant skull where bone has not yet formed
_____ 8. bone marrow	h. lining of the bone marrow canal
_____ 9. medullary canal	i. elements which make bones hard and durable
_____ 10. early embry- onic period	j. end structure of a long bone
	k. bone cells or osteocytes
	l. bone covering which contains blood vessels, lymph vessels, and nerves

PARTS OF THE SKELETON

KEY WORDS

acetabulum
appendicular
  skeleton
articular process
axial skeleton
bipedal
body of
  vertebrae
calcaneous
cervical
clavicle
coccyx
costal
  cartilage
ethmoid
femur
fibula
foramen
frontal bone
glenoid fossa
humerus

hyoid bone
ilium
innominate bones
intervertebral
  disc
ischium
longitudinal arch
lumbar
manubrium
metacarpal
metatarsal
occipital bone
olecranon process
opposable thumb
ossa carpi
paranasal sinus
parietal bone
patella
phalange
pubis
quadripedal

radius
sacral
sacroiliac joint
scapula
sesamoid bone
spinous process
sphenoid
suture
symphysis pubis
talus
tarsus
temporal bone
thoracic
tibia
transverse arch
transverse
  process
true ribs
ulna
vertebrae
xiphoid process

OBJECTIVES

- Name the components of the two main parts of the human skeleton
- Describe the functions of the main bone structures
- Locate the bones in the human skeleton
- Define the Key Words that relate to this unit of study

The skeletal system is comprised of two main parts. The *axial skeleton* consists of the skull, spinal column, ribs, breastbone and hyoid bone. The **hyoid bone** is a U-shaped bone in the neck. The tongue is attached to it. The **appendicular skeleton** includes the upper extremities: shoulder girdles, arms, wrists, hands, and the lower extremities: hip girdle, legs, ankles and feet, figure 10–1.

AXIAL SKELETON

The skull is composed of the cranium and facial bones. The cranium houses and protects

the delicate brain, while the facial bones guard and support the eyes, ears, nose and mouth. Some of the facial bones, such as the nasal bones, are made of bone and cartilage. For example, the upper part of the nose (bridge) is bone, while the lower part is cartilage.

Cranial bones are thin and slightly curved. During infancy, these bones are held snugly together by an irregular band of connective tissue called a **suture**. As the child grows, this connective tissue ossifies and turns into hard bone. Thus the cranium becomes a highly efficient, dome-shaped shield for the brain. The dome shape affords better protection than

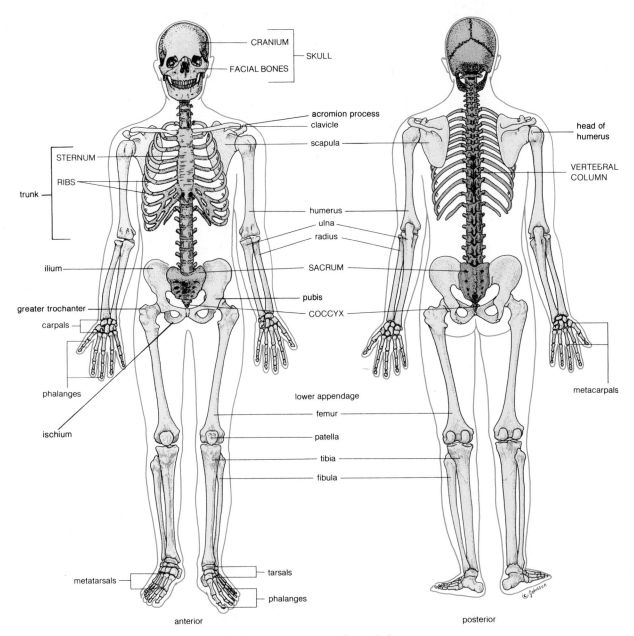

Figure 10-1   Bones of the skeleton

a flat surface, deflecting blows directed toward the head. However, it is not invulnerable and a particularly hard blow may fracture it. This can lead to a concussion: if the bone is depressed, serious injury to brain tissue may result. A depressed fracture may require surgery to relieve the pressure from the brain.

Collectively, there are twenty-two bones in the skull. Eight bones are in the cranium: **frontal bone,** left and right **parietal, occipital,** left and right **temporal, sphenoid** and **ethmoid.** The remaining fourteen are facial bones. Of these, the mandible (lower jaw) is the largest and aids in chewing. The smallest bones are the three within the ear: the hammer, anvil, and stirrup; they play a vital role in hearing, see color plates 4 and 5.

The skull contains large spaces (cavities) within the facial bones, referred to as **paranasal sinuses.** These sinuses are lined with mucous membranes. When a person suffers from a cold, flu or hayfever, the membranes become inflamed and swollen, producing a copious amount of mucus. This may lead to sinus pain and a "stuffy" nasal sensation.

Spine

The spine, or vertebral column, is strong and flexible. It supports the head and provides for the attachment of the ribs. The spine also encloses the spinal cord of the nervous system.

The spine consists of small bones called **vertebrae** which are separated from each other by pads of cartilage tissue called **intervertebral disks.** The vertebral column is divided into five sections from the first to the last vertebrae: **cervical** (neck) **thoracic** (chest), **lumbar** (lower back), **sacral** (hip) and **coccyx** (tail), figure 10–2(a). The first vertebra is the atlas, which supports the skull. The second is called the

axis: it makes rotation of the skull possible as the atlas turns upon the axis.

There are 33 separate vertebrae within the developing embryo. Before birth, several will fuse together, leaving only 26. These include seven cervical, twelve thoracic, five lumbar vertebrae, five fused sacral vertebrae, and four coccygeal vertebrae, figure 10–2(b).

When you study a model of the human skeleton, you will notice that the spine is curved instead of straight. A curved spine has more strength than a straight one would have. Furthermore, its shape provides the proper balance for human **bipedal** (two-footed) posture, as opposed to the **quadripedal** four-footed) posture of most animals. Before birth, the thoracic and sacral regions are convex curves. As the infant learns to hold up its head, the cervical region becomes concave. When the child learns to stand, the lumbar region also becomes concave. This completes the four curves of a normal, adult human spine. Sometimes the spine does not form normally as illustrated in figure 10–3.

A typical vertebra, as seen in figure 10–4 on page 94, contains three basic parts: body, foramen and (several) processes. The large, solid part of the vertebra is known as the **body;** the central opening for the spinal cord is called the **foramen.** Above the foramen protrude two wing-like bony structures called **transverse processes.** The roof of the foramen contains the **spinous process** (spine) and the **articular processes.**

Ribs and Sternum

The thoracic area of the body is protected and supported by the thoracic vertebrae, ribs, and sternum.

The breastbone (sternum) is divided into three parts: the upper region (**manubrium**), the

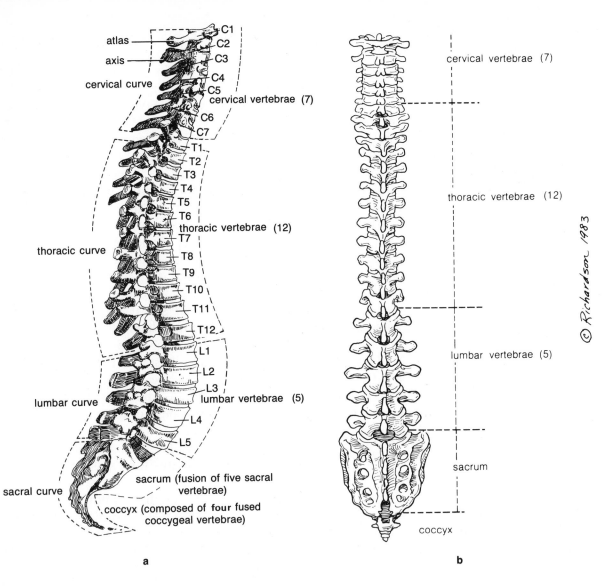

atlas
axis
cervical curve
C1
C2
C3
C4
C5
cervical vertebrae (7)
C6
C7
T1
T2
T3
T4
T5
T6
thoracic vertebrae (12)
T7
thoracic curve
T8
T9
T10
T11
T12
L1
L2
L3
lumbar curve
lumbar vertebrae (5)
L4
L5
sacrum (fusion of five sacral vertebrae)
sacral curve
coccyx (composed of **four** fused coccygeal vertebrae)

cervical vertebrae (7)

thoracic vertebrae (12)

© Richardson 1983

lumbar vertebrae (5)

sacrum

coccyx

a

b

Figure 10-2   (a) Lateral view of the spine; (b) dorsal view of the spine

body, and a lower cartilaginous part called the **xiphoid process.** Attached to each side of the upper region of the sternum, by means of ligaments, are the two **clavicles** (collar bones).

Seven pairs of **costal cartilages** join seven pairs of ribs directly to the sternum. These are known as **true ribs.** The human body contains twelve pairs of ribs. The first seven pairs are true ribs. The next three pairs are "false ribs" because their costal cartilages are attached to the seventh rib instead of directly to the sternum. Finally, the last two pairs of ribs, connected neither to the costal cartilages nor the sternum, are floating ribs, figure 10–5.

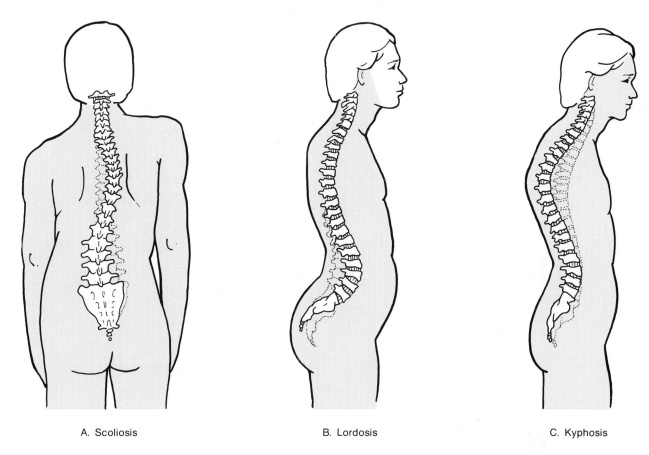

A. Scoliosis   B. Lordosis   C. Kyphosis

Figure 10-3   Abnormal curvature of the spine: (a) Scoliosis, (b) Lordosis, (c) Kyphosis

THE APPENDICULAR SKELETON

The appendicular skeleton includes the bones in the upper and lower extremities; the axial includes bones of the head and trunk. There are 126 bones in the appendicular skeleton.

Shoulder Girdle

The shoulder girdle consists of four bones: two curved clavicles and two triangular **scapulae** (shoulder bones). Using a model of the human skeleton, we observe two broad, flat triangular surfaces (scapulae) on the upper posterior surface. They permit the attachment of muscles which assist in arm movement, while also serving as a place of attachment for the arms. The two clavicles, attached at one end to the scapulae and at the other to the sternum, help to brace the shoulders and prevent excessive forward motion.

Arm

The bone structure of the arm consists of the humerus, the radius, and the ulna. The **humerus** is located in the upper arm and the **radius** and **ulna** in the forearm.

A typical vertebra

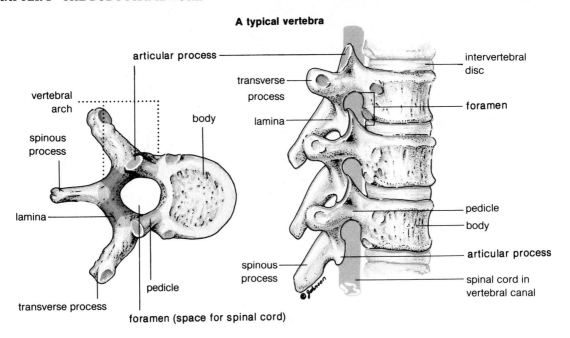

a. **Superior view**

b. **Right lateral view**

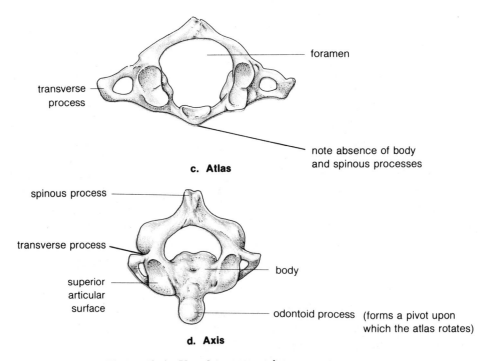

c. **Atlas**

d. **Axis**

Figure 10-4 Vertebrae comparison

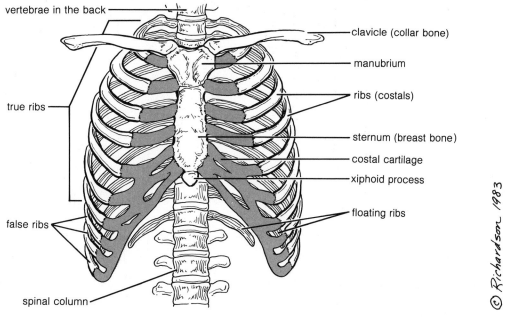

vertebrae in the back

clavicle (collar bone)

manubrium

ribs (costals)

true ribs

sternum (breast bone)

costal cartilage

xiphoid process

floating ribs

false ribs

spinal column

© Richardson 1983

Figure 10-5 Ribs and breastbone

The humerus, the only bone in the upper arm, is the second largest bone in the body. The upper end of the humerus has a smooth, round surface called the head, which articulates with the scapula. The upper humerus is attached to the scapula socket (**glenoid fossa**) by muscles and ligaments. These muscles are the biceps and triceps brachii.

The forearm is composed of two bones: the radius and the ulna. The **radius** is the bone running up the thumb side of the forearm. Its name derives from the fact that it can rotate the ulna. This is an important characteristic, permitting the hand to rotate freely and with great flexibility. The ulna, by contrast, is far more limited. It is the largest bone in the forearm; at its upper end, it produces a projection called the **olecranon process,** forming the elbow, figure 10–6.

Hand

The human hand is a remarkable piece of skeletal engineering and dexterity. It contains more bones for its size than any other part of the body. Collectively, the hand has twenty-seven bones and an opposable thumb, figure 10–7.

The wrist bone, or **ossa carpi,** is comprised of eight small bones arranged in two rows. They are held together by ligaments which permit sufficient movement to allow the wrist a great deal of mobility and flexion. However, there is very little lateral (side) movement of these carpal bones. On the palmar side of the hand are attached a number of short muscles which supply mobility to the little finger and thumb.

The hand is composed of two parts: the palmar surface with five **metacarpal bones,** and five fingers comprised of fourteen **phalanges** (singular, phalanx). Each finger, except for the thumb, has three phalanges, whereas the thumb has two. There are hinge joints between each phalanx, allowing the fingers to be bent easily. The thumb is the most flexible finger because the end of the metacarpal bone is

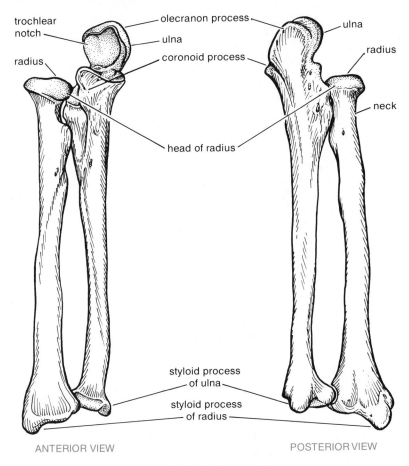

trochlear notch
olecranon process
ulna
radius
ulna
coronoid process
radius
head of radius
neck
styloid process of ulna
styloid process of radius
ANTERIOR VIEW
POSTERIOR VIEW

Figure 10-6   Radius and ulna

more rounded, and there are muscles attached to it from the hand itself. Thus the thumb can be extended across the palm of the hand. Only man and other primates possess such a digit known as an **opposable thumb.**

Pelvic Girdle

In youth, the pelvic girdle (**innominate bones**) consists of three bones. Found on either side of the midline of the body, the innominate bones include the **ilium** (plural, **ilia**), the **ischium** (plural, **ischia**) and the **pubis** (plural, **pubes**). However, these bones eventually fuse with the sacrum to form a bowl-shaped struc-

ture called the pelvic girdle, figure 10–8. Eventually these two sets of innominate bones form a joint with the bones in front, called the **symphysis pubis** and with the sacrum in back, as the **sacroiliac joint.**

The pelvic girdle serves as an area of attachment for the bones and muscles of the leg. It also provides support for the viscera (soft organs) of the lower abdominal region. There is an obvious anatomical difference between the male and female pelvis. The female pelvis is much wider than that of the male. This is necessary for childbearing (pregnancy) and childbirth. In addition, the *pelvic inlet* is wider in the female, and the pelvic bones are lighter and smoother than those of the male.

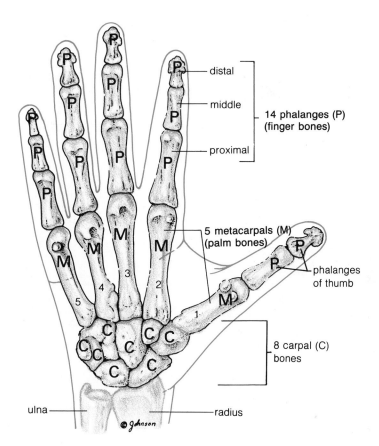

distal

middle

14 phalanges (P)
(finger bones)

proximal

5 metacarpals (M)
(palm bones)

phalanges
of thumb

8 carpal (C)
bones

ulna

radius

© Johnson

Figure 10-7   Diagram showing the 27 bones of the right hand—dorsal view

Upper Leg

The upper leg contains the longest and strongest bone in the body, the thigh bone or **femur.** The upper part of the femur has a smooth rounded head, figure 10–9. It fits neatly into a cavity of the ilium known as the **acetabulum,** forming a ball-and-socket joint. The femur is an amazingly strong bone. A direct compressible force applied to the *top* of the femur of from 15,000–19,000 pounds per square inch is required to break it. How then, do fractures occur? In the event of a side blow or twisting motion, a few hundred pounds of pressure per square inch is enough to break the femur.

Lower Leg

The lower leg consists of two bones: the **tibia** and the **fibula.** The tibia is the largest of the two lower leg bones. The **patella** (kneecap) is found in front of the knee joint. It is a flat, triangular, **sesamoid bone.** The patella is formed in the tendons of the large muscle in front of the femur (quadriceps femoris). In females, it appears at around two or three years of age; in males, at about six. The patella, attached to the tibia by a ligament, ossifies as early as puberty. Surrounding the patella are four bursae, which serve to cushion the knee joint.

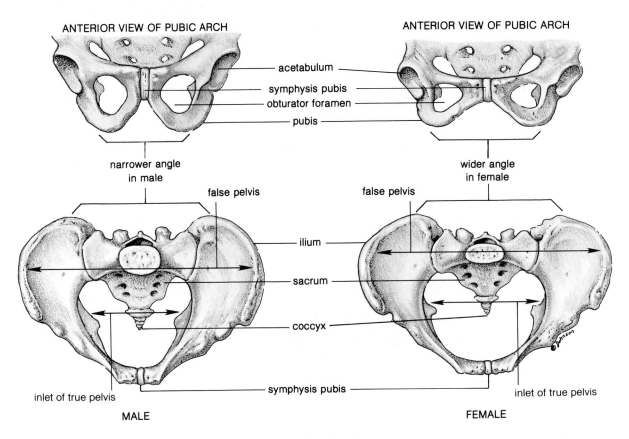

ANTERIOR VIEW OF PUBIC ARCH

ANTERIOR VIEW OF PUBIC ARCH

acetabulum
symphysis pubis
obturator foramen
pubis

narrower angle
in male

wider angle
in female

false pelvis

false pelvis

ilium

sacrum

coccyx

inlet of true pelvis

inlet of true pelvis

symphysis pubis

MALE

FEMALE

Figure 10-8   Comparison of the female and male pelvises

The Ankle

The ankle (**tarsus**) contains seven tarsal bones. These bones provide a connection between the foot and leg bones. The largest ankle bone is the heel bone or **calcaneous.** The tibia and fibula articulate with a broad tarsal bone called the **talus.** Ankle movement is a sliding motion, allowing the foot to extend and flex when walking.

The Foot

The foot has five **metatarsal bones** which are somewhat comparable to the metacarpals of the hand. But, there is an important differ-

ence between the metatarsals and the metacarpals within the palm of the hand. The metatarsal and tarsal bones are arranged to form two distinct arches, which of course are not found in the palm. One arch runs longitudinally from the calcaneus to the heads of the metatarsals; it is called the **longitudinal arch.** The other, which lies perpendicular to the longitudinal arch in the metatarsal region, is known as the **transverse arch.** Strong ligaments and leg muscle tendons help to hold the foot bones in place to form those two arches. In turn, arches strengthen the foot and provide flexibility and springiness to the stride. In certain cases, these arches may "fall" due to weak foot ligaments

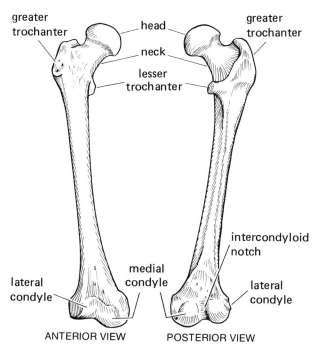

greater trochanter — head — greater trochanter

neck

lesser trochanter

intercondyloid notch

medial condyle

lateral condyle

lateral condyle

ANTERIOR VIEW   POSTERIOR VIEW

Figure 10-9   Anterior and posterior views of the femur

and tendons. Then downward pressure by the weight of the body slowly flattens them, causing "fallen arches" or "flatfeet." Flatfeet cause a good deal of stress and strain on the foot muscles, leading to pain and fatigue. Factors which may lead to flatfeet include improper prenatal nutrition, dietary or hormonal imbalances, fatigue, overweight, poor posture, and shoes which do not fit properly.

The toes are similar in composition to the fingers. There are three phalanges in each, with the exception of the big toe which has only two. Since the big toe is not opposable like the thumb, it cannot be brought across the sole. There are a total of fourteen phalanges in each foot, figure 10–10.

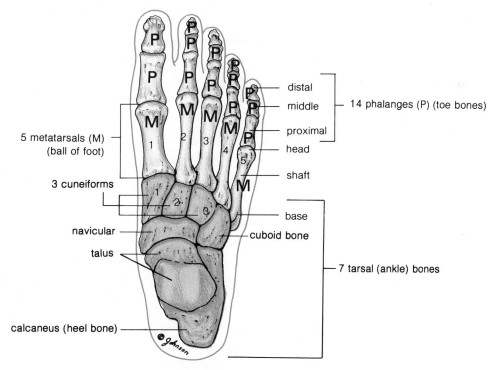

5 metatarsals (M) (ball of foot)

3 cuneiforms

navicular

talus

calcaneus (heel bone)

distal
middle
proximal
head
shaft

14 phalanges (P) (toe bones)

base
cuboid bone

7 tarsal (ankle) bones

Figure 10-10   Dorsal view of the right foot and its 26 bones

Further Study and Discussion

- Using a model of the human skeleton, identify the following structures:
  — the cranium, the zygomatic arch, maxilla, and the frontal bone
  — shoulder girdle, clavicle and scapula
  — sternum, manubrium and xiphoid process
  — pelvic girdle, ilium, ischium and the pubis
  — spinal column, the atlas, the axis, the cervical vertebra, the thoracic vertebra, the lumbar vertebra, the sacrum and the coccyx
  — arms, humerus, radius and the ulna
  — legs, femur, patella, fibula and the tibia
  — foot, calcaneous, talus, metatarsals and the phalanges

- Find out why the two lowest pairs of ribs are called floating ribs

- Explain why the first vertebra in the spinal column is called the atlas and why it has no body like other vertebra do.

Assignment

A. Complete the following statements.

  1. The two main parts of the skeletal system are the _____ skeleton and the _____ skeleton.

  2. Two main areas of the skull consist of the _____ and the _____ .

  3. The largest of the fourteen facial bones is the _____ .

  4. The three tiny bones of the ear which assist in the hearing function are the _____ , _____ , and _____ .

  5. The spinal or vertebral column consists of small bones separated from each other by pads of _____ called

     _____ _____ .

  6. The odontoid process is an important structure of the second vertebra, the _____ .

  7. The flat bone lying between the ribs in the front of the chest is the

     _____ .

  8. The bones which form the pelvic girdle are called the _____ bones.

9. The individual bones which form the pelvis are the _____ ,

    _____ , _____ , _____

    and _____ .

10. The largest bone in the body is the _____ or

    _____ bone.

11. The bones of the skull are the _____ , _____ ,

    _____ , and _____ bones.

12. The sutures of the skull are the _____ , _____ ,

    and _____ sutures.

13. The spinal column has five main vertebral sections, the _____ ,

    _____ , _____ , _____ ,

    and _____ .

14. The first vertebra which supports the skull is the _____ .

15. The odontoid process forms a pivot upon which the _____
    vertebra rotates.

B. Answer the following questions.

    1. What is the function of the hyoid bone?

    2. Explain why the cranium is dome-shaped.

    3. Why is the spinal column curved instead of straight?

    4. What is the function of a foramen?

5. Describe the anatomical differences between the male and female pelvic girdle.

6. What does the term "opposable thumb" mean?

7. Explain what is meant by "flatfeet." How does this condition occur?

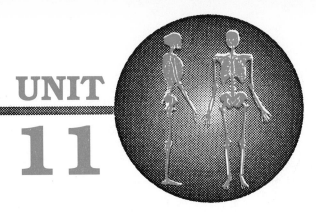

UNIT 11

REPRESENTATIVE DISORDERS OF THE BONES AND JOINTS

KEY WORDS

ankylosis
arthritis
bunion
bursitis
chondrosarcoma
closed fracture
clubfoot (talipes)
comminuted
  fracture
dislocation
Ewing's sarcoma
fracture
gout (gouty
  arthritis)

greenstick
  fracture
kyphosis
lordosis
lumbago
microcephalus
neoplasm
open fracture
osteitis
osteoarthritis
osteogenic
  sarcoma
osteoma
osteomalacia

osteoporosis
reduction
rickets
rheumatoid
  arthritis
scoliosis
spina bifida
spondylitis
spondylolisthesis
sprain
subluxation
webbed or extra
  fingers and toes

OBJECTIVES

■ Define four types of bone fractures
■ Identify common bone and joint injuries
■ Identify common bone and joint disorders
■ Define the Key Words that relate to this unit of study

The most common injury to a bone is a **fracture,** or break. When this occurs, there is swelling due to injury and bleeding tissues. The process of restoring the fractured bone to its original position is known as **reduction.** A cast is applied to hold the fracture in place and at rest. Healing takes place and the bone knits, or grows together again. The following outline identifies the common types of fractures, figure 11–1.

• **Closed** — The bone is broken, but the broken ends *do not* pierce through the skin forming an external wound.

• **Open** — This is the most serious type of fracture, where the broken bone ends pierce and protrude through the skin. This can cause infection of the bone and of the neighboring tissues.

• **Greenstick** — Here we have the simplest type of fracture. The bone is partly bent, but it never completely separates. The break is similar to that of a young, sap-filled woodstick, where the fibers separate lengthwise when bent. Such fractures are common among children because their bones contain flexible cartilage.

• **Comminuted** — The bone is splintered or broken into many pieces that can become embedded in the surrounding tissue.

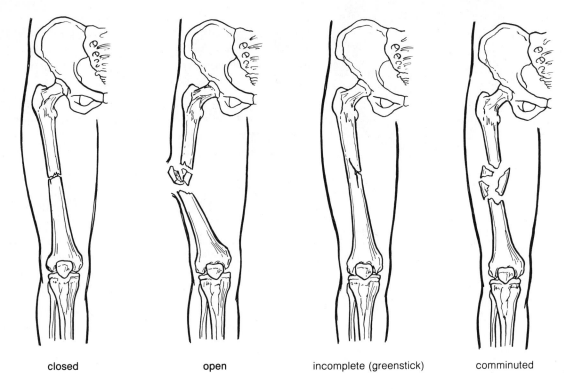

© Richardson 1983

| closed | open | incomplete (greenstick) | comminuted |

Figure 11-1   Types of fractures

BONE AND JOINT INJURIES

A **dislocation** occurs when a bone is displaced from its proper position in a joint. This may result in the tearing and stretching of the ligaments. Reduction or return of the bone to its proper position is necessary, along with rest to allow the ligaments to heal.

A **sprain** is an injury to a joint caused by any sudden or unusual motion, such as "turning the ankle." The ligaments are either torn from their attachments to the bones or torn across, but the joint is not dislocated. A sprain is accompanied by rapid swelling and acute pain in the area. Treatment consists of supporting the joint until the ligaments heal. This is usually done with adhesive strapping or an Ace bandage.

Ankylosis occurs when a joint becomes completely immobile because the bones have fused solid.

Arthritis is an inflammatory condition of one or more joints, accompanied by pain and often by changes in bone position. There are several types, the most common being rheumatoid arthritis, osteoarthritis, and gouty arthritis:

- **Rheumatoid arthritis** is a chronic systemic disease affecting the connective tissues and joints. There is acute inflammation of the connective tissue, thickening of the synovial membrane, and ankylosis of joints. The joints are badly swollen and painful. The pain, in turn, causes muscle spasms which may lead to deformities in the joints. In addition, the cartilage that separates the joints will degenerate, and hard calcium fills the spaces. When the joints become stiff and immobile, muscles attached to these joints slowly atrophy. This disease affects aproximately three times more women than men. Its cause is unknown, although everything from emotional factors to endocrine and metabolic disorders has been cited.

- **Osteoarthritis** is a degenerative joint disease where the cartilage softens and degenerates, stimulating the formation of new bone at the joints. The joints affected are those receiving a great deal of wear and tear, particularly the lower extremity joints and the spine. Individuals over 45 years of age are most commonly affected.

- **Gouty arthritis (gout)** is caused by a faulty uric acid metabolism. The level of uric acid is elevated in the bloodstream. Eventually uric acid crystals deposit in the joints, especially the metatarsophalangeal joint of the big toe.

A **bunion** is the swelling of the bursa of the foot, usually of the metatarsophalangeal joint in the big toe. (A bursa is a small sac between parts that move on each other.) Bunions result from poorly fitting shoes, poor walking posture, or a genetic tendency. The big toe then becomes adducted.

Rickets is a disease of the bones which is caused by a lack of vitamin D. Portions of the bones are soft, due to lack of calcification. The soft bones bend, causing such deformities as bowlegs and pigeon breast. The disease may be prevented by providing a growing child with sufficient quantities of calcium, vitamin D, and exposure to sunshine.

Clubfoot (talipes) is a congenital (existing at birth) malformation. It may involve one or both feet. The deformity may take one of several forms: the body weight may rest on the heel or ball of the foot only, or the inner or outer side of the sole may touch the ground.

Microcephalus is a congenital or hereditary (inborn) condition in which there is a marked diminution in the size of the cranium due to early ossification of the sutures of the skull. This is usually accompanied by arrested mental development.

Spina bifida is a congenital condition in which the vertebral column, which contains the spinal cord, does not develop completely and unite properly. This disorder usually affects the lumbar and sacral regions. Frequently, the contents of the spinal cord protrude out of the spinal cavity.

Osteoporosis, or softening of the bones, is caused by a deficiency in male or female hormones. The bones fracture easily because of brittleness. Replacement of hormones and increased mineral intake may slow the process.

Bursitis is the acute inflammation of the synovial bursa, which cushions a joint during motion. It can be caused by local or systemic inflammation or excess tension. Calcium deposits may form within the elbow, knee, and shoulder joints. This accumulation of calcium impedes movement of the joint.

Webbed *and* **extra fingers and toes** are congenital conditions which must be corrected by early surgery.

Scoliosis is a side-to-side or lateral curvature of the spine.

Kyphosis ("hunchback") is a humped curvature in the thoracic area of the spine.

Lordosis ("swayback") is an exaggerated inward curvature in the lumbar region of the spine just above the sacrum.

Subluxation is the most common problem associated with neck injuries. In this condition, a vertebra is displaced from its normal position, or normal range of movement, without having been completely dislocated. A subluxated neck vertebra can result from an automobile injury, especially whiplash, or other sudden, unexpected body movements. A sharp blow to the chin, face or head, even an uncontrolled coughing fit or a violent sneeze can subluxate a vertebra, figure 11–2.

OTHER MEDICALLY RELATED DISORDERS

Bone disorders also occur with tuberculosis, osteomyelitis, and benign or malignant *tumors,* to name a few. Rheumatic fever causes the inflammation of connective tissue, notably in the heart and blood vessels, and around joints, synovial tissues and tendons. A common clinical symptom is arthritis.

Lumbago is a backache in the lower lumbar and lumbosacral area of the spinal column.

Neoplasms are various types of tumors. Neoplasms can occur in bone. The common benign tumors include the following:

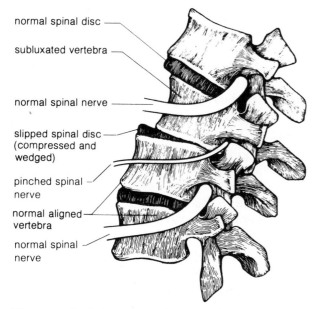

normal spinal disc

subluxated vertebra

normal spinal nerve

slipped spinal disc (compressed and wedged)

pinched spinal nerve

normal aligned vertebra

normal spinal nerve

Figure 11-2 Subluxation of a vertebra. The second vertebra is out of alignment. Note the effect on the spinal disc and nerve. (Courtesy of CPR, Teaneck, New Jersey)

- **Osteomas** (exostoses) are benign bony tumors seen specifically in the membrane bones of the skull. They have a tendency to extend into the orbit (eye) or nasal sinuses (cavities).

- **Giant cell tumors** are very distinctive bone tumors. They are thought to arise from nonbony connective tissue or marrow. They make their appearance after the second decade of life. These tumors occur near the end of long limb bones, and it causes thinning of the compact bone.

Some malignant tumors are:

- **Osteogenic sarcoma**

- **Ewing's sarcoma** — A malignant tumor of bone marrow.

- **Chondrosarcoma** — A malignant tumor made from malignant chondrocytes or cartilage cells.

Osteitis is an inflammation of bone tissue. In osteitis deformanis (Paget's disease), loss of calcium and bone softening occurs. This is followed by calcium deposition that causes bony thickening and abnormalities. Its cause is unknown.

Osteomalacia is a softening of bones as a result of a lack of Vitamin D in the diet or not enough exposure to sunlight. The mineral content of bone is lowered due to inadequate absorption of calcium and phosphorus from the intestine. Osteomalacia is also called "adult rickets."

Spondylitis is an inflammation of the vertebrae.

Spondylolisthesis is the forward displacement of one vertebra upon the one below it. It commonly happens between the fifth lumbar vertebra and the sacrum or the fourth lumbar over the fifth lumbar vertebra.

Further Study and Discussion

• Make drawings of the different types of fractures as they would look if the leg were broken.

Assignment

1. What is the difference between a closed and open fracture?

2. Explain why a child with rickets would have bowlegs and other bone deformities. How can this disease be prevented?

3. What is a sprain? How can a sprain be treated?

4. Why is any form of arthritis considered to be a degenerative process?

5. State three congenital bone disorders and name the part of the body affected by each.

6. What is bursitis?

7. What is a neoplasm?

8. What are two types of benign bony tumors and what specific parts of the skeleton will it affect?

9. What causes osteomalacia and what is another name for it?

10. What bony disorder can cause bony thickening and abnormalities? What is it caused by?

THE BODY FRAMEWORK

A. Match each term in column I with its correct description in column II.

	Column I	Column II
_____	1. atlas	a. also called innominate bones
_____	2. axis	b. bone of the upper arm
_____	3. femur	c. fibrous band which joins bone to bone
_____	4. frontal bone	
_____	5. humerus	d. contents of medullary canal
_____	6. ligament	e. necessary for growth and repair of bone tissue
_____	7. mandible	
_____	8. pelvic girdle	f. name for thigh bone
_____	9. periosteum	g. vertebra on which skull rests
_____	10. red marrow of bone	h. name for forehead
_____	11. tendon	i. name of lower jaw
_____	12. yellow marrow of bone	j. vertebra on which head rotates
		k. makes red blood cells
		l. joins a muscle to a bone
		m. name of upper jaw

B. List five functions of the skeletal system.

C. State the difference between a dislocation and a sprain.

D. Explain the location and functions of the periosteum and Haversian canals.

E. Briefly answer the following questions.
  1. What is a neoplasm?
  2. What causes osteomalacia and what is another name for it?

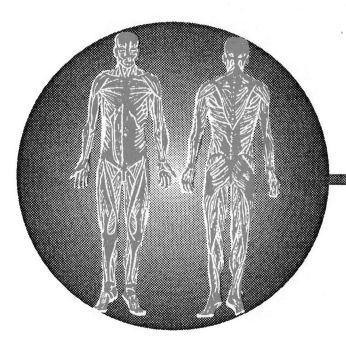

CHAPTER 3

BODY MOVEMENT

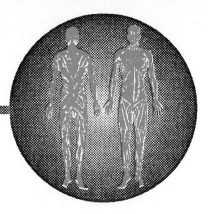

INTRODUCTION TO THE MUSCULAR SYSTEM

KEY WORDS

cardiac
  muscle
locomotion
multinucleate
myoglobin

red muscle
skeletal (striated)
  muscle
smooth (visceral)
  muscle

sphincter
syncytium
white muscle

OBJECTIVES

- Describe the functions of muscles
- Describe each of the three muscle types
- Define the Key Words related to this unit of study

The ability to move is an essential activity of the living human body which is made possible by the unique function of contractility in muscles.

Muscles comprise a large part of the human body; nearly half our body weight comes from muscle tissue. If you weigh 140 pounds, about 60 pounds of it comes from the muscles attached to your bones. Collectively, there are over 650 different muscles in the human body. These muscles allow us to move our bodies from place to place (**locomotion**) as well as move individual parts of the body. They help the body stay erect and determine posture, while producing most of the body's heat. Muscles also participate in the less obvious movements of the internal organs. In addition to playing a role in movement, muscles give the body its characteristic form. The skeleton determines the overall body shape, but the muscles that drape the skeleton produce the contours we perceive as beautiful and graceful.

TYPES OF MUSCLES

All body movements are determined by three principle types of muscles. They are skeletal, smooth, and cardiac muscle. These muscles are also described as striated, spindle-shaped, and nonstriated because of the way their cells look under the ordinary compound light microscope.

Skeletal muscles are attached to the bone of the skeleton. They have cross bandings (striations) of alternating light and dark bands running perpendicular to the length of the muscle, figure 12–1. Because of this appearance, they are called **striped** or **striated** muscle; also voluntary muscle, because they contain nerves under voluntary control. Skeletal muscle is composed of bundles of muscle cells. Each cell is **multinucleate** (containing many nuclei). This special type of cell is called a **syncytium.**

The fleshy body parts are made of skeletal muscles. They provide movement to the limbs, but contract quickly, fatigue easily and

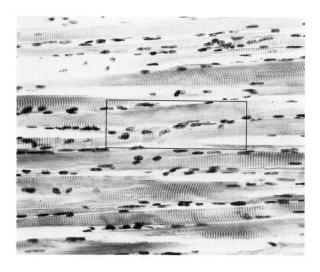

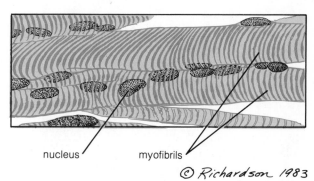

nucleus myofibrils

© Richardson 1983

Figure 12-1 Voluntary or striated (skeletal) muscle cells (Photograph courtesy of Armed Forces Institute of Pathology, negative 72-13786)

lack the ability to remain contracted for prolonged periods. Blinking the eye, talking, breathing, dancing, eating and writing are all produced by the motion of these muscles.

There are two kinds of skeletal muscle. We can readily see this when we examine chicken that has been cooked. There are two kinds of meat: the so-called "dark meat" and "light meat," or **red muscle** and **white muscle.** The difference in color is due to the presence of the red pigment **myoglobin.** Myoglobin is

richer in red muscle and turns brown when heated, resulting in dark meat. Myoglobin is a protein, which can bind to oxygen molecules. It is similar to the hemoglobin found in red blood cells. When oxygen is plentiful, skeletal muscle binds and stores myoglobin until needed, as during vigorous muscle contraction.

Smooth (visceral) muscle cells are small and spindle-shaped. There is only one nucleus, located at the center of the cell. They are called

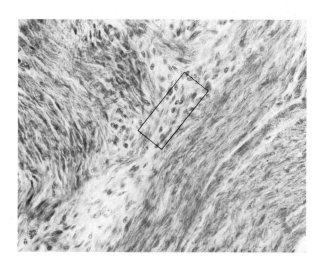

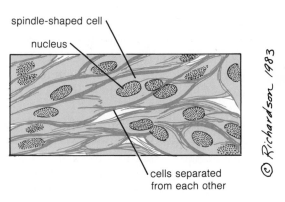

spindle-shaped cell

nucleus

© Richardson 1983

cells separated from each other

Figure 12-2 Involuntary or smooth muscle cells (Photograph courtesy of Armed Forces Institute of Pathology, negative 71-9163)

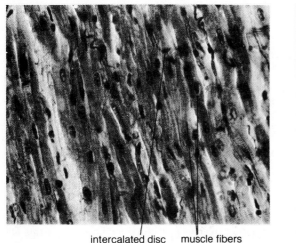
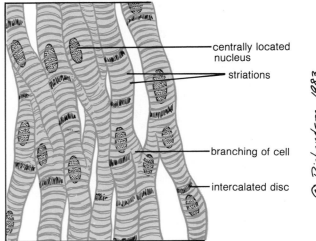

intercalated disc   muscle fibers

centrally located nucleus

striations

branching of cell

intercalated disc

© Richardson 1983

Figure 12-3 Cardiac muscle cells (Photograph reprinted, by permission, from Joan G. Creager, *Human Anatomy and Physiology*, 97)

smooth muscles because they are unmarked by any distinctive striations. Unattached to bones, they act slowly, do not tire easily, and can remain contracted for a long time, figure 12–2 on page 113.

Smooth muscles are not under conscious control; for this reason they are also called involuntary muscles. Their actions are controlled by the autonomic (automatic) nervous system. Smooth muscles are found in the walls of the internal organs, including the stomach, intestines, uterus, and blood vessels. Thus they help push food along the length of the alimentary canal, contract the uterus during labor and childbirth, and control the diameter of the blood vessels as the blood circulates throughout the body.

Cardiac muscle is found only in the heart. Cardiac muscle cells are striated and branched, and they are involuntary, figure 12–3. Healthy cardiac muscle contracts rapidly and is very strong. It is well suited to a lifetime function of pumping blood throughout the body. When the heart beats normally, it holds a rhythm of about 72 beats per minute. However, the activity of various nerves leading to the heart can increase or decrease its rate. Cardiac muscle requires a continuous supply of oxygen to function. Should its oxygen supply be cut off for as little as thirty seconds, it would stop beating.

Sphincter muscles are special circular muscles in the walls of the anus and the urethra. They open and close to control the passage of substances.

Table 12–1 summarizes the characteristics of the three major muscle types.

Table 12–1 Summary of the Characteristics of the Three Major Muscle Types

MUSCLE TYPE	LOCATION	STRUCTURE	FUNCTION
Skeletal muscle (striated, voluntary)	Attached to the skeleton and also located in the wall of the pharynx and esophagus.	A skeletal muscle fiber is long, cylindrical, multinucleated, and contains alternating light and dark striations. Nuclei located at edge of fiber.	Contractions occur voluntarily and may be rapid and forceful.
Smooth muscle (nonstriated, involuntary)	Located in the walls of tubular structures and hollow organs, such as in the digestive tract, urinary bladder, and blood vessels.	A smooth muscle fiber is long and spindle-shaped with no striations.	Contractions occur involuntarily and are rhythmic and slow.
Cardiac (heart) muscle	In the heart	Short, branching fibers with a centrally located nucleus; striations not distinct	Contractions occur involuntarily and are rhythmic and automatic.

Further Study and Discussion

- Observe prepared slides of muscle tissue or bring several types of uncooked meat to class (tripe, steak and heart). Using dissecting needles, place a few fibers in a drop of water on a slide. Observe each under the compound microscope. Notice the different kinds of fibers. Draw and label these fibers. Describe how they differ in appearance.

- Make up a chart listing the 3 muscle types and give several examples of each type.

Assignment

A. Place the most correct answer in the space or spaces provided.

1. Muscles help to keep the body erect and therefore determine our

   _____ .

2. Muscles produce most of the _____ that is generated in the body.

3. The action of muscles upon bones is responsible for movements of our _____ .

4. A specialized muscle, the heart, is responsible for _____ throughout the body.

5. Muscle tissue helps get carbon dioxide out and oxygen into the body through the _____ .

6. Three principal types of muscle tissue are the _____ , _____ , and the _____ .

7. Cardiac muscle is an _____ muscle.

B. Answer the following questions.

1. What is myoglobin?

2. What is meant by "red muscle"?

3. List three characteristics of smooth muscle.

4. What part of the nervous system controls involuntary muscle actions?

5. Name four actions that are controlled by skeletal muscles.

ATTACHMENT OF MUSCLES

KEY WORDS

abduction
adduction
antagonist
belly of muscle
biceps
contractibility
depressor

dilator muscle
elasticity
extensibility
extensor
flexor
insertion
levator

muscle fatigue
muscle tone
origin
pronation
sphincter muscle
supination
triceps

OBJECTIVES

- List the characteristics of muscles
- Describe how pairs of muscles work together
- Describe how muscles are attached
- Describe how muscles are ready for action
- Define the Key Words relating to this unit of study

All muscles, whether they are skeletal, smooth or cardiac, have three characteristics in common. One is **contractibility,** a quality possessed by no other body tissue. When a muscle shortens or contracts, it reduces the distance between the parts of its contents, or the space it surrounds. The contraction of skeletal muscles which connect a pair of bones brings the attachment points closer together. This causes the bone to move. When cardiac muscles contract, they reduce the area in the heart chambers, pumping blood from the heart into the blood vessels. Likewise, smooth muscles surround blood vessels and the intestines, causing the diameter of these tubes to decrease upon contraction.

Another property of muscles is **extensibility** (the ability to be stretched). When we bend our forearm, the muscles on the back of it are extended or stretched. Finally, muscles exhibit **elasticity** (ability of a muscle to return to its original length when relaxing). Collectively,

these three properties of muscles — contractibility, extensibility and elasticity — produce a veritable mechanical device capable of complex, intricate movements.

ANTAGONISTIC MUSCLE PARTS

There are over 600 different muscles in the body. For any of these muscles to produce movement in any part of the body, it must be able to exert its force upon a movable object. In other words, muscles must be attached to bones for leverage in order to have something to pull against.

Muscles are attached to the bones of the skeleton by nonelastic cords called tendons. Bones are connected by joints. Skeletal muscles are attached in such a way as to bridge these joints. So, when a skeletal muscle contracts, the bone to which it is attached will move.

117

Muscles are attached at both ends to bones, cartilage, ligaments, tendons, skin and sometimes to each other. The **origin** is the part of a skeletal muscle that is attached to a fixed structure or bone; it moves least during muscle contraction. The **insertion** is the other end, attached to a movable part; it is the part that moves most during a muscle contraction. The **belly** is the central body of the muscle, figure 13–1.

The muscles of the body are arranged in pairs. One produces movement in a single direction, the other does so in the opposite direction. This arrangement of muscles with opposite actions is known as an **antagonist** pair.

By example, upper arm muscles are arranged in antagonist pairs, figure 13–1. The muscle located on the front part of the upper arm is the **biceps.** One end of the biceps is attached to the scapula and humerus (its origin). When the biceps contracts, these two bones remain stationary. The opposite end of the biceps is attached to the radius of the lower arm (its insertion); this bone moves upon contraction of the biceps.

The muscle on the back of the upper arm is the **triceps.** Try this simple demonstration: Bend your elbow. With your other hand, feel the contraction of the belly of the biceps. At the same time, stretch your fingers out (around the arm) to touch your triceps; it will be in a relaxed state. Now extend your forearm; feel the simultaneous contraction of the triceps and relaxation of the biceps. Now bend the forearm halfway and contract the biceps and triceps. They cannot move, since both sets of muscles are contracting at the same time.

The biceps is a **flexor** muscle, because it flexes or bends a joint, in this case the elbow. The triceps is an **extensor** muscle, since it extends or straightens a joint. In addition to the elbow joint, antagonistic flexors and extensors are located at the ankle, knee, wrist and several other areas, figure 13–2. There are other types of antagonistic movements controlled by skeletal muscles. **Adduction** moves parts of the body toward the midline of the body; *abduction* moves parts of the body away from the midline. **Levator** and **depressor** muscles raise and lower body parts, as in raising and lower-

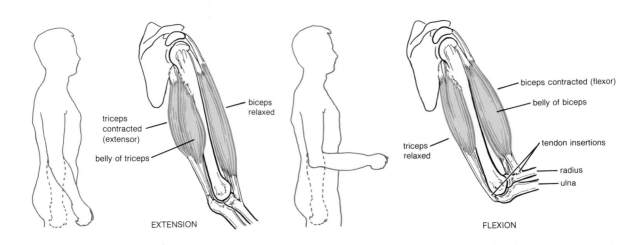

triceps contracted (extensor)

belly of triceps

biceps relaxed

EXTENSION

biceps contracted (flexor)

belly of biceps

triceps relaxed

tendon insertions

radius

ulna

FLEXION

Figure 13-1   Coordination of antagonistic muscles

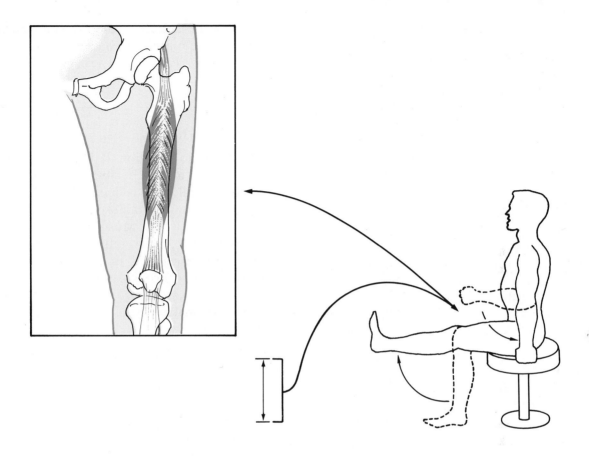

Figure 13-2 Extension of lower leg at the knee joint by contraction of the *rectus femoris*

ing the mandible when chewing or speaking. Then we have **pronation** and **supination**: pronation rotates the forearm so that the palm of the hand is turned towards the body, while supination turns the palm away. Finally, there are **sphincter muscles** and **dilators** — which decrease or increase openings — such as the muscles around the anus and the mouth.

The blood delivers oxygen and glucose, which are necessary for muscle function, to muscle cells. In addition, the liver and the muscle cells themselves store glucose in the form of glycogen. This starch can be converted back to glucose when additional energy is required for muscle contraction.

Skeletal muscle, in addition to helping us move, maintains our posture and produces heat. Living human beings must constantly maintain their body temperature within a rather narrow range (98.6°F or 37°C). As a result of catabolism, muscles produce heat and wastes. Since skeletal muscles make up close to half our total body weight, they generate much of the body's heat.

MUSCLE FATIGUE

Muscle fatigue is caused by an accumulation of lactic acid in the muscles. During periods of vigorous exercise, the blood is unable to transport enough oxygen for the complete oxidation of glucose in the muscles. This causes the muscles to contract anaerobically (without oxygen).

Aerobic oxidation is a chemical process whereby energy and pyruvic acid are released from sugar. The pyruvic acid eventually is converted to CO_2 and waste, which is then excreted from the body. However, in anaerobic (insufficient oxygen) oxidation of muscles, the pyruvic acid is converted into lactic acid. The lactic acid normally leaves the muscle, passing into the bloodstream. But if vigorous exercise continues, the lactic acid level in the blood rises sharply. In such cases, lactic acid accumulates within the muscle. This impedes muscular contraction, causing muscle fatigue and cramps.

MUSCLE TONE

In order to function rapidly and well, muscles should always be slightly contracted and ready to pull. This is **muscle tone.** People in good health have firm muscles which are always ready to work. Muscle tone can be achieved through proper nutrition and regular exercise. Each muscle is in contact with the nervous system through the motor nerve which carries messages from the brain to the muscles and makes them always ready for action.

Further Study and Discussion

- Ask your butcher for a chicken leg with the foot still intact. Cut open the skin and free the ends of the tendons. Pull the tendons in the front of the leg, then those behind it. What happened to the toes? Did the tendons stretch?

- Discuss what happens to muscles that are not used.

- Make arrangements for a physiotherapist to speak about maintaining muscle tone in the elderly patient.

Assignment

A. Complete the following sentences.

   1. Muscles are arranged in _____ , one muscle being _____ to the other and performing an action _____ to that of the other.

   2. A muscle which bends a joint is called a _____ .

   3. The muscle which bends a joint appears thicker and shorter than the one that straightens the joint, called an _____ .

4. Muscles may be attached to _____ , _____ ,
   _____ , _____ , _____ , and sometimes to _____ _____ .

5. The end of the muscle which moves least during muscle contraction
   is the _____ .

6. The end of the muscle moving the most is the _____ .

7. The nourishment necessary for the work of the muscle cells is fur-
   nished by the _____ and carried by the _____ .

8. Muscles and the liver store _____ which may be converted
   to glucose.

9. Muscle fatigue is caused by an accumulation of _____ , a
   result of _____ _____ of stored sugar.

10. Oxidation is the main _____ _____ by which
    _____ is released from the sugar in the cells.

B. Answer the following questions.

1. List the three properties of muscles.

2. Explain what is meant by an antagonistic muscle pair.

3. Describe how a muscle becomes fatigued.

PRINCIPAL SKELETAL MUSCLES

KEY WORDS

appendicular
  muscle group
axial muscle
  group
femur

humerus
intramuscular
mandible
mastication
physiotherapy

sarcoplasm
scapula
strength

OBJECTIVES

- Locate the important skeletal body muscles
- Describe the function of these muscles
- Identify the muscles using the technical names
- Discuss how sports training can alter skeletal muscles
- Identify the sites of intramuscular injection
- Define the Key Words relating to this unit of study

The skeletal or voluntary muscles are made up of all the muscles that are attached to and help to move the skeleton. These muscles line the walls of the oral, abdominal, and pelvic cavities. Skeletal muscles also control the movement of the following structures—the eyeballs, the eyelids, the lips, the tongue, and the skin.

Figures 14–1 and 14–2 show the principal skeletal muscles. The skeletal muscles can be classified into two major muscle groups:

- **Axial muscle group.** These are the head, face, neck, and trunk muscles.

- **Appendicular muscle group.** These are the extremity muscles.

There are 656 muscles in the human body. This breaks down to 327 antagonistic muscle pairs and 2 unpaired muscles. These 2 unpaired muscles are the orbicularis oris and the diaphragm. The 656 muscles can be divided and subdivided into the following muscle regions.

A. *Head muscles*

1. Muscles of expression
2. Muscles of **mastication** (chewing)
3. Muscles of the tongue
4. Muscles of the pharynx
5. Muscles of the soft palate

B. *Neck muscles*

1. Muscles moving the head
2. Muscles moving the hyoid bone and the larynx

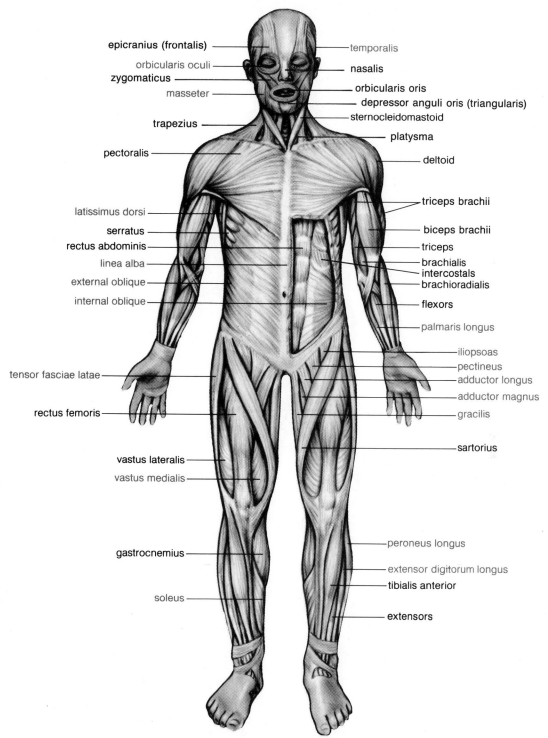

epicranius (frontalis)
orbicularis oculi
zygomaticus
masseter
trapezius
pectoralis
latissimus dorsi
serratus
rectus abdominis
linea alba
external oblique
internal oblique
tensor fasciae latae
rectus femoris
vastus lateralis
vastus medialis
gastrocnemius
soleus

temporalis
nasalis
orbicularis oris
depressor anguli oris (triangularis)
sternocleidomastoid
platysma
deltoid
triceps brachii
biceps brachii
triceps
brachialis
intercostals
brachioradialis
flexors
palmaris longus
iliopsoas
pectineus
adductor longus
adductor magnus
gracilis
sartorius
peroneus longus
extensor digitorum longus
tibialis anterior
extensors

Figure 14-1   Principle skeletal muscles of the body—anterior view

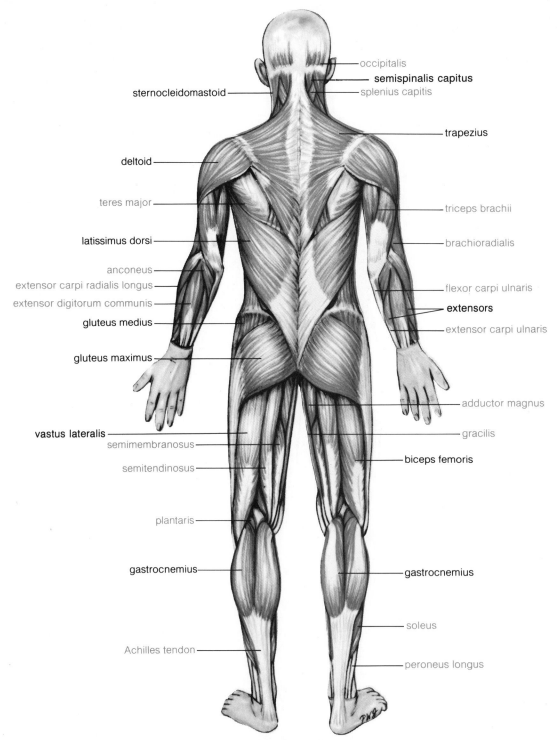

occipitalis

semispinalis capitus

splenius capitis

sternocleidomastoid

trapezius

deltoid

teres major

triceps brachii

latissimus dorsi

brachioradialis

anconeus

extensor carpi radialis longus

extensor digitorum communis

flexor carpi ulnaris

extensors

gluteus medius

extensor carpi ulnaris

gluteus maximus

adductor magnus

vastus lateralis

gracilis

semimembranosus

biceps femoris

semitendinosus

plantaris

gastrocnemius

gastrocnemius

soleus

Achilles tendon

peroneus longus

Figure 14-2   Principle skeletal muscles of the body—posterior view

3. Muscles moving the upper ribs

C. *Trunk and extremity muscles*

1. Muscles that move the vertebral column
2. Muscles that move the scapula
3. Muscles of breathing
4. Muscles that move the humerus
5. Muscles that move the forearm
6. Muscles that move the wrist, hand, and finger digits
7. Muscles that act on the pelvis
8. Muscles that move the femur
9. Muscles that move the leg
10. Muscles that move the ankles, the foot, and the toe digits

The following tables give a listing of some representative skeletal muscles that are involved in various types of bodily movements.

MUSCLES OF THE HEAD

Muscles controlling facial expression. These control human facial expressions such as anger, fear, grief, joy, pleasure, and pain. Refer to table 14–1.

Muscles of mastication. These muscles control the **mandible** (lower jaw), raising it to close the jaw and lowering it to open the jaw. Refer to table 14–2.

MUSCLES OF THE NECK

Muscles that move the head. Extension, flexion, and rotation are the major movements of the head. Refer to table 14–3.

Table 14–1 Representative Muscles of Facial Expression

MUSCLE	EXPRESSION	LOCATION	FUNCTION
Epicranius (occipito frontalis)	Surprise	On either side of the forehead	Raises eyebrow and wrinkles forehead
Depressor anguli oris	Doubt, disdain, contempt	Found along the side of the chin	Depresses corner of mouth
Orbicularis oris	Doubt, disdain, contempt	Ring-shaped muscle found around the mouth	Compresses and closes the lips
Platysma (broad sheet muscle)	Horror	Broad, thin muscular sheet covering the side of the neck and lower jaw	Draws corners of mouth downward and backward
Zygomaticus major	Laughing or smiling	Extends diagonally upward from corner of mouth	Raises corner of mouth
Nasalis	Muscles of the nose	Found over the nasal bones	Closes and opens the nasal openings
Orbicularis oculi	Sadness	Surrounds the eye orbit underlying the eyebrows	Closes the eyelid and tightens the skin on the forehead

Table 14–2 Representative Muscles of Mastication

MUSCLE	LOCATION	FUNCTION
Masseter	Covers the lateral surface of the ramus (angle) of the mandible	Closes the jaw
Temporalis	Located on the temporal fossa of the skull	Raises the jaw and closes the mouth and draws the jaw backward

Table 14–3 Representative Muscles of the Neck

MUSCLE	LOCATION	FUNCTION
Sternocleidomastoid (two heads)	Large muscles extending diagonally across sides of neck	Flexes head; rotates the head toward opposite side from muscle
Semispinalis capitis	A band of muscle composed of several strips lying along the cervical and thoracic spines.	Extends the head and rotates it to the opposite side
Splenius capitis	Extends diagonally across the posterolateral side of the neck	When both contract, pulls head backward; when only one contracts, rotates head and tips the face upward

MUSCLES OF THE UPPER EXTREMITIES

These muscles help to move the shoulder (**scapula**) and arm (**humerus**) and the forearm, wrist, hand, and fingers. Refer to table 14–4.

MUSCLES OF THE TRUNK

The trunk muscles control breathing and the movements of the abdomen and the pelvis. Refer to table 14–5.

MUSCLES OF THE LOWER EXTREMITIES

The muscles of the lower extremities assist in the movement of the thigh (**femur**), the leg, the ankle, the foot, and the toes. Refer to table 14–6.

Exercise and training will alter the size, structure, and strength of a muscle.

HOW SPORTS TRAINING AND WORK CHANGES MUSCLES

Exercise and training will alter the size, structure, and strength of a muscle.

Size and Muscle Structure

Skeletal muscles that are not used will atrophy and those that are used excessively will hypertrophy. The hypertrophy is caused by changes in the **sarcoplasm** (cytoplasm found in the individual skeletal muscle fibers) and *not* to an increase in the number of muscle fibers. Muscles that have been injured can regenerate only to a limited degree. If the muscle damage is extensive, then the muscle tissue is replaced by connective (scar) tissue. Muscles that are overexercised or worked will have a tremendous increase of connective tissue between the muscle fibers. This causes the skeletal muscle to become tougher.

Table 14–4 Representative Muscles of the Upper Extremities

MUSCLE	LOCATION	FUNCTION
Trapezius	A large triangular muscle located on upper surface of back	Moves the shoulder; extends the head
Deltoid	A thick triangular muscle that covers the shoulder joint	Abducts the upper arm
Pectoralis major	Anterior part of the chest	Flexes the upper arm and helps to adduct the upper arm
Serratus	Anterior chest	Moves scapula forward and helps to raise the arm
Biceps brachii	Upper arm to radius	Flexes the lower arm
Triceps brachii	Posterior arm to ulna	Extends the lower arm
Extensor and flexor carpi muscle groups	Extends from the anterior and posterior fore-arm to the hand	Moves the hand
Extensor and flexor digitorum muscle groups	Extends from the anterior and posterior fore-arm to the fingers	Moves the fingers

Table14–5 Representative Muscles of the Trunk

MUSCLE	LOCATION	FUNCTION
External intercostals	Found between the ribs	Raises the ribs to help in breathing
Diaphragm	A dome-shaped muscle separating the thoracic and abdominal cavities	Helps to control breathing
Rectus abdominis	Extends from the ribs to the pelvis	Compresses the abdomen
External oblique	Anterior inferior edge of the last eight ribs	Depresses ribs, flexes the spinal column, and compresses the abdominal cavity
Internal oblique	Found directly beneath the external oblique, its fibers running in the opposite direction	Same as above

Effect of Training on Muscle Strength

Strength (capacity to do work) is increased by proper training. Training can have the following effects on skeletal muscles:

- Increase in muscle size

- Improved antagonistic muscle coordination, where antagonistic muscles are relaxed at the right moment and do not interfere with the functioning of the working muscle

- Improved functioning in the cortical brain region, where the nerve impulses that start muscular contraction

Table 14–6 Representative Muscles of the Lower Extremities

MUSCLE	LOCATION	FUNCTION
Gluteus maximus	Buttocks	Extends femur and rotates it outward
Gluteus medius	Extends from the deep femur to the buttocks	Abducts and rotates the thigh
Pectineus	Found on the inner side of the thigh	Adducts and flexes the femur
Tensor fasciae latae	A flat muscle found along the upper lateral surface of the thigh	Flexes, abducts, and medially rotates the thigh
Rectus femoris	Anterior thigh	Flexes thigh and extends the lower leg
Sartorius (Tailor's muscle)	A long, straplike muscle that runs diagonally across the anterior and medial surface of the thigh	Flexes and rotates the thigh and leg
Gracilis	A long, thin muscle on the medial surface of the thigh	Adducts and flexes the thigh, rotates thigh medially, and flexes leg at knee
Gastrocnemius	Calf muscle	Points toes and flexes the lower leg
Soleus	A broad flat muscle found beneath the gastrocnemius	Extends foot
Peroneus longus	A superficial muscle found on the lateral side of the leg	Extends and everts the foot and supports arches

Effect of Training on Muscle Efficiency

The following will occur:

- Improved coordination of all muscles involved in a particular activity

- Improvement of the respiratory and circulatory system to supply the needs of an active muscular system

- Elimination or reduction of excess fat

- Improved joint movement involved with that particular muscle activity

MASSAGE MUSCLES

Occasionally a health care professional must give either a total body massage or a massage to a specific body area to a patient. The correct type of massage is essential in either providing the proper **physiotherapy*** or a general sense of comfort and well-being to a patient.

The health care professional must be aware of the specific skeletal muscles involved in therapeutic massage. The importance of these skeletal muscles comes from their proximity to the body's surface and their relatively large size. Table 14–7 gives the names of these superficial skeletal muscles and their general locations. It is essential for the health care professional to be able to locate these skeletal muscles not only on the muscle diagrams but also on the living bodies of patients with different physiques: scrawny, muscular, thin, fat, male, and female.

---

*Physiotherapy is the treatment of disease and injury by physical means using light, heat, cold, water, electricity, massage, and exercise.

Table 14–7 Skeletal Muscles Involved In Massage

NAME OF SKELETAL MUSCLE	LOCATION
Sternocleiodomastoid	Side of the neck
Trapezius	Back of the neck and upper back
Latissimus dorsi	Lower back
Pectoralis major	Chest
Serratus anterior	Lateral ribs
External oblique	Anterior and lateral abdomen
Deltoid	Shoulder
Biceps brachii	Anterior aspect of arm
Triceps brachii	Posterior aspect of arm
Brachioradialis	Anterior and proximal forearm
Gluteus maximus	Buttock
Tensor fascia latae	Lateral and Proximal Thigh
Sartorius	Anterior thigh
Quadriceps femoris group (rectus femoris, vastus lateralis, vastus medialis, vastus intermedius)	Anterior thigh
Hamstring group (biceps, femoris, semitendinosus, semimembranosus)	Posterior thigh
Gracilis	Medial thigh
Tibialis anterior	Anterior leg
Gastrocnemius	Posterior leg
Soleus	Posterior (Deep) leg
Peroneus longus	Lateral leg

INTRAMUSCULAR INJECTIONS

A health care professional occasionally has to administer an **intramuscular** (into the muscle) injection into the patient. Therefore, a working knowledge of the major skeletal muscles and the underlying anatomy of the area to be injected is needed. If an intramuscular injection is required, and the amount to be injected is less than 5 milliliters, the deltoid muscle is the best location, figure 14–3. The hypodermic needle is inserted into the deltoid about two-fingers' width below the acromion process of the scapula. If the amount to be injected is more than 5 milliliters, the gluteal area is used. The intramuscular injection is made into the gluteus medius muscle. When injecting into the gluteus medius muscle, the gluteal blood vessels and the sciatic nerve must be avoided.

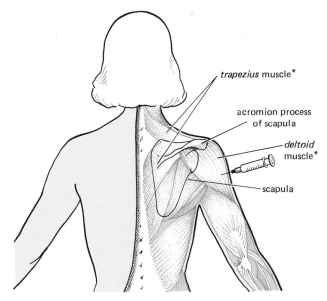

trapezius muscle*

acromion process of scapula

deltoid muscle*

scapula

Figure 14-3 The two superficial muscles* involved in intramuscular injections

Further Study and Discussion

- Identify the muscles which seem to work in pairs.
- Discuss the effect of massage on muscles.

Assignment

A. Give the general function of the listed muscles.
 1. Deltoid

 2. Intercostals

 3. Rectus Femoris

 4. Gluteus Maximus

 5. Triceps (brachii)

 6. Pectoralis major

 7. Sartorius

 8. Extensors

 9. Trapezius

 10. Tibialis anterior

B. Briefly answer the following questions.

1. What is sarcoplasm?

2. What happens to overexercised or overworked muscles?

3. What effects will training have on muscle efficiency?

4. What are the two sites for intramuscular injection?

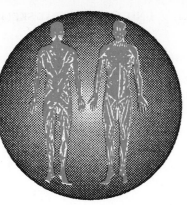

UNIT 15

REPRESENTATIVE MUSCULOSKELETAL DISORDERS

KEY WORDS

abdominal hernia
charley horse
flatfeet (talipes)
inguinal hernia
muscle atrophy
muscle fatigue
muscle
  hypertrophy

muscle spasms
muscular
  dystrophy
myalgia
myasthenia
  gravis
myokymia
myositis

pleurodynia
poliomyelitis
rehabilitation
stiff neck
tetanus (lockjaw)

Muscular coordination is very important if a person is to perform his/her daily functions efficiently. Injuries and diseases which may affect muscles sometimes interfere with these functions. The retraining of injured or unused muscles is a type of **rehabilitation** called therapeutic exercise.

Muscle atrophy can occur to muscles which are infrequently used; they shrink in size and lose muscle strength. An example is **poliomyelitis** (polio), where there is damage or paralysis of nerves carrying nerve messages to the muscles. The muscles are understimulated, and gradually waste away. Muscle atrophy due to nerve paralysis may reduce a muscle up to 25% of its normal size. The wasted muscle is replaced by non-contractile connective tissue. Muscle atrophy can also be caused by prolonged bedrest or the immobilization of a limb in a cast. Muscle atrophy can be minimized by direct electrical stimulation, massage, or special exercise.

Flatfeet (fallen arches or **talipes**) result from a weakening of the leg muscles that support the arch. The downward pressure on the foot eventually flattens out the arches. Muscle strength can be increased by exercise, massage, and electrical stimulation.

An **abdominal hernia**, or rupture, may occur in a weak place in the muscular abdominal wall. It is caused by bulging of the intestine through an opening in the wall of the abdominal cavity normally containing it. The **inguinal hernia** is the most frequent type of hernia. It appears in the groin area.

Muscle hypertrophy is a condition in which a muscle enlarges and grows stronger. It results from overworking or overexercising. This leads to an increase in the diameter or size of muscle cells, as opposed to an increase in the number of muscle cells. So a change in girth increases the total force of the muscle's contraction.

Muscle fatigue may occur from the temporary overuse of a muscle. Fatigue lessens the muscle's ability to perform work. (Review unit 13.)

Stiff neck may be due to an inflammation of the trapezius muscle. The rigidity is the result of unusual overuse of the muscle.

Muscle spasms are sudden and violent contractions caused by sudden overworking of the muscle or by poor circulation to the localized area.

Tetanus (lockjaw) is an infectious disease, usually fatal, characterized by continuous spasms of the voluntary muscles. It is caused by a toxin from a tetanus bacillus, *Clostridium tetani*, which can enter the body through any open wound (especially a puncture wound).

Muscular dystrophy is a chronic wasting disease of the muscles. It often appears during childhood and is thought to result from some genetic disturbance.

Myasthenia gravis leads to progressive muscular weakness and paralysis, sometimes even death. The cause is still unknown, but many researchers believe it may be due to a defect in the immune system, affecting myoneural function. In extreme cases, it can be fatal due to the paralysis of the respiratory muscles.

A **charley horse** is an injury that is common amongst athletes in which a muscle is torn or bruised. It is accompanied by severe pain and cramps.

Myalgia is muscular pain.

Myokymia is a muscular condition characterized by chronic contraction of a muscle when at rest or the widespread twitching of muscle strips independent of each other.

Myositis is a condition where there is an abnormally slow relaxation of the muscle after voluntary muscle contraction.

Pleurodynia is a pain that occurs in the chest area, specifically in the intercostal area.

Further Study and Discussion

- Visit a physical rehabilitation center. Report on the success of muscle retraining in this program.

- Discuss how neglectful patient care can lead to muscular atrophy.

- Invite a physical therapist to discuss rehabilitation with your class.

Assignment

Match each term in column I with its correct description in column II.

	Column I	Column II
_____	1. muscular atrophy	a. the retraining or rehabilitation of muscle use
		b. the temporary overuse of a muscle
_____	2. muscular dystrophy	c. chronic wasting of the muscle tissue
		d. sudden and violent muscle contraction

_____ 3. paralysis

_____ 4. stiff neck

_____ 5. muscle fatigue

_____ 6. muscle hypertrophy

_____ 7. muscle spasm

_____ 8. hernia

_____ 9. therapeutic exercise

_____ 10. tetanus

_____ 11. pleurodynia

_____ 12. charley horse

_____ 13. myositis

e. continuous spasm caused by a toxin

f. immobility caused by blocked nerve messages

g. bulging of an organ through a muscular wall

h. major loss of muscle strength and size

i. rigidity often caused from inflammation of the trapezius muscle

j. muscle enlargement due to overworking of the muscle

k. condition resulting from weak arch muscles

l. abnormally slow relaxation of a voluntary muscle after contraction

m. chest pain

n. injury common to athletes

BODY MOVEMENT

A.   Match each term in column I with its correct function in column II.

Column I	Column II
_____ 1. biceps	a. extends upper arm
_____ 2. diaphragm	b. assists in breathing
_____ 3. gastrocnemius	c. flexes lower arm
_____ 4. gluteus medius	d. extends spinal column and moves trunk
_____ 5. latissimus dorsi	e. moves foot and leg
_____ 6. sacrospinalis	f. closes body openings
_____ 7. serratus	g. abducts and rotates thigh
_____ 8. sphincter	h. moves shoulder
	i. moves the head

B.   Define the following terms.

1. Flatfoot

2. Bursitis

3. Hernia, or rupture

4. Muscular atrophy

5. Paralysis

6. Tetanus

C. Briefly answer the following questions.

1. What happens to overexercised muscles?

2. What are the two sites for intramuscular injection?

3. What is a charley horse and its symptoms?

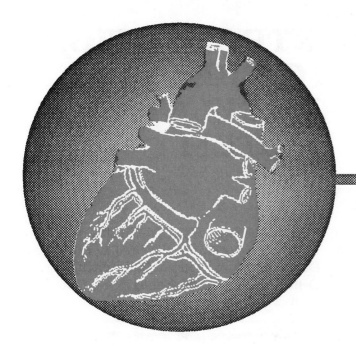

CHAPTER 4

TRANSPORT OF BLOOD AND OXYGEN

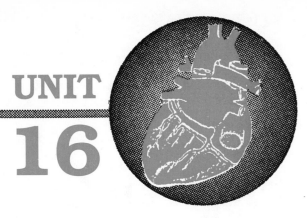

UNIT 16

INTRODUCTION TO THE CIRCULATORY SYSTEM

KEY WORDS

acid
acid-base balance
alkali
base
bicarbonate
blood
closed circulatory
  system

phosphate
plasma
platelets
pulmonary
  circulation

red blood cells
systemic
  (general)
  circulation
white blood cells

OBJECTIVES

- Describe the functions of the circulatory system
- List the components of the circulatory system
- Describe the two routes of blood circulation
- Define the Key Words relating to this unit of study

Blood is an essential life supportive fluid, transported throughout the body through a system of blood vessels. This is known as a **closed circulatory system,** a major characteristic of vertebrates.

The circulatory system is the largest organ of the body. If one were to lay all of the blood vessels in a single human body end to end, they would stretch one fourth the way from earth to the moon, a distance of some 60,000 miles.[1]

FUNCTIONS OF BLOOD

Blood performs numerous functions in helping the body to maintain a stable internal environment. This environment is essential to the functioning of the body's various activities.

Blood is a liquid tissue, composed of a fluid component (plasma), and a solid compo-

nent (blood cells). Blood cells include red blood cells, white blood cells, and platelets. The **red blood cells** convey oxygen to the cells for oxidation, and carbon dioxide away for excretion. **White blood cells** protect against disease by engulfing and digesting bacteria and foreign matter which has invaded the body. The **platelets** help the blood to clot whenever internal or external bleeding occurs.

Plasma suspends blood cells and transports them throughout the body. In addition to bringing dissolved nutrients to the cells, plasma also carries metabolic waste products from the cells to the various excretory organs, where they are excreted or converted into compounds useful for other purposes. Endocrine glands, which synthesize chemical compounds called hormones, secrete these hormones into the plasma. The plasma then circulates them to various body parts in order to help regulate bodily functions.

Blood also helps the body to maintain its water content and body temperature. It is es-

---

1. I. Sherman and V. Sherman, *Biology: A Human Approach* (New York: Oxford University Press, 1979).

sential that the body's temperature does not rise too far above 98.6°F or 37°C. High body temperature will disrupt important chemical reactions in the cells. Generally, highly active muscle tissue creates a good deal of heat that can raise the body's temperature. To counter this effect, blood then circulates more quickly through the tissue to diffuse the heat. This excess heat is subsequently given off over the body's surface through the skin.

Finally, blood helps to maintain the body's internal **acid-base balance.** Chemicals in the bloodstream, known as **bicarbonates** and **phosphates,** neutralize small amounts of **acids** or **alkalis** (basic compounds).

The various functions of blood are summarized in table 16–1.

COMPONENTS OF THE CIRCULATORY SYSTEM

As mentioned earlier, the blood itself contains plasma, red blood cells, white blood cells, and platelets. They are transported within a **closed circulatory system.** In such a system, blood does not, under normal circumstances, leave the blood vessels to flow among the tissues. Rather, it remains inside the blood vessels and is transported throughout the body to form a closed circuit of blood. This blood circuit is composed of arteries arterioles, veins, venules, and capillaries. Blood is pumped through the blood vessels by the action of a muscular pump, which we know as the heart.

The circulatory system also includes the lymphatic system. This consists of the lymph and tissue fluid derived from the blood and the lymphatic vessels, which return the lymph to the blood. The spleen is considered a part of the circulatory system. It provides a reservoir for blood and is active in destroying microorganisms in the blood.

Table 16–1 Summary of the Various Functions of Blood

FUNCTION	EFFECT ON BODY
Nutritive	Transporting nutrient molecules (glucose, amino acids, fatty acids, and glycerol) from the small intestine or storage sites to the tissues
Respiratory	Transporting oxygen from the lungs to the tissues and carbon dioxide from the tissues to the lungs
Excretory	Transporting waste products (lactic acid, urea, and creatinine) from the cells to the excretory organs
Regulatory	Transporting hormones and other chemical substances that control the proper functioning of many organs
	Circulating excess heat to the body surfaces and to the lungs, through which it is lost (controls body temperature)
	Maintains water balance and a constant environment for tissue cells
Protective	Circulating antibodies and defensive cells throughout the body to combat infection and disease

MAJOR BLOOD CIRCUITS

Blood leaves the heart through arteries and returns by veins.* The blood uses two circulation routes:

1. The **general** (or **systemic**) **circulation** carries blood throughout the body, figure 16–1.

2. The **pulmonary circulation** carries blood from the heart to the lungs and back, figure 16–2.

---

*With the exception of pulmonary circulation.

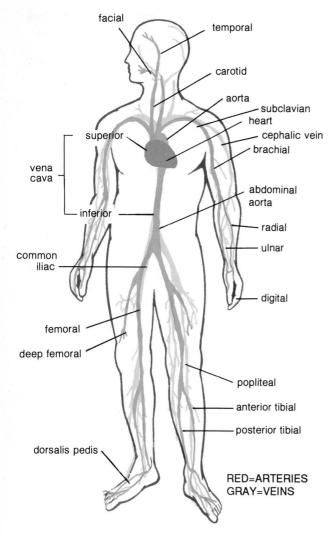

facial

temporal

carotid

aorta

subclavian

heart

cephalic vein

brachial

superior

vena cava

inferior

abdominal aorta

radial

ulnar

common iliac

digital

femoral

deep femoral

popliteal

anterior tibial

posterior tibial

dorsalis pedis

RED=ARTERIES
GRAY=VEINS

Figure 16-1   General or systemic circulation

CHANGES IN THE COMPOSITION OF CIRCULATING BLOOD

The major substances added to and removed from the blood as it circulates through organs along the various sites of the circulatory system are outlined in Table 16–2. (This table includes only the major changes in the blood as it passes through certain specialized organs or structures.)

Table 16–2   Changes in the Composition of the Blood

ORGANS	BLOOD LOSES	BLOOD GAINS
Digestive glands	Raw materials needed to make digestive juices and enzymes	Carbon dioxide
Kidneys	Water, urea, and mineral salts	Carbon dioxide
Liver	Excess glucose, amino acids, and worn-out red blood cells	Released glucose, urea, and plasma proteins
Lungs	Carbon dioxide and water	Oxygen
Muscles	Glucose and oxygen	Lactic acid and carbon dioxide
Small intestinal villi	Oxygen	End products of digestion (glucose and amino acids)

Further Study and Discussion

- If available, observe blood cells circulating through capillaries in the web of a frog's foot, or in the tail of a goldfish. Note the direction of the bloodflow.

- Discuss how blood from the general circulation is oxygenated by blood from the pulmonary circulation.

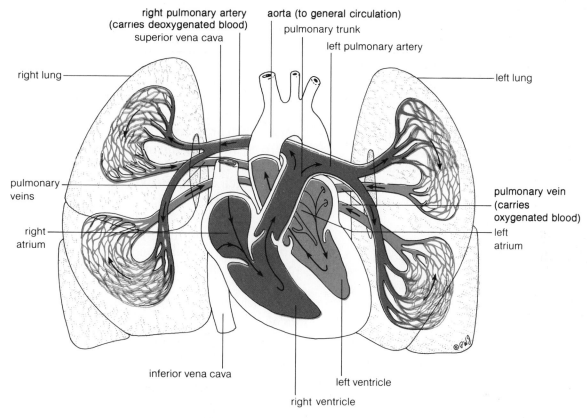

Figure 16-2 Pulmonary circulation

Assignment

A. Briefly answer the following questions.

 1. Describe the chief functions of the circulatory system.

 2. What is the name of the large vein which returns blood to the heart from the general circulation?

 3. What is meant by a closed circulatory system?

 4. What is the composition of blood? List the components of the circulatory system.

B. Match each term in column I with its description or function in column II.

	Column I	Column II
_____	1. pulmonary artery	a. vein which carries freshly oxygenated blood from the lung to the heart
_____	3. lymphatic system	b. circulation route which carries blood to and from the heart and lungs
_____	3. pulmonary vein	
_____	4. spleen	c. organ which provides a reservoir for blood, destroys microorganisms in the blood, and removes worn out blood cells
_____	5. pulmonary circulation	
_____	6. left ventricle	d. artery which carries deoxygenated blood from the heart to the lung
_____	7. general circulation	e. system which consists of lymph and tissue fluid derived from the blood
_____	8. right ventricle	
_____	9. aorta	f. blood from the pulmonary vein which re-enters the heart through the right atrium
		g. artery which carries blood with nourishment, oxygen and other materials from the heart to all parts of the body
		h. ventricle from which the aorta receives blood
		i. circulation which carries blood throughout the body
		j. ventricle from which the pulmonary artery leaves the heart

UNIT 17

THE HEART

KEY WORDS

aortic semilunar
  valve
apex
atrioventricular
  bundle (bundle
  of His)
atrioventricular
  node
atrioventricular
  valve
atrium
auricle
bicuspid (mitral)
  valve
cardiac arrest
cardiac
  arrhythmia

cardiopulmonary
  resuscitation
  (CPR)
congenital
deoxygenated
endocardium
fibrous
  pericardium
foramen ovale
histocompatibility
immuno-
  suppressants
Jarvick-7
myocardium
myogenic
oxygenated
pericardial fluid

pericardium
pulmonary
  semilunar valve
Purkinje network
semilunar valves
septum
serous
  pericardium
sinoatrial node
  (pacemaker)
stethoscope
tricuspid valve
ventricle

OBJECTIVES

- Describe the structure of the heart
- Describe the function of various parts of the heart
- Locate and identify various parts of the heart
- Discuss the major problem that heart transplant patients encounter
- Discuss the value of the development of the artificial heart
- Define Key Works relating to this unit of study

The blood's circulatory system, like other systems of the body, is extremely efficient. The main organ responsible for this efficiency is the heart, a tough, simply-constructed muscle about the size of a closed fist

The adult human heart is about 5 inches long and 3.5 inches wide, weighing less than a pound (12–13 oz.). The importance of a healthy, well-functioning heart is obvious: to circulate life-sustaining blood throughout the body. When the heart stops beating, life stops as well! To explain further, if the blood flow to the brain ceases for 5 seconds or more, the subject loses consciousness. After 15–20 seconds, the muscles twitch convulsively; after 9 minutes without blood flow, the brain cells are irreversibly damaged.

The heart is located in the thoracic cavity. This places the heart between the lungs, behind the sternum, in front of the thoracic vertebrae and above the diaphragm. Although the heart is centrally located, its axis of symmetry is not along the midline. The heart's **apex** (conical tip) lies on the diaphragm and points to the left of the body. It is at the apex where the heartbeat is most easily felt and heard through the **stethoscope.**

Try this simple demonstration: place the disk or bowl of a stethoscope over the heart's apex. This is the area between the fifth and sixth ribs, along an imaginary line extending from the middle of the left clavicle. Since the heartbeat is felt and heard so easily at the apex, this gives rise to the popular but incorrect no-tion that the heart is located on the left side of the body.

Knowledge of the correct position of the heart can make all the difference in the treatment of **cardiac arrest.** Using the heel of the hand, one applies a series of sharp, forceful, pushing motions to the lower sternum of the victim so as to restart the heartbeat. During such a medical emergency, the combination of manual heart compression and artificial respiration can save a life. This life-saving technique is known as **cardiopulmonary resuscitation (CPR)** and should be performed only by those specifically trained in CPR.

STRUCTURE OF THE HEART

The heart is a hollow, muscular, double pump which circulates the blood through the blood vessels to all parts of the body. At rest, the heart pumps two ounces of blood with each beat, five quarts per minute, seventy-five gallons per hour.

Surrounding the heart is a double layer of fibrous tissue called the **pericardium.** Between these two pericardial layers is a space filled with a lubricating fluid called **pericardial fluid.** This fluid prevents the two layers from rubbing against each other and creating friction. The thin inner layer covering the heart is the **serous pericardium.** The tough outer membrane is the **fibrous pericardium.**

Cardiac muscle tissue, or **myocardium,** makes up the wall of the heart. On the inner lining lies a smooth tissue called the **endocardium.** The endocardium covers the heart valves and lines the blood vessels providing smooth transit for the flowing blood.

A frontal view of the human heart reveals a thick, muscular wall separating it into a right half and a left half. This partition, known as the **septum** completely separates the blood in the one half from that in the other half, see color plate 6.

In the human fetus, however, there is an opening in the septum, **foramen ovale,** which connects the two sides of the heart. This condition exists uniquely in the human fetus and in the newborn infant. The opening allows blood to flow freely from the left side to the right side without passing through the lungs for oxygen. Only after birth do the lungs begin to function as an oxygen source, whereupon the foramen ovale closes, forming the solid septum. After this, the right side of the heart carries only **deoxygenated*** (without oxygen) blood and the left side carries only **oxygenated** (with oxygen) blood.

The human heart is separated into right and left halves by the septum. In turn, each half is divided into two parts, thus creating four chambers. The two upper chambers are called the **right atrium** and the **left atrium** (pl. atria). The atrium is also referred to as the **auricle.** The lower chambers are the **right ventricle** and the **left ventricle,** figure 17–1.

The heart has two **atrioventricular valves** and two **semilunar valves** which permit the blood to flow in one direction only. These valves keep the blood from flowing backwards into the chambers.

- The **tricuspid valve** is positioned between the right atrium and the right ventricle. Its name comes from the fact that there are three points, or cusps, of attachment (on the floor of the right ventricle). It allows blood to flow from the right atrium into the right ventricle, but not in the opposite direction.

- The **mitral bicuspid valve** is located between the left atrium and the left ventricle. Blood flows from the left atrium into the left ventricle, while backflow from

---

*Note: Venous blood is said to be deoxygenated, meaning that it contains a large amount of carbon dioxide. However, a small amount of oxygen is present.

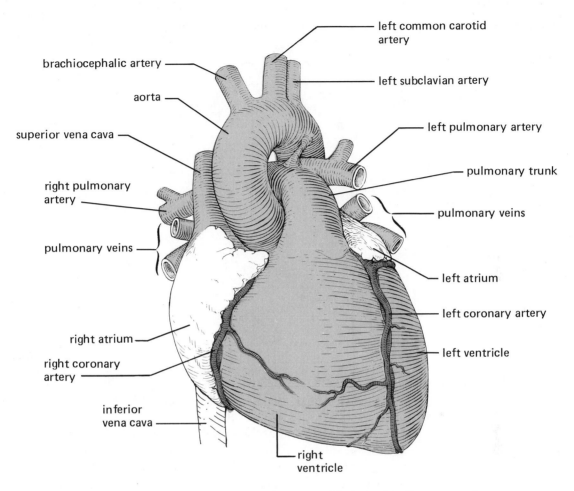

brachiocephalic artery

aorta

superior vena cava

right pulmonary
artery

pulmonary veins

right atrium

right coronary
artery

inferior
vena cava

left common carotid
artery

left subclavian artery

left pulmonary artery

pulmonary trunk

pulmonary veins

left atrium

left coronary artery

left ventricle

right
ventricle

Figure 17-1   Anterior view of the heart with the pericardium removed

the left ventricle to the left atrium is prevented.

- The **pulmonary semilunar valve** is found at the orifice (opening) of the pulmonary artery. It lets blood travel from the right ventricle into the pulmonary artery, and then into the lungs.

- The **aortic semilunar valve** is at the orifice of the aorta. This valve permits the blood to pass from the left ventricle into the aorta, but not backwards into the left ventricle. See figure 17–2.

CONTROL OF HEART CONTRACTIONS

A heart completely removed from the body will continue to beat rhythmically if it is supplied with a proper nutrient media. This shows that heartbeat generates in the heart muscle itself. It is therefore said to be **myogenic** (myo—muscle; gennan—to produce; Gk.). The myocardium contracts rhythmically in order to perform its duty as a forceful pump. See color plate 7.

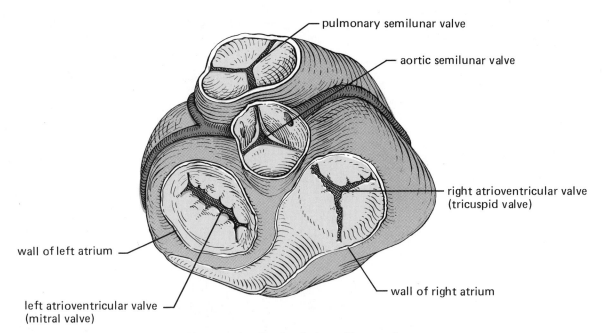

pulmonary semilunar valve

aortic semilunar valve

right atrioventricular valve
(tricuspid valve)

wall of left atrium

wall of right atrium

left atrioventricular valve
(mitral valve)

Figure 17-2 Overhead view of heart valves

Control of heart muscle contractions is found within a group of conducting cells located at the opening of the superior vena cava into the right atrium. These cells are known as the **sinoatrial (S-A) node,** or **pacemaker.** The S-A node can only be identified by microscopic examination of the cardiac tissue. It sends out an electrical impulse which spreads out over the atria, making them contract simultaneously. This causes blood to flow downward from the upper atrial chamber to the atrioventricular openings. The electrical impulse eventually reaches the **atrioventricular (A-V) node**, which is another conducting cell group located between the atria and ventricle.

From the A-V node, the electrical impulse is carried to conducting fibers in the septum. These conducting fibers are known as the **atrioventricular bundle** or the **bundle of His.** It divides into a right and left branch; each branch then subdivides into a fine network of branches spreading throughout the ventricles, called the **Purkinje network.** The electrical impulse shoots along the Purkinje fibers, until it reaches the heart's apex.

The combined action of the S-A and A-V nodes is instrumental in the cardiac cycle. The cardiac cycle comprises one complete heartbeat, with both atrial and ventricular contractions.

1. The S-A node stimulates the contraction of both atria. Blood flows from the atria into the ventricles through the open tricuspid and mitral valves. At the same time, the ventricles are relaxed, allowing them to fill with the blood. At this point, since the semilunar valves are closed, the blood cannot enter the pulmonary artery or aorta.

2. The A-V node stimulates the contraction of both ventricles so that the

blood in the ventricles is pumped into the pulmonary artery and the aorta through the semilunar valves which are now open. At this point the atria are relaxed and the tricuspid and mitral valves closed.

3. The ventricles relax; the semilunar valves are closed to prevent the blood flowing back into the ventricles. The cycle begins again with the signal from the S-A node.

HEART TRANSPLANTS

A heart transplant is needed in cases where the individual's own heart can no longer function properly. This happens when someone has suffered repeated heart attacks, and there is irreparable damage to the heart muscle, valves, or blood vessels leading to and from the heart. Occasionally, a baby or young child might need a heart transplant because of a **congenital** (occurring at birth) heart defect.

There are always problems that follow even the most "successful" of heart transplants, however. The problem is one of **histocompatibility** (matching of tissue type) and organ rejection. Heart transplants that occur between two unrelated people must be monitored carefully. When the heart from the donor is placed into the recipient's body, the recipient's body chemically recognizes the donated heart as a "foreign" donated heart. Thus, the recipient's immune system starts to reject the transplanted heart.

Medical science has counteracted the rejection by developing chemicals called **immunosuppressants.** These drugs suppress the recipient's immune system so it will not form antibodies to reject the donated heart. Unfortunately, the effect of these chemicals is not permanent. Also, suppressing the recipient's immune system indefinitely is not medically wise because he or she will be more susceptible to disease and infection. Often times a heart transplant patient dies not from problems arising from the donated heart but from a case of pneumonia! So the science and technology of heart transplants is still in its formative stages. However, a heart transplant can perhaps prolong the life and maybe even improve the quality of life for an individual with a chronic heart problem.

ARTIFICIAL HEART

The major problem arising from human transplants between two unrelated people is one of histocompatibility. Also, the availability of a healthy heart at the precise moment when it is needed is another problem. In the search to solve these two problems, scientists have developed an artificial heart.

A permanent artificial heart was installed in a human for the first time in medical history on December 3, 1982. The recipient was Dr. Barney Clark, a retired dentist. The artificial heart was an air-powered polyurethane heart called the Jarvick-7 artificial heart. Installation of the Jarvick-7 heart was necessary when Dr. Clark's own heart no longer responded to regular cardiac care. Dr. Clark remained alive for 112 days after the Jarvick-7 implant. In that time period, the Jarvick-7 heart had beaten almost 13 million times. The artificial heart actually worked normally until it was disconnected after Dr. Clark's death. Dr. Clark died from a multiorgan system failure. The development and improvement of artificial hearts like the Jarvick-7 holds promise for the improvement of the quality of life for many chronically suffering heart patients.

Further Study and Discussion

- If laboratory facilities are available, obtain a calf or sheep heart to examine. Notice the pericardium which is the tissue-like covering around the heart. Locate the atria, ventricles and identify the four valves.
- On Figure 17–3 locate and label the various structures of the heart. Also include valves, vessels, and nodes.

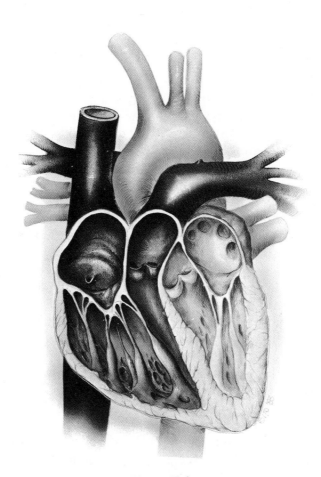

Figure 17-3

Assignment

A. Briefly answer the following questions.

  1. What is the pericardium? Describe its function.

  2. Describe the endocardium and list its functions.

  3. Name the four chambers of the heart.

  4. Name each valve, then locate its position by identifying the structure or area on both sides of the valve.

  5. What function does a valve perform?

  6. Who would be a likely candidate for either a human heart or artificial heart transplant?

7. What is the major problem encountered in human heart transplants?

8. What are immunosuppressants?

9. What was the name of the artificial heart implanted into Dr. Clark's chest?

B. Complete the following statements.
   1. The heart or cardiac muscle is called the _____ .
   2. The _____ is the smooth lining of the heart.
   3. The structure known as the _____ stimulates the contraction of the ventricles.
   4. The ventricle with the thickest muscular structure is on the _____ side of the heart.
   5. The _____ is also called the pacemaker of the heart.

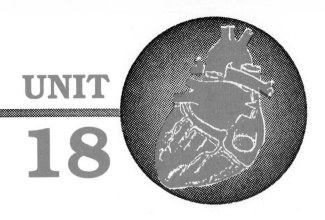

UNIT 18

FUNCTION AND PATH OF GENERAL CIRCULATION

KEY WORDS

aorta
aortic arch
arteriole
bifurcate
brachiocephalic
    artery
coronary
    artery
coronary
    circulation

coronary sinus
coronary vein
hepatic portal
    vein
inferior vena cava
left common
    carotid artery
left subclavian
    artery
portal circulation

portal vein
pulmonary artery
pulmonary vein
renal artery
renal circulation
renal vein
superior vena
    cava
venule

OBJECTIVES

■ Trace the path of the general circulation
■ Describe the four main functions of general circulation
■ Name some specialized circulatory systems
■ Define the Key Words relative to this unit of study

The function of the general (systemic) circulation is fourfold: it circulates nutrients, oxygen, water, and secretions to the tissues and back to the heart; it carries products such as carbon dioxide and other dissolved wastes away from the tissues; it helps equalize body temperature; it aids in protecting the body from harmful bacteria.

THE GENERAL CIRCULATION

Let us trace a drop of blood through the human circulatory system. The blood can return to the heart from the arms or legs. Blood flowing from the upper part of the body (head, neck, and arms) returns to the right side of the heart via the **superior vena cava.** The superior vena cava is one of the two largest veins in the body. Blood from the lower part of the body (legs and trunks) enters the heart through the **inferior vena cava** (the other of the largest veins).

From both these veins, blood enters the right atrium, which then contracts, forcing the blood through the tricuspid valve into the right ventricle. This chamber contains deoxygenated blood from the tissues. Deoxygenated blood contains very little oxygen but a good deal of carbon dioxide.

The right ventricle then contracts to push the deoxygenated blood through the pulmonary semilunar valve into the pulmonary trunk. The pulmonary trunk **bifurcates** (divides in two). It branches into the **right pulmonary artery**, bringing deoxygenated blood to the right lung, and into the **left pulmonary artery,** bringing blood to the left lung.

Inside the lungs, the pulmonary arteries branch into countless small arteries called **arterioles**. The arterioles connect to dense beds of capillaries lying in the alveoli lung tissue. Here, gaseous exchange takes place: carbon dioxide leaves the red blood cells and is discharged into the air in the alveoli, to be ex-

151

creted from the lungs. Oxygen, in turn, combines with hemoglobin in the red blood cells. From these capillaries the blood travels into small veins or **venules.**

Venules from the right lung eventually form two larger **pulmonary veins,** known as the right pulmonary veins. These veins carry oxygenated blood from the right lung back to the heart and into the left atrium.

From the left lung, blood also enters the left atrium via the two left pulmonary veins. Then the left atrium contracts, sending the blood through the bicuspid, or mitral valve, into the left ventricle. This chamber, then, acts as a pump for newly oxygenated blood. When the left ventricle contracts, it sends oxygenated blood through the aortic semilunar valve, then into the **aorta.**

The aorta is the largest artery in the body. As the aorta emerges (ascending aorta) from the anterior (upper) portion of the heart, it forms an arch. This arch is known as the **aortic arch.** Three branches come from this arch: the **brachiocephalic,** the **left common carotid,** and the **left subclavian** arteries, see color plate 8A. These arteries and their branches carry blood to the arms, neck and head.

From the aortic arch, the aorta descends along the mid-dorsal wall of the thorax and abdomen. Many arteries branch off from their descending aorta, carrying oxygenated blood throughout the body. The first branch from the descending aorta is the **coronary artery.** It carries blood to the heart's muscular wall.

As the desending aorta proceeds posteriorly, it sends off additional branches to the body wall, stomach, intestines, liver, pancreas, spleen, kidneys, reproductive organs, urinary bladder, legs, and so forth. Each of these arteries subdivides into still smaller arteries, then into arterioles, and finally into numerous capillaries embedded in the tissues. This is where hormones, nutrients, oxygen and other materials are transferred from the blood into the tissue.

In turn, metabolic waste products, such as carbon dioxide and nitrogenous wastes, are picked up by the blood. Hormones secreted by specialized tissues, and nutrients from the small intestines and liver, are also absorbed by the blood. Blood then runs from the capillaries first into tiny veins, through increasingly larger veins, and finally into one (or more) of the veins which exit from the organ. Eventually it empties into one of two largest veins in the body, see color plate 8B.

Deoxygenated venous blood, returning from the lower parts of the body, empties into the inferior vena cava. Venous blood from the upper body parts (arms, neck and head) passes into the superior vena cava. Both the inferior and superior vena cavae empty their deoxygenated blood into the right atrium.

Coronary Circulation

Some circulatory routes within the general circulation are called by special names. The **coronary circulation,** which brings oxygenated blood to the heart, is a part of the general circulation. It has two branches, the left and right coronary arteries. These branches come off from the aorta just above the heart. The branches encircle the heart muscle, with many tiny branches going to all parts of the heart muscle. Blood returns to the right atrium by a pocket or trough in the wall of the right atrium, the **coronary sinus** into which the **coronary veins** empty, see color plates 9 and 10.

Renal Circulation

The **renal circulation** is that part of the general circulation which carries blood from the aorta through the **renal artery** to the kidneys and then through the renal vein back into the heart by way of the inferior vena cava. This **renal vein** carries limited amounts of cell waste since many of them have been removed from the blood in the kidneys.

Portal Circulation

The **portal circulation** is a branch of the general circulation. Veins from the pancreas, stomach, small intestine, colon and spleen empty their blood into the **portal vein** in the liver.

It is very important that venous blood makes a detour through the liver before returning to the heart. After meals, blood reaching the liver contains a higher than normal concentration of glucose. The liver removes the excess glucose, converting it to storage glycogen. In the event of vigorous exercise, work or prolonged periods without nourishment, gly-

cogen reserves will be changed back into glucose for energy. This detour insures that the blood's glucose concentration is kept within a relatively narrow range.

The liver also detoxifies (neutralizes) drugs and toxins, degrades hormones no longer useful to the body, and produces urea during the catabolism of amino acids. The liver also removes worn-out red blood cells from circulation.

Deoxygenated venous blood leaves the liver through the **hepatic portal vein,** which carries it to the inferior vena cava. From the inferior vena cava, blood enters the right atrium, see color plate 11. The red blood cell debris is then carried with bile from the liver into the intestine and is removed from the body in the feces.

Further Study and Discussion

- Starting from the right ventricle trace the path of a red blood cell out of the heart, into the lungs for oxygenation and back to the left ventricle and out of the heart into the abdomen.

Assignment

A. Briefly answer the following questions.

1. Describe the chief functions of the general circulatory system.

2. Name the special circulatory system which is responsible for each of the following functions.
    a. Carries water to the kidneys

    b. Nourishes the heart

    c. Serves the digestive organs

B. Complete the following statements.

   1. The blood leaves the heart from the _____ventricle through the _____ , the largest artery in the body.

   2. The deoxygenated blood re-enters the heart through the _____ _____ and into the _____ atrium.

C. Match each term in column I with its correct description in column II.

Column I	Column II
_____ 1. coronary circulation	a. a part of the general circulation which is made up of veins and carries digested food and water to the liver
_____ 2. renal vein	
_____ 3. portal circulation	b. that part of the general circulation which carries blood from aorta to the kidneys and back to the heart
_____ 4. renal circulation	
_____ 5. hepatic portal vein	c. the part of the general circulation which nourishes the heart
	d. the great vein of the general circulatory system
	e. carries limited amounts of cellular waste back to the heart by way of the inferior vena cava
	f. the vein which goes from the liver to the inferior vena cava heavily supplied with nutrients

UNIT 19

PULMONARY CIRCULATION

OBJECTIVES

- Trace the route of the pulmonary circulation
- Describe the function of the pulmonary circulation
- Compare the general and pulmonary circulatory system

The pulmonary circulation carries blood from the heart to the lungs and back to the heart. The blood carried by the pulmonary trunk is deoxygenated blood which is a darker red than when it leaves the lungs. There are also waste products in this blood. One of the waste products carried by the blood from the cells is carbon dioxide. It is exchanged for a new supply of oxygen in the lungs. The now oxygenated blood is bright red.

The pulmonary circulation starts its circuit by leaving the right ventricle of the heart through the pulmonary trunk, figure 19–1. The pulmonary trunk, carrying deoxygenated blood, bifurcates into a right pulmonary artery going to the right lung, and a left pulmonary artery to the left lung. These two arteries eventually branch out into capillaries inside the lungs. Here, the exchange of carbon dioxide for oxygen takes place. The blood, freshly supplied with oxygen, returns to the heart by way of the right and left pulmonary veins. It enters the left atrium of the heart (the opposite side from which it left). It is now ready to make its circuit throughout the body by way of the general circulation to distribute a fresh supply of oxygen.

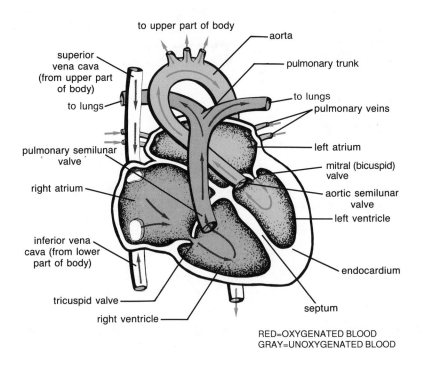

Figure 19-1   Schematic of pulmonary circulation

Further Study and Discussion

- Research and discuss what is meant by a "blue baby." Why does the baby have a bluish appearance? What can be done for this baby to help it survive?

Assignment

Briefly answer the following questions.

1. Which two main organs are involved in the pulmonary circulation?

2. Which pulmonary vessel carries deoxygenated blood?

3. Name the major waste material present in deoxygenated blood.

4. What functions do the capillaries perform in the alveoli of the lungs?

5. Name the chamber of the heart from which the blood enters the lungs and the chamber to which the oxygenated blood returns.

UNIT 20

BLOOD VESSELS

KEY WORDS

arteries
arteriole
arteriosclerosis
capillary
diastolic blood
  pressure
endothelial cell
metarteriole

precapillary
  sphincter
pulse
reflux
systolic blood
  pressure
tunica adventitia
  (externa)

tunica intima
tunica media
valves (in
  veins)
vein
venule

OBJECTIVES

- List the five types of blood vessels
- Describe the particular function of each type of blood vessel
- Identify the principal blood vessels of the body
- Define the Key Words relating to this unit of study

The heart pumps the blood to all parts of the body through a remarkable system of three types of blood vessels: arteries, capillaries, and veins.

ARTERIES

Arteries carry oxygenated blood away from the heart to the capillaries. (There is one exception — the pulmonary arteries — which carry deoxygenated blood from the heart to the lungs). The arteries transport blood under very high pressure; they are thus elastic, muscular and thick-walled. The thickness of the arteries makes them the strongest of the three types of blood vessels. Table 20–1 lists the principal arteries and the areas they serve.

As seen in color plate 12, the arterial walls are composed of three layers. The outer layer is called the **tunica adventitia** or **externa.** This layer is composed of loose connective tissue,

scattered throughout with bundles of smooth muscle cells. These bundles of smooth muscle cells lend great elasticity to the arteries. This elasticity allows the arteries to withstand sudden large increases in internal pressure, created by the large volume of blood forced into them at each heart contraction. When arteries become hardened, as in **arteriosclerosis,** the **systolic blood pressure** increases greatly.

The **tunica media** is the middle arterial layer. It is composed of muscle cells arranged in a circular pattern. This layer controls the artery's diameter, thus regulating the blood flow through the artery. The tunica media has the most important function, making the arteries very compliant. In this way, the dilation and constriction of the arteries allows for the free flow of blood. This keeps the blood flow steady and even and reduces the heart's work.

An inner layer **(tunica intima)** consists of three smaller layers. The layer lining, facing

Table 20–1 Principal Arteries

NAME	AREA SERVED
Common carotid Innominate Right and left coronary Lateral thoracic Pulmonary Aortic arch Right and left subclavian Thoracic aorta	Neck, head and chest
Right and left palmar digital Right and left ulnar Right and left radial Right and left brachial	Arms and hands
Abdominal aorta Celiac Superior mesenteric Renal	Abdominal region
Common iliac Right and left external iliac	Abdomen and legs
Right and left deep femoral Right and left femoral Right and left popliteal Right and left anterior tibial Right and left posterior tibial Right and left dorsal pedis	Legs and feet

the lumen of the artery, is made of **endothelial cells.** They give the arterial lining a smooth surface that does not obstruct blood flow. The next layer consists of delicate connective tissue, found only in arteries with a very large diameter. An elastic layer, composed of a membrane of elastic fibers, is the third layer. This helps to strengthen the arterial walls.

The pulmonary trunk and the aorta (the largest artery in the body) lead away from the heart and branch into smaller arteries. These smaller arteries, in turn, branch into **arterioles.** Arterioles give rise to the smallest blood vessels, the **capillaries,** figure 20–1.

CAPILLARIES

Capillaries are microscopic in size; they are so small they can only be seen through a compound microscope. Capillaries connect the arterioles with tiny veins, called **venules.** Capillaries are branches of the finest arteriole divisions, known as **metarterioles.** The metarterioles have lost most of their connective tissue and muscle layers. Eventually the last traces of these two tissues disappear, and there remains only a simple endothelial cell layer. This endothelial cell layer constitutes the capillaries.

The capillary walls are extremely thin, so as to allow for the selective permeability of various cells and substances. Thus, nutrient molecules and oxygen can pass out of the capillaries and into the surrounding tissues. Consequently, metabolic waste products like carbon dioxide and nitrogenous wastes pass back into the bloodstream for excretion at their proper sites.

Tiny openings in the capillary walls allow white blood cells to leave the bloodstream and enter the tissue spaces to help destroy invading bacteria. In the capillaries, too, some of the plasma diffuses out of the bloodstream and into the tissue spaces. This fluid is called interstitial fluid and is returned to the bloodstream in the form of lymph via the lymphatic vessels.

The internal diameter of a capillary is so small that red blood cells often pass through them in single file. Sometimes the diameter of red blood cells exceeds that of the capillaries; they become compressed and distorted as they flow through the capillary.

Blood flow through the capillaries can be controlled, despite the fact that muscle cells do not line the capillary walls. This is achieved by the action of small muscular bands called **precapillary sphincters.** These bands are found at the region where the capillary branches from an arteriole, or metarteriole.

Although capillaries are ultimately responsible for transporting blood to all tissues, not all capillaries are open simultaneously.

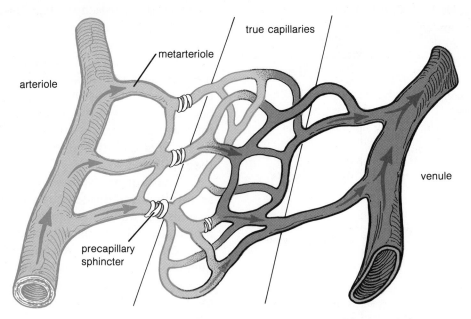

Figure 20-1 Capillary bed connecting an arteriole with a venule

This system allows for regulation of blood flow to so-called "active" tissues. In the human brain, for instance, most of the capillaries remain open. However, in a resting muscle, only 1/20 to 1/50 of the capillaries transport blood to the muscle cells. Compare this to an actively contracting muscle where as many as 190 capillaries per square millimeter are open. If the same muscle is not active, there may be as few as five capillaries open per square millimeter.

VEINS

The **veins** carry deoxygenated blood away from the capillaries to the heart in venules. (A venule is a small vein). The smallest venules are hardly larger than a capillary, but they contain a muscular layer which is not present within capillaries. Table 20–2 lists the principal veins and the areas they serve.

The vein's structure is comparable to that of the artery; however, veins are considerably

Table 20–2 Principal Veins

NAME	AREA SERVED
Internal jugular External jugular Right and left innominate Right and left subclavian Pulmonary Superior vena cava Inferior vena cava Right and left axillary	Head, Neck, Chest
Right and left cephalic Right and left basilic	Arms
Hepatic Portal Splenic Common iliac	Abdominal region
Right and left great saphenous Right and left femoral Right and left popliteal Right and left posterior tibial Right and left anterior tibial Right and left dorsal venous arch	Legs

less elastic and muscular. Also the walls of the veins are much thinner than those of the arteries since they do not have to withstand such high internal pressures. This is because pressure from the heart's contraction is greatly diminished by the time the blood reaches the veins for its return journey. Thus the thinner walled veins can collapse easily when not filled with blood. Finally, veins have *valves* along their length. These valves allow blood to flow only in one direction, towards the heart. This prevents **reflux** (backflow) of blood toward the capillaries, figure 20–2. Valves are found in abundance in veins, where there is a greater chance for reflux. So, there are many valves in the lower extremities, where blood has to oppose the force of gravity.

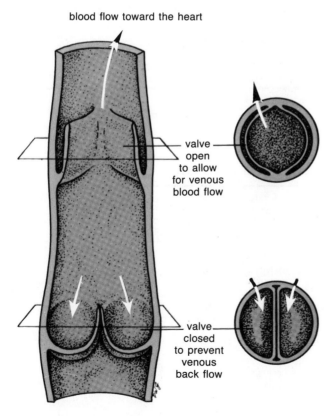

blood flow toward the heart

valve open to allow for venous blood flow

valve closed to prevent venous back flow

Figure 20-2   Valves in the vein

Eventually, all the venules converge to make up larger veins, which ultimately form the body's largest veins, the vena cavae. Venous blood from the upper part of the body returns to the right atrium via the superior vena cava; blood from the lower body parts is conducted to the heart via the inferior vena cava.

BLOOD PRESSURE

Initially, when the heart pumps blood into the arteries, the surge of blood filling the vessels creates pressure against their walls. The pressure at the moment of contraction is the **systolic blood pressure,** caused by the rush of blood which follows contraction of the ventricles. The lessened force of the blood (when the ventricles are relaxed) is called **diastolic pressure.** The pressure present in the arteries that are close to the initial surge of blood is greatest and gradually decreases as the blood travels further away from the pumping action.

PULSE

If you touch certain areas of the body, such as the radial artery at the wrist, you will feel alternating, beating throbs. These throbs represent your body's pulse points. A **pulse** is the alternating expansion and contraction of an artery as blood flows through it.

Try this simple demonstration: place your fingertips (except for the thumb) over an artery which is near the surface of the skin and over a bone. There are six locations where you can conveniently feel your pulse:

- **Brachial artery** — located at the crook of the elbow, along the inner border of the biceps muscle.

- **Common carotid artery** — found in the neck, along the front margin of the sternocleidomastoid muscle, near the lower edge of the thyroid cartilage.

- **Dorsalis pedis artery** — on the anterior surface of the foot, below the ankle joint.

- **Facial artery** — at the lower edge of the mandible, on a line with the corners of the mouth.

- **Radial artery** — at the wrist, on the posterior surface of the radius.

- **Temporal artery** — slightly above the outer edge of the eye.

Further Study and Discussion

- Investigate and be prepared to discuss the following questions: What is blood pressure? Where is it usually taken? How is it measured? What instruments are used for taking blood pressure?

- Try the following experiment with a classmate and discuss the findings.
    Take the pulse for 30 seconds while the student is seated.
    Take the pulse for 30 seconds while the student is standing
    Ask the student to jump up and down 25 times, being sure that the knees are well flexed.
      a. Check the pulse immediately after the exercise
      b. Check the pulse one minute after exercise
      c. Check the pulse two minutes after exercise

Assignment

Match each term in column I with its description in column II.

Column I	Column II
_____ 1. arteries	a. small arteries which lead to capillaries
_____ 2. capillaries	b. permit blood to flow in only one direction
_____ 3. valves	c. enter the right atrium of the heart
_____ 4. veins	d. blood vessels which carry blood back to the heart
_____ 5. arterioles	e. connect arterioles with venules
	f. large, thick, muscle-walled blood vessels that carry blood away from the heart

UNIT
21

THE BLOOD

OBJECTIVES

- List the important components of the blood
- Describe the function of each component
- Recognize the significance of the various blood types
- Define the Key Words relating to this unit of study

The average adult has eight to ten pints of blood in his or her body. Loss of more than two pints at any one time leads to a serious condition.

Blood is the transporting fluid of the body. It carries nutrients from the digestive tract to the cells, oxygen from the lungs to the cells, waste products from the cells to the various organs of excretion, and hormones from secreting cells to other parts of the body. It aids in the distribution of heat formed in the more active tissues (such as the skeletal muscles) to all parts of the body. Blood also helps to regulate the acid-base balance, and to protect against infection. Consequently, it is a vital fluid to our life and health.

BLOOD COMPOSITION _____

Blood is composed of a liquid portion called **plasma,** which contains various types of dissolved chemicals and several different kinds of blood cells, see color plate 13. Although most of the cells are red blood cells, there are various types of white blood cells as well. The blood also contains large numbers of platelets.

BLOOD PLASMA _____

Plasma is a straw colored, complex liquid, comprising about 55% of the blood volume and containing the following substances in solution:

1. **Water** — Water makes up about 92% of the total volume of plasma. This percentage is maintained by the kidneys, and by water intake and output.

2. **Blood proteins** — There is a protein found in red blood cells known as hemoglobin, which comprises about two-thirds of the blood proteins. Plasma proteins (discussed next) make up approximately one-third.

3. **Plasma proteins** — These three proteins are the most abundant of those found in plasma: fibrinogen, serum albumin and serum globulin.

    a. **Fibrinogen** is necessary for blood clotting. Without fibrinogen, the slightest cut or wound would bleed profusely. It is synthesized in the liver, and makes up about 4% of the total plasma proteins.

    b. **Serum albumin** is the most abundant of all the plasma proteins. It constitutes some 53% of the total plasma proteins. Another product of the liver, serum albumin helps to maintain the blood's osmotic pressure and volume. It provides the "pulse pressure" needed to hold and pull water from the tissue fluid back into the blood vessels. This is important because metabolic waste, like carbon dioxide, can be excreted from the cells. Normally, plasma proteins do not pass through the capillary walls, since their molecules are relatively large. Since they are colloidal substances, they can give up, or take up, water-soluble substances, thus regulating the osmotic pressure within the blood vessels.

    c. **Serum globulin** — It makes up about 43% of the total volume of plasma proteins. It is formed not only in the liver, but also in the lymphatic system (discussed in unit 22). **Gamma globulin** has been fractionated (separated) from serum albumin. This portion helps in the synthesis of antibodies, which destroy or render harmless various disease-causing organisms. **Prothrombin** is yet another globulin, formed continually in the liver, which helps blood to coagulate. Vitamin K is necessary in aiding the process of prothrombin synthesis.

4. **Nutrients** — Nutrient molecules are absorbed from the digestive tract. Glucose, fatty acids, cholesterol and amino acids are dissolved in the blood plasma.

5. **Mineral salts** — These are also called **electrolytes,** the most abundant being

sodium chloride (NaCl). The others are potassium chloride (KCl), phosphates, sulphates, bicarbonates, etc. These come from foods and chemical processes occurring in the body. They act as chemical buffers in helping to maintain the acid-base balance of the blood.

6. **Hormones, vitamins, and enzymes —** These three substances are found in very small amounts in the blood plasma. They generally help the body to control its chemical reactions.

7. **Metabolic waste products —** All of the body's cells are actively engaged in chemical reactions to maintain homeostasis. As a result of this, waste products are formed and subsequently carried by the plasma to the various excretory organs.

RED BLOOD CELLS

Red blood cells, or **erythrocytes,** are biconcave, disc-shaped cells. They are caved in on both sides, with a thin center and thicker margins. When viewed from above, they appear to have a doughnut shape, see color plate 13.

Hemoglobin

Erythrocytes contain a red pigment (coloring agent) called **hemoglobin,** which provides its characteristic color. Hemoglobin is composed of a protein molecule called **globin,** and an iron compound called **heme.** A single red blood cell contains several million molecules of hemoglobin. Hemoglobin is vital to the function of the red blood cell, helping it to transport oxygen to the tissues and carbon dioxide away from the tissues.

Function

In the capillaries of the lung, erythrocytes pick up oxygen from the inspired air. The oxygen chemically combines with the hemoglobin, forming the compound **oxyhemoglobin.** The oxyhemoglobin-laden erythrocytes circulate to the capillaries of tissues. Here oxygen is released to the tissues, and carbon dioxide is picked up by the hemoglobin, forming **carboxyhemoglobin.** The red blood cells circulate back to the lungs to give up the carbon dioxide and absorb more oxygen. The oxyhemoglobin and caboxyhemoglobin are responsible for the blood's color. Except for pulmonary arteries, blood cells that travel in the arteries carry oxyhemoglobin, which gives blood its bright red color. Except for pulmonary veins, blood cells in the veins contain carboxyhemoglobin, which is responsible for the dark, crimson-blue color characteristic of venous blood.

Erythropoiesis

Erythropoiesis, or synthesis of red blood cells, occurs in the red bone marrow of essentially all bones, until adolescence. (In the fetus, red blood cells are also produced by the spleen and liver.) As one grows older, the red marrow of the long bones is replaced by fat marrow; erythrocytes are thereafter formed only in the short and flat bones.

Erythrocytes come from primitive cells in the red bone marrow called **hemocytoblasts.** As the hemocytoblast matures into an erythrocyte, it loses its nucleus and cytoplasmic organelles. The hemocytoblast also becomes smaller, gains hemoglobin, develops a biconcave shape, and enters into the bloodstream. To aid in erythropoiesis, vitamin B_{12}, folic acid, copper, cobalt, iron, and proteins are needed.

Since erythrocytes are **enucleated** (contain no nucleus), they only live about 120 days. Destruction occurs as the cells age, rendering them more vulnerable to rupturing. They are broken down by the spleen and liver. Hemoglobin breaks down into globin and heme; the iron content of heme is used to make new red blood cells. The normal count of red blood cells ranges from 5,500,000 to 7,000,000 per cubic millimeter of blood for men; 4,500,000 to 6,000,000 per cubic millimeter for women.

Hemolysis

Under certain conditions, the erythrocyte membrane is disrupted. This causes the hemoglobin to escape into solution in the blood plasma. This is called **hemolysis,** or **laking.** When laking occurs, the red blood cells become colorless "ghosts." Hemolysis occurs when a hypotonic solution is given intravenously, from antibody-antigen reactions between the erythrocyte antigens and plasma agglutinins or from **autoimmune** (self-produced) antibodies against the erythrocytes.

WHITE BLOOD CELLS

White blood cells are known as **leukocytes.** They are larger than the erythrocytes, ranging from 1 1/4 to 2 times their diameter. They are granular, translucent, and ameboid in shape. Leukocytes are synthesized in both red bone marrow and in lymphatic tissue.

Types of Leukocytes

Leukocytes are classified into two major groups of cells: the **granulocytes (granular leukocytes)** and the **agranulocytes (agranular leukocytes).** This classification is due to their cytoplasmic granules, nuclear structure, and reactions to stains like Wright's stain. Granulocytes are synthesized in red bone marrow from cells called **myeloblasts.** Granulocytes are destroyed as they age and as a result of partici-

pating in bacterial destruction. The life-span of white blood cells is variable, but most granulocytes live only a few days.

There are three types of granulocytes: neutrophils, eosinophils, and basophils. Neutrophils are also called **polymorphonuclear leukocytes.**

Neutrophils phagocytize bacteria with lysosomal enzymes in the leukocyte. (**Phagocytosis** is a process that surrounds, engulfs and digests harmful bacteria.) **Eosinophils** phagocytize the remains of antibody-antigen reactions. They also increase in great numbers in allergic conditions, malaria, and in worm infestation. **Basophils** also undergo phagocytosis, and their count increases during chronic inflammation and during the healing from an infection.

Agranulocytes are divided into lymphocytes and monocytes. **Lymphocytes** are further subdivided into **B-lymphocytes,** which are synthesized in the bone marrow, and **T-lymphocytes** from the thymus gland (unit 44). Still others are formed by the lymph nodes and spleen. Their life-span ranges from a few days to several years. They basically help the body by synthesizing and releasing antibody molecules and by protecting against the formation of cancer cells.

Monocytes are formed in bone marrow. They assist in phagocytosis, and are able to leave the bloodstream to attach themselves to tissues; here they become tissue **macrophages,** or **histiocytes.** During an inflammation, histiocytes help to wall off and isolate the infected area.

The aforementioned types of leukocytes (basophils, neutrophils, eosinophils, and monocytes) which can undergo phagocytosis are called **phagocytes.** Unlike erythrocytes, they can move through the intercellular spaces of the capillary wall into neighboring tissue. This process is known as **diapedesis.**

A normal leukocyte count averages from 5000 to 9000 cells per cubic millimeter of blood (1 leukocyte for every 100 erythrocytes).

To summarize, leukocytes help protect the body against infection and injury. This is achieved through: (1) phagocytosis and destruction of bacteria, (2) synthesis of antibody molecules, (3) "cleaning up" of cellular remnants at the site of inflammation, and (4) the walling off of the infected area. See tables 21–1 and 21–2.

INFLAMMATION

If living tissue is damaged in any way, the body usually responds to the damage by either neutralizing or eliminating the cause of the damage. When this happens, the damaged body part goes through an inflammation process. **Inflammation** occurs when tissues are subjected to chemical or physical trauma (cut or heat). Invasion by **pathogenic** (disease-causing) microorganisms like bacteria, fungi, protozoa, and viruses also can cause inflammation.

The characteristic symptoms of inflammation are redness, local heat, swelling, and pain. This is due to irritation by bacterial toxins, to increased blood flow, to congestion of blood vessels, and to the collection of blood plasma in the surrounding tissues (**edema**). This results from the release of **histamine** (compound responsible for the dilation and increased permeability of blood vessels) from the mast cells (which are tissue basophils) of connective tissue during bacterial infection. Histamine and other chemical substances increase blood flow to the injured area as well as increasing capillary permeability. Thus, large amounts of blood plasma and fibrinogen enter the damaged area. The damaged area is walled off as a result of the clotting action of fibrinogen on the damaged tissue and macrophage action. (A **macrophage** is a large white blood cell that devours bacteria and dead cells.)

Neutrophils move very quickly to the damaged area by **chemotaxis.*** Then the neutrophils move through the capillary walls by diapedesis and begin phagocytosis of the pathogenic microorganisms. Macrophages also will participate in phagocytosis.

In most inflammations, a cream-colored liquid called **pus** forms. Pus is a combination

---

Chemotaxis is a response of an organism or a cell to a chemical stimulus by either moving towards or away from the chemical stimulus. Moving towards a chemical stimulus is classified as positive chemotaxis and away as negative chemotaxis.

Table 21–1 The Different Types of Leukocytes and Their Sizes

MAJOR TYPES OF LEUKOCYTES	SPECIFIC KINDS OF LEUKOCYTES	SIZE
Granulocytes 60-70%	Neutrophils Eosinophils Basophils	9-12 mu 10-14 mu 8-10 mu
Agranulocytes Lymphocytes 20-30%	Small Large	7-10 mu up to 20 mu
Monocyte 5-8%	Mononuclear Transitional	9-12 mu 9-12 mu

Table 21–2 Characteristics And Functions Of The Leukocytes

LEUKOCYTE	WHERE FORMED	TYPE OF NUCLEUS	CYTOPLASM	FUNCTION
Agranular leukocytes 1. Lymphocyte	Lymph glands and nodes, bone marrow, spleen	One large, spherical nucleus; may be indented Sharply defined and stains pale blue	Cytoplasm stains a pale blue and contains scattered violet granules	Helps to form antibodies at a site of inflammation; protects against cancer
2. Monocyte (macrophage)	Lymph glands and nodes, bone marrow, spleen	One lobulated or horseshoe-shaped nucleus that stains blue	Abundant cytoplasm that stains a gray-blue	Phagocytosis of cellular debris and foreign particles
Granular leukocytes 1. Neutrophil	Formed in bone marrow from neutrophilic myelocytes	Lobulated: contains 1 to 5 or more lobes, stains deep blue	Cytoplasm has a pink tinge with very fine granules.	Displays marked phagocytosis toward bacteria during infections and inflammations. Contributes to pus formation.
2. Eosinophil	Formed in bone marrow from eosinophilic myelocytes	Irregularly shaped with 2 lobes, stains blue, but less deeply than neutrophils	Cytoplasm has a sky-blue tinge with many coarse, uniform, round or oval bright-red granules.	Marked increase during parasitic, worm infections
3. Basophil (mast cell)	Formed in bone marrow from basophilic myelocytes	Centrally located, slightly lobulated nucleus, stains a light purple and hidden by granules	Cytoplasm has a mauve color with many large deep-purple granules.	Phagocytosis; releases histamine and promotes the inflammatory response.

of dead tissue, dead and living bacteria, dead leukocytes, and blood plasma. If the damaged area is below the epidermis, an **abscess** (pus-filled cavity) forms. If it is on the skin or a mucosal surface, it is called an **ulcer**. In many inflammations, chemical substances called **pyrogens** are formed. Some of these pyrogens are absorbed into the bloodstream and circulated to the hypothalamus. In the hypothalamus, the pyrogens affect the temperature-control center, which raises the body's temperature causing fever or **pyrexia**.

In addition to the inflammation, there is an increased production of neutrophils by bone marrow. In many severe infections, a **leukocytosis-inducing factor (LIF)** develops. LIF stimulates the production and release of neutrophils into the bloodstream, and thus the leukocyte count rises. If the white blood cell count exceeds 10,000 cells per cubic milliliter (mm^3), a condition called **leukocytosis** exists. Following healing, the leukocyte count returns to normal, which is from 5,000 to 9,000 white blood cells per mm^3. Sometimes, a decrease in the number of white blood cells occurs. This is called **leukopenia**. Leukopenia can be caused by taking marrow-depressant drugs, by pathologic conditions, or by radiation.

THROMBOCYTES (BLOOD PLATELETS)

Thrombocytes are the smallest of the solid components of blood. They are ovoid-shaped structures, synthesized from the larger **megakaryocytes** in red bone marrow. Thrombocytes are actually fragments of the megakaryocytes cytoplasm, see color plate 13.

The normal blood platelet count ranges from 250,000 to 450,000 per cubic millimeter of blood. Platelets function in the initiation of the blood-clotting process. When a blood vessel is damaged, as in a cut or wound, the vessel's collagen fibers come into contact with the platelets. The platelets are then stimulated to produce sticky projecting structures, allowing them to stick to the collagen fibers. The platelets secrete adenosine diphosphate (ADP), which affects adjacent platelets, making them sticky as well. This reaction occurs countless times, creating a "platelet plug" to stop the bleeding. Subsequently, the blood clotting process follows to "harden" the platelet plug. Old platelets eventually disintegrate in the bone marrow.

Coagulation

Blood clotting or **coagulation** is a complicated and essential process which depends in large part on thrombocytes. When a cut or other injury ruptures a blood vessel, clotting must occur to stop the bleeding. On the other hand, unnecessary clotting can clog vessels, cutting off the vital supply of oxygen.

Although the exact details of this process are not clear, there is a general agreement that the following reaction occurs. Whenever a blood vessel or tissue is injured, as in a cut, a substance called **thromboplastin** is produced. An injury to a blood vessel makes the lining rough; as blood platelets flow over the roughened area, they disintegrate, releasing thromboplastin.

Thromboplastin is a complex substance that can only cause coagulation if calcium ions and prothrombin are present. Prothrombin is a plasma protein synthesized in the liver,

The thromboplastin and calcium ions act as enzymes in a reaction that converts prothrombin into **thrombin.** This reaction occurs only in the presence of bleeding, because normally there is no thrombin in the blood plasma.

In the second stage of coagulation, the thrombin just formed acts as an enzyme, changing **fibrinogen** (a plasma protein) into **fibrin.** These gel-like fibrin threads layer themselves over the cut, creating a fine, meshlike network. This fibrin network entraps the red blood cells, platelets, and plasma, creating a blood clot. At first, serum (a pale yellow fluid) oozes out of the cut. As the serum slowly dries, a crust (scab) forms over the fibrin threads, completing the common clotting process.

In order for coagulation to occur successfully, two **anticoagulants** (substances preventing coagulation) must be neutralized. These are called **antithromboplastin** and **antiprothrombin (heparin)**; they are neutralized by thromboplastin. Thromboplastin is released when platelets disintegrate and tissues are injured.

Prothrombin supply, which is necessary to blood-clotting, is dependent on vitamin K. Vitamin K is a catalyst in the synthesis of prothrombin by liver cells. It is synthesized in the body by a type of bacteria found in the intestines. Some vitamin K may be found in the diet, for example, cabbage, cauliflower, spinach, and soybeans. See Figure 21–1 for a summary of the coagulation process.

Clotting Time. The time it takes for blood to clot is known as its **clotting time.** The clotting time for humans is from four to six minutes.

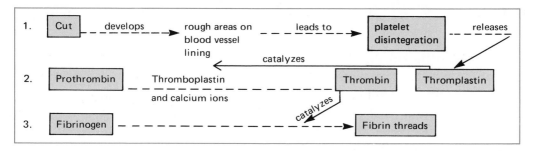

Figure 21-1   Summary of blood clotting reactions

This information is quite useful prior to surgery.

BLOOD TYPES

There are four major groups, or types of blood: A, B, AB and O. Blood type is inherited from one's parents. It is determined by the presence — or absence — of the blood glyco-protein called **agglutinogen,** on the surface of the red blood cell. People with type A blood have the A agglutinogen on their red blood cells. Type B blood has the type B agglutinogen; type AB has both A and B agglutinogen; and type O has *neither* of the agglutinogens.

There is a protein present in the plasma, known as **agglutinin**. An individual with type A blood has *b* agglutinin in the blood plasma. Type B blood possesses *a* agglutinin; type O contains *both* a and b agglutinin; and type AB contains *no* agglutinins.

Knowledge of one's correct type is important in cases of blood transfusions and surgery. Agglutinins react with the agglutinogens of the same type, causing the red blood cells to clump together, figure 21–2. The clumping of blood clogs up the blood vessels, impeding circulation, thus causing death.

By way of example, if a person with type A blood needs a transfusion, he *must receive only type A blood.* Should he receive type B, the B agglutinogens of the type B blood would clump with the b agglutinins of the person's type A blood. This would prove fatal! However, persons with type A blood can receive both types A and O blood. How is this possible? Because the red blood cells of type O contain no A or B agglutinogens. Therefore they cannot clump with the B agglutinins of type A nor the A agglutinins of type B. Thus blood type O can be donated to all four blood types, for which reason it is known as the **universal donor.**

Conversely, type AB, having no agglutinins in its plasma, can receive all four blood types. The reason is that, lacking agglutinins, AB cannot agglutinate the red blood cells of any donor. It is thus called the **universal recipient.** Table 21–3 provides a summary of pertinent facts about blood types.

RH FACTOR

Human red blood cells, in addition to containing agglutinogens A and B, also contain the Rh antigen. This antigen was first discovered in the Rhesus monkey, in 1940, by Karl Landsteiner and Alexander Wierner. We know it as the **Rh factor.** The Rh factor is found on the surface of red blood cells. So people possessing the Rh factor are said to have Rh positive (Rh^+) blood. Those without the Rh factor have Rh negative (Rh^-) blood.

CLUMPING PATTERN

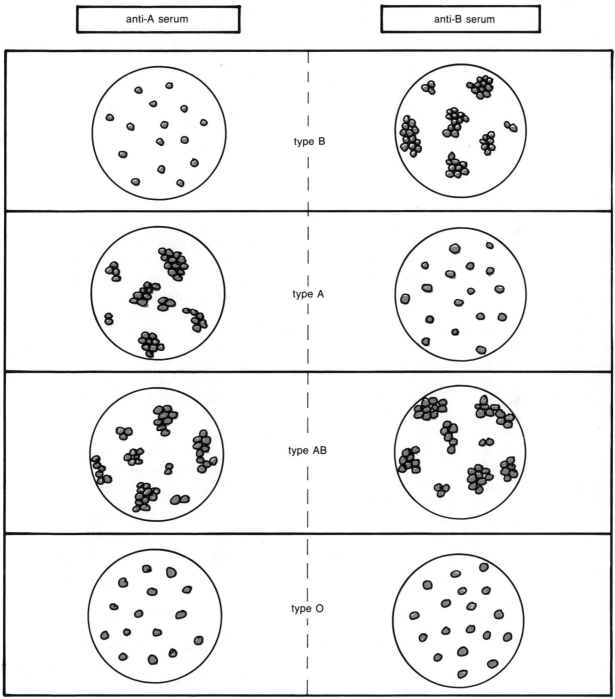

Figure 21-2 Blood types

Table 21–3 Blood Types

BLOOD TYPE	PERCENT OF US POPULATION	AGGLUTINOGEN ON RED BLOOD CELLS	AGGLUTININ IN PLASMA	CAN RECEIVE	CAN DONATE TO
A	41%	A	b	A or O only	A or AB only
B	12%	B	a	B or O only	B or AB only
AB	3%	A and B	none	A, B, AB, O	AB only
O	44%	None	a and b	O only	A, B, AB, O

About 85% of North Americans are Rh positive, 15% Rh negative. Neither Rh negative nor Rh positive blood contains antibodies, or agglutinins in its plasma. However, if an Rh negative individual receives a transfusion of Rh positive blood, he or she will develop antibodies to it. The antibodies take two weeks to develop. Generally there is no problem with the first transfusion. But, if a second transfusion of Rh positive blood is given, the accumulated Rh antibodies will clump with the Rh antigen (agglutinogen) of the blood being received. So, both blood type and Rh factor must be taken into account for safe and successful transfusions.

The same problem arises when an Rh negative mother is pregnant with an Rh positive fetus. The mother's blood can develop anti-Rh agglutinins to the fetus' Rh agglutinogens. The firstborn child will normally suffer no harmful effects. However, subsequent pregnancies will be affected, because the mother's accumulated anti-Rh agglutinins will clump the baby's red blood cells. If the condition is left untreated, the baby will usually be born anemic.

BLOOD NORMS

Tests have been devised to use physiological blood norms in diagnosing and following the course of certain diseases. Some of these norms are listed in table 21–4.

As stated earlier, prothrombin is a factor found in blood plasma. It is needed for coagulation. The test to determine the prothrombin concentration in the blood plasma is made before and after the administration of vitamin K. If such concentration takes longer to appear than the time shown in table 21–4, liver damage or failure to absorb vitamin K is suspected as a cause.

Sedimentation rate is the time required for erythrocytes to settle to the bottom of an

Table 21–4 Blood Tests

TEST	NORMAL RANGE
Bleeding time	1 to 3 minutes
Coagulation time	6 to 12 minutes
Hemoglobin count	14 to 16 gms per 100 mL
Platelet count	250,000 to 450,000 per cubic millimeter (mm³)
Prothrombin time (quick)	10 to 15 seconds
Sedimentation rate (Westergren) in first hour	Men: 0 to 12 millimeters Women: 0 to 20 millimeters
Red blood cell count	Men: 5.5 to 7.0 million/mm³ Women: 4.5 to 6.0 million/mm³
White blood cell count	5000 to 9000/mm³

upright tube at room temperature. It indicates whether disease is present and is very valuable in observing the progression of inflammatory conditions. The Westergren method shows the normal rate for women is slightly higher than for men.

Further Study and Discussion

• If laboratory facilities are available, practice determining hemoglobin count. Clean the tip of your finger with alcohol (70%). Prick it with a sterile needle. Place a large drop of blood on a piece of filter paper. As soon as the fluid is absorbed, compare it with the color scale which your instructor will have available. What is your hemoglobin? What is the normal hemoglobin count?

• Prepare a slide using a few drops of your own blood. Examine it under the microscope. Note the red and white blood cells.

• Before a transfusion may be given, blood must be typed and cross-matched. Discuss why this is necessary.

Assignment

A. Briefly answer the following questions.

1. Name the three major types of blood cells.

2. What name is given to the straw-colored liquid portion of the blood?

3. What five proteins are contained in the blood?

4. Which part of the red blood cell is responsible for carrying oxygen?

5. Which body structure is the primary site for red blood cell production?

6. Which type of blood cell protects the body against infection?

7. Which blood cell initiates the blood-clotting process?

8. Name the gel-like substance that forms the tangled threads of the clot.

9. Name six blood tests often relied upon to diagnose and follow the course of blood disorders.

10. Which two organs of the body break down red blood cells?

11.   What is hemolysis?

12.   What are the symptoms of inflammation?

13.   What does LIF stand for and what is its function?

B. Select the letter which most correctly completes the statement.
  1.   Blood of the universal donor is
      a. type B   c. type AB
      b. type A   d. type O
  2.   Blood of the universal recipient is
      a. type B   c. type AB
      b. type A   d. type O
  3.   Negative Rh blood is found in
      a. 5% of the population   c. 15% of the population
      b. 10% of the population   d. 20% of the population
  4.   The blood type found in the largest percent of the population is
      a. type O   c. type AB
      b. type A   d. type B
  5.   The prothrombin in the blood-clotting process is dependent upon
      a. vitamin A   c. vitamin P
      b. vitamin K   d. vitamin D

C. Select the most appropriate answer.
  1.   One of the following is not a blood cell.
      a. erythrocyte   c. neurocyte
      b. leukocyte   d. phagocyte

2. Erythrocytes contain all but one of the following elements.
   a. Rh factor
   b. leukocytes
   c. hemoglobin
   d. globin and heme

3. What characteristic is not true of normal thrombocytes?
   a. They average 4500 for each cubic millimeter of blood
   b. They are also called platelets
   c. They are plate-shaped cells
   d. They initiate the blood-clotting process

4. The normal leukocyte cell
   a. can only be produced in the lymphatic tissue
   b. goes to the infection site to engulf and destroy microorganisms
   c. is too large to move through the intracellular spaces of the capillary wall
   d. exists in numbers which amount to an average of 12,000 cells per cubic millimeter of blood

5. The blood-clotting process
   a. requires a normal platelet count which is 5000 to 9000 for each cubic millimeter of blood
   b. is delayed by the rupture of platelets which produces thromboplastin
   c. occurs in less time with persons having type O blood
   d. requires vitamin K for the synthesis of prothrombin

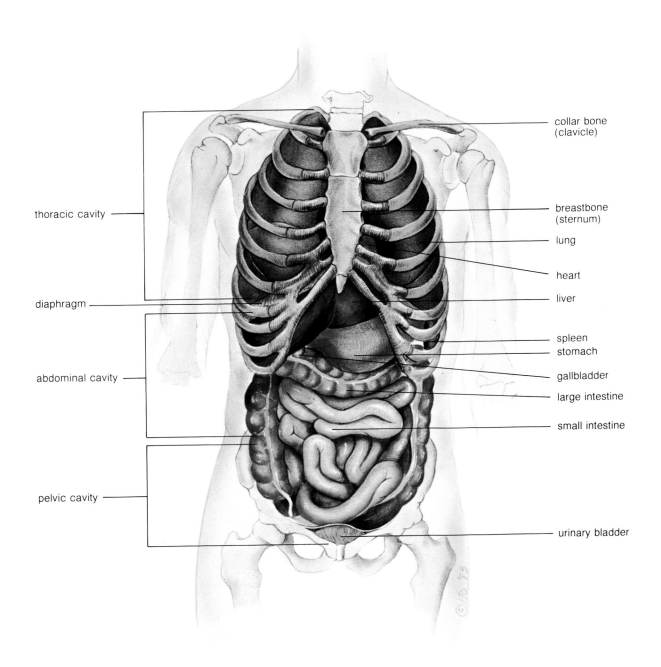

collar bone
(clavicle)

breastbone
(sternum)

lung

heart

liver

spleen

stomach

gallbladder

large intestine

small intestine

urinary bladder

thoracic cavity

diaphragm

abdominal cavity

pelvic cavity

Plate 1 The ventral cavity

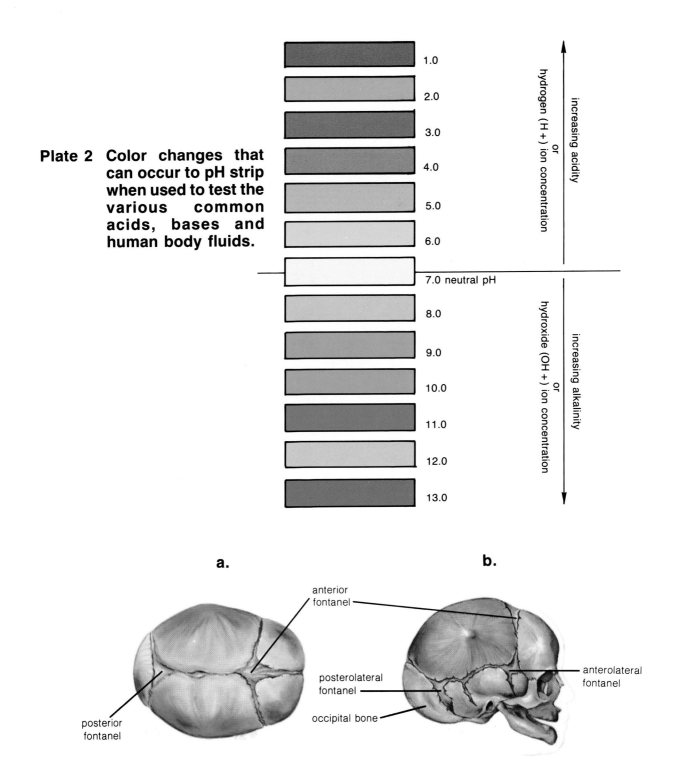

Plate 2 Color changes that can occur to pH strip when used to test the various common acids, bases and human body fluids.

1.0

2.0

3.0

4.0

5.0

6.0

7.0 neutral pH

8.0

9.0

10.0

11.0

12.0

13.0

increasing acidity
or
hydrogen (H +) ion concentration

increasing alkalinity
or
hydroxide (OH +) ion concentration

a.

b.

anterior fontanel

posterolateral fontanel

occipital bone

anterolateral fontanel

posterior fontanel

Plate 3 Top (a) and side (b) views of an infant's skull. The soft cartilage spots on an infant's head are called fontanels.

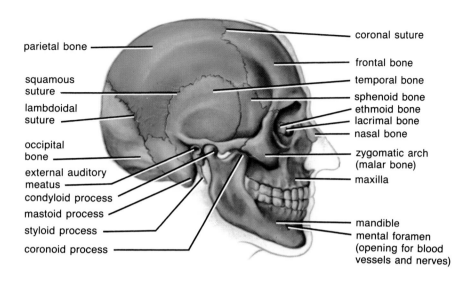

parietal bone

coronal suture

frontal bone

temporal bone

squamous suture

sphenoid bone

lambdoidal suture

ethmoid bone

lacrimal bone

nasal bone

occipital bone

zygomatic arch (malar bone)

external auditory meatus

maxilla

condyloid process

mastoid process

styloid process

coronoid process

mandible

mental foramen (opening for blood vessels and nerves)

Plate 4   Side view of the adult skull

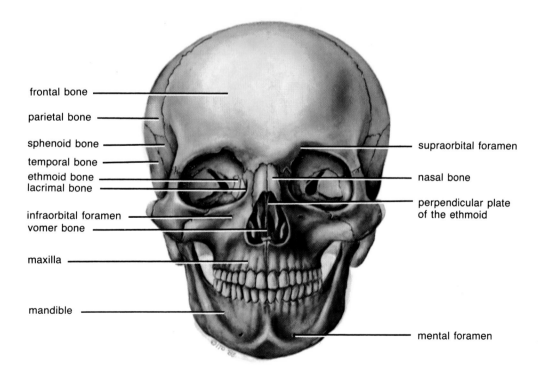

frontal bone

parietal bone

sphenoid bone

supraorbital foramen

temporal bone

ethmoid bone

nasal bone

lacrimal bone

infraorbital foramen

perpendicular plate of the ethmoid

vomer bone

maxilla

mandible

mental foramen

Plate 5   Front view of the adult skull

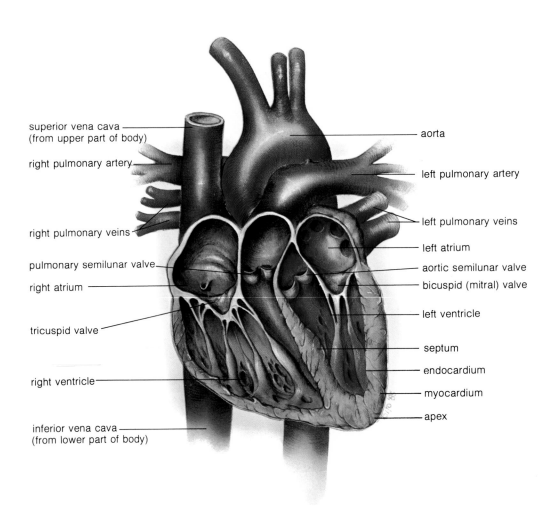

superior vena cava
(from upper part of body)

right pulmonary artery

right pulmonary veins

pulmonary semilunar valve

right atrium

tricuspid valve

right ventricle

inferior vena cava
(from lower part of body)

aorta

left pulmonary artery

left pulmonary veins

left atrium

aortic semilunar valve

bicuspid (mitral) valve

left ventricle

septum

endocardium

myocardium

apex

Plate 6   The heart and its valves

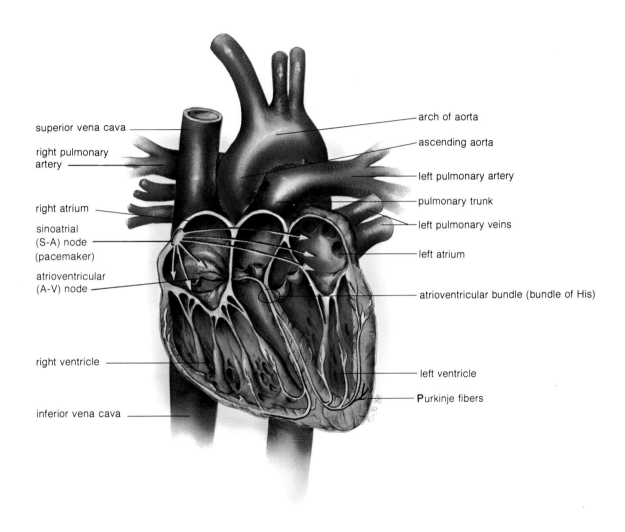

superior vena cava

right pulmonary artery

right atrium

sinoatrial (S-A) node (pacemaker)

atrioventricular (A-V) node

right ventricle

inferior vena cava

arch of aorta

ascending aorta

left pulmonary artery

pulmonary trunk

left pulmonary veins

left atrium

atrioventricular bundle (bundle of His)

left ventricle

Purkinje fibers

Plate 7   Conductive pathway of an electrical impulse in a heart contraction

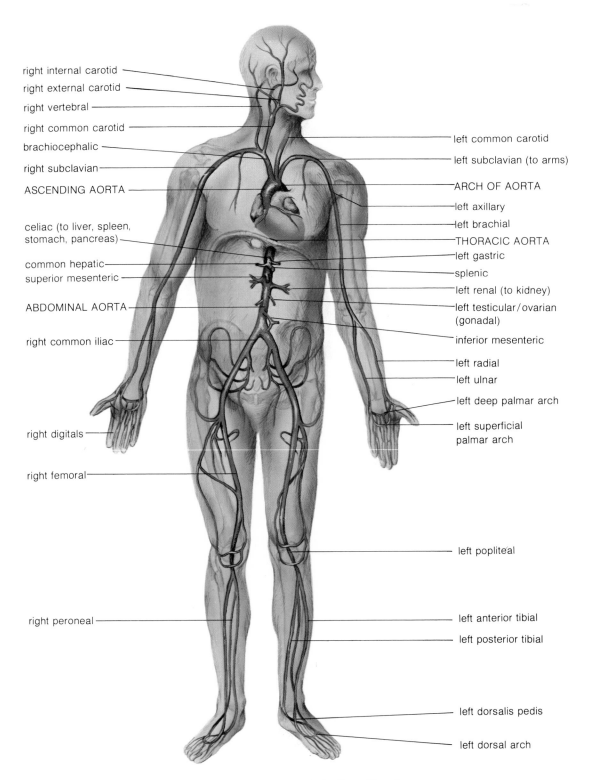

right internal carotid

right external carotid

right vertebral

right common carotid

brachiocephalic

right subclavian

ASCENDING AORTA

celiac (to liver, spleen, stomach, pancreas)

common hepatic

superior mesenteric

ABDOMINAL AORTA

right common iliac

right digitals

right femoral

right peroneal

left common carotid

left subclavian (to arms)

ARCH OF AORTA

left axillary

left brachial

THORACIC AORTA

left gastric

splenic

left renal (to kidney)

left testicular/ovarian (gonadal)

inferior mesenteric

left radial

left ulnar

left deep palmar arch

left superficial palmar arch

left popliteal

left anterior tibial

left posterior tibial

left dorsalis pedis

left dorsal arch

Plate 8A   Arterial distribution

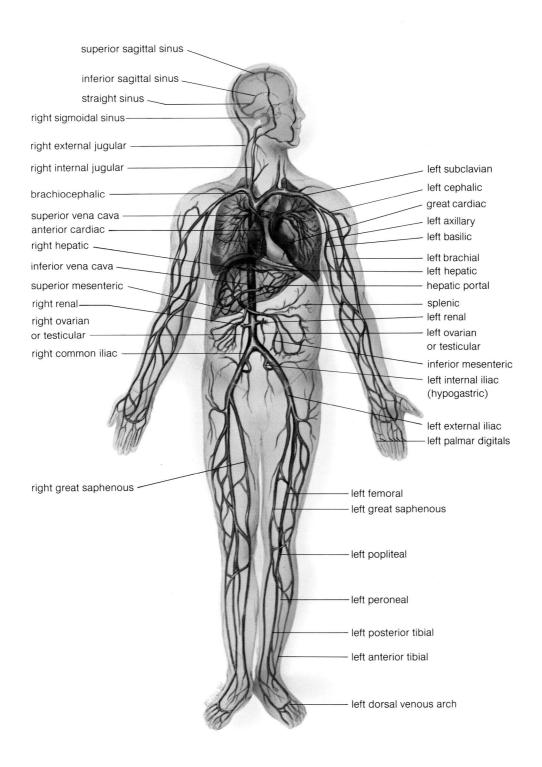

superior sagittal sinus

inferior sagittal sinus

straight sinus

right sigmoidal sinus

right external jugular

right internal jugular

brachiocephalic

superior vena cava

anterior cardiac

right hepatic

inferior vena cava

superior mesenteric

right renal

right ovarian
or testicular

right common iliac

right great saphenous

left subclavian

left cephalic

great cardiac

left axillary

left basilic

left brachial

left hepatic

hepatic portal

splenic

left renal

left ovarian
or testicular

inferior mesenteric

left internal iliac
(hypogastric)

left external iliac

left palmar digitals

left femoral

left great saphenous

left popliteal

left peroneal

left posterior tibial

left anterior tibial

left dorsal venous arch

Plate 8B   Venous distribution

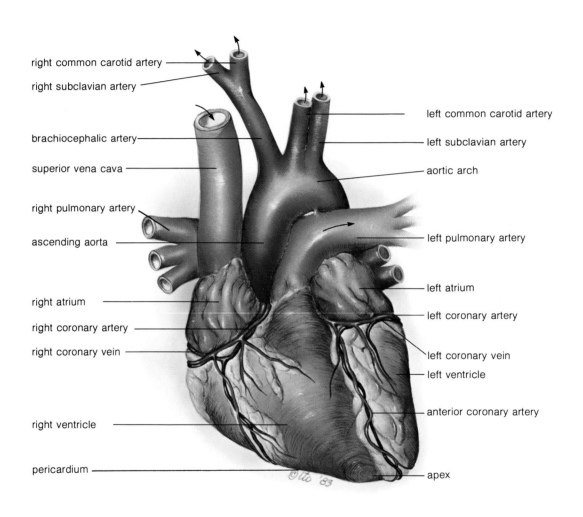

right common carotid artery

right subclavian artery

brachiocephalic artery

superior vena cava

right pulmonary artery

ascending aorta

right atrium

right coronary artery

right coronary vein

right ventricle

pericardium

left common carotid artery

left subclavian artery

aortic arch

left pulmonary artery

left atrium

left coronary artery

left coronary vein

left ventricle

anterior coronary artery

apex

Plate 9   Front view of the heart

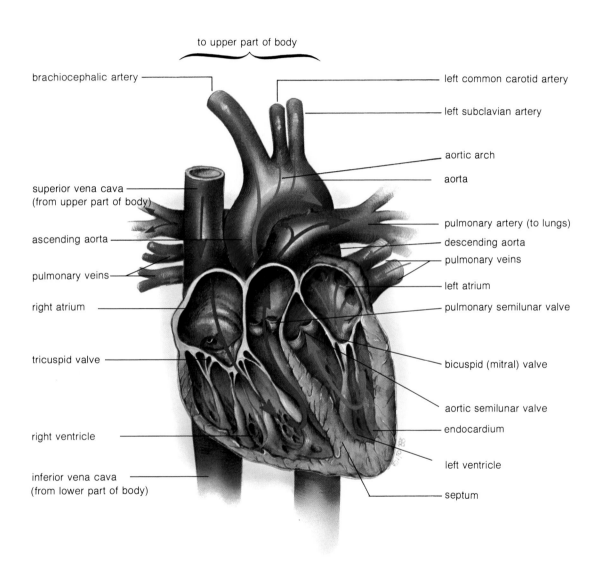

to upper part of body

brachiocephalic artery

left common carotid artery

left subclavian artery

aortic arch

aorta

superior vena cava
(from upper part of body)

pulmonary artery (to lungs)

ascending aorta

descending aorta

pulmonary veins

pulmonary veins

left atrium

right atrium

pulmonary semilunar valve

tricuspid valve

bicuspid (mitral) valve

aortic semilunar valve

endocardium

right ventricle

left ventricle

inferior vena cava
(from lower part of body)

septum

Plate 10   Blood flow into, around, and out of the heart

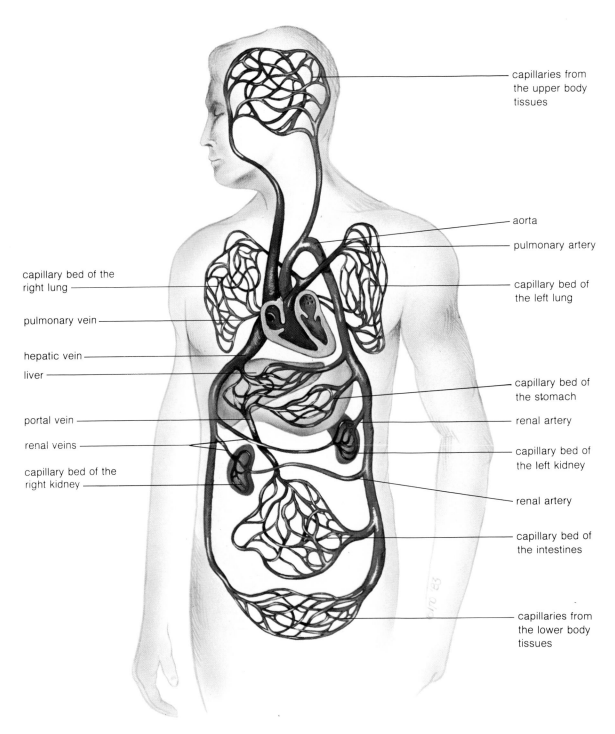

capillaries from
the upper body
tissues

aorta

pulmonary artery

capillary bed of
the left lung

capillary bed of the
right lung

pulmonary vein

hepatic vein

liver

capillary bed of
the stomach

renal artery

portal vein

renal veins

capillary bed of
the left kidney

capillary bed of the
right kidney

renal artery

capillary bed of
the intestines

capillaries from
the lower body
tissues

**Plate 11   The systemic, pulmonary, renal, and portal
blood circuits**

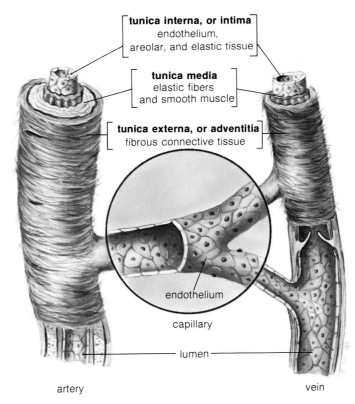

tunica interna, or intima
endothelium,
areolar, and elastic tissue

tunica media
elastic fibers
and smooth muscle

tunica externa, or adventitia
fibrous connective tissue

endothelium

capillary

lumen

artery

vein

a. Types of blood vessels and their general structure

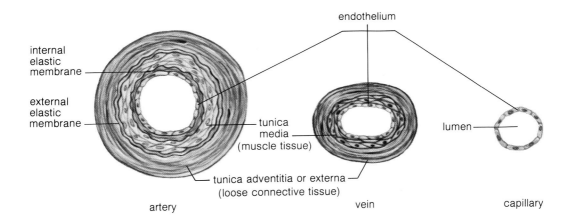

endothelium

internal
elastic
membrane

external
elastic
membrane

tunica
media
(muscle tissue)

tunica adventitia or externa
(loose connective tissue)

lumen

artery

vein

capillary

b. Cross section of blood vessels

Plate 12   Different types of blood vessels and their cross-sectional views

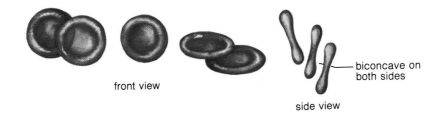

biconcave on
both sides

front view

side view

a. Red blood cells (erythrocytes)

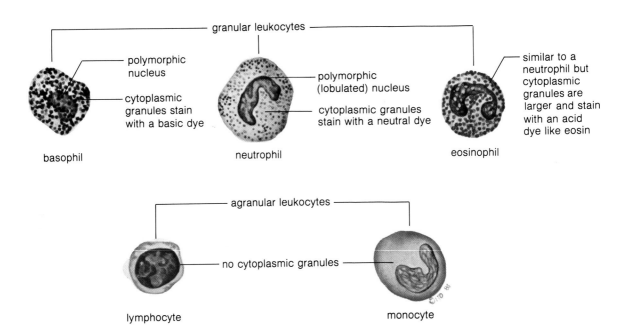

granular leukocytes

polymorphic
nucleus

cytoplasmic
granules stain
with a basic dye

basophil

polymorphic
(lobulated) nucleus

cytoplasmic granules
stain with a neutral dye

neutrophil

similar to a
neutrophil but
cytoplasmic
granules are
larger and stain
with an acid
dye like eosin

eosinophil

agranular leukocytes

no cytoplasmic granules

lymphocyte

monocyte

b. White blood cells (leukocytes)

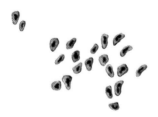

c. Platelets (non-cellular cytoplasmic fragments)

Plate 13   Blood cells and platelets

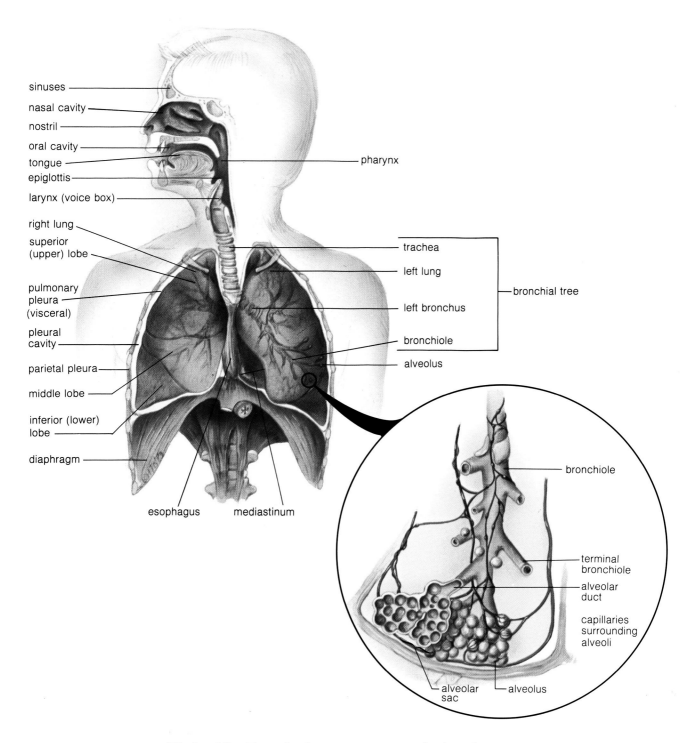

sinuses

nasal cavity

nostril

oral cavity

tongue

epiglottis

larynx (voice box)

right lung

superior (upper) lobe

pulmonary pleura (visceral)

pleural cavity

parietal pleura

middle lobe

inferior (lower) lobe

diaphragm

esophagus   mediastinum

pharynx

trachea

left lung

left bronchus

bronchiole

alveolus

bronchial tree

bronchiole

terminal bronchiole

alveolar duct

capillaries surrounding alveoli

alveolar sac   alveolus

Plate 14   Respiratory organs and structures

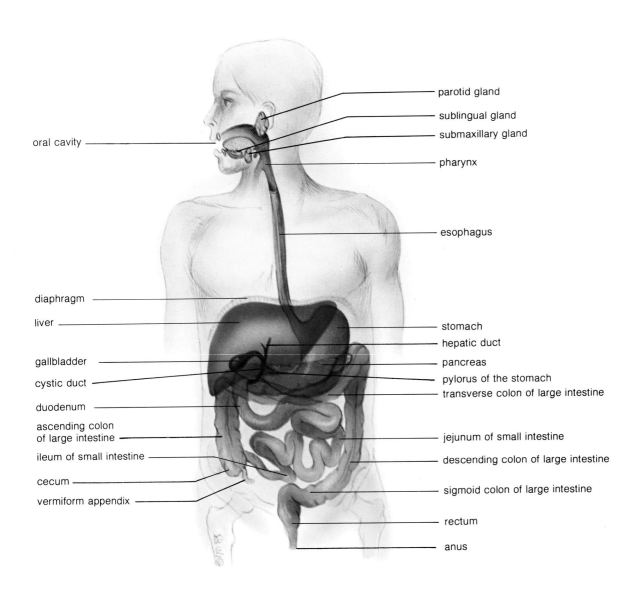

parotid gland

sublingual gland

submaxillary gland

oral cavity

pharynx

esophagus

diaphragm

liver

stomach

hepatic duct

gallbladder

pancreas

cystic duct

pylorus of the stomach

transverse colon of large intestine

duodenum

ascending colon
of large intestine

jejunum of small intestine

ileum of small intestine

descending colon of large intestine

cecum

sigmoid colon of large intestine

vermiform appendix

rectum

anus

Plate 15   Alimentary canal and accessory organs

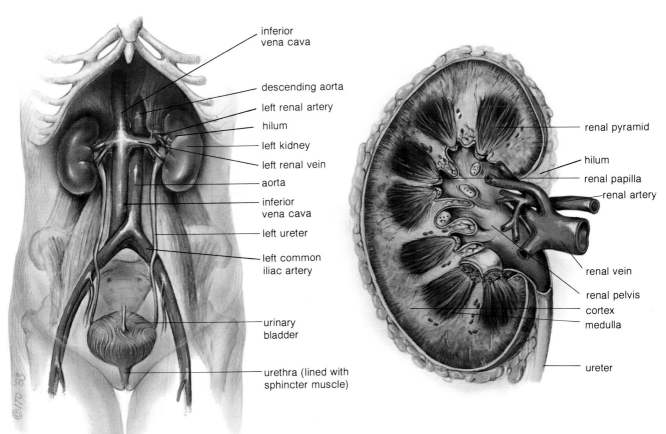

inferior vena cava

descending aorta

left renal artery

hilum

left kidney

left renal vein

aorta

inferior vena cava

left ureter

left common iliac artery

urinary bladder

urethra (lined with sphincter muscle)

renal pyramid

hilum

renal papilla

renal artery

renal vein

renal pelvis

cortex

medulla

ureter

Plate 16A The urinary system

Plate 16B Cross section of the kidney

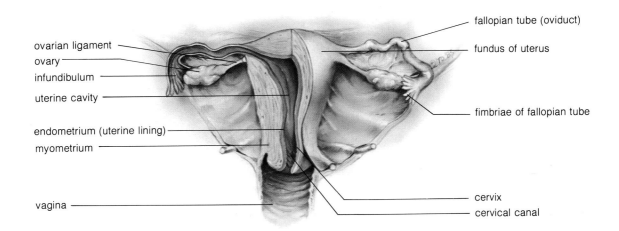

ovarian ligament

ovary

infundibulum

uterine cavity

endometrium (uterine lining)

myometrium

vagina

fallopian tube (oviduct)

fundus of uterus

fimbriae of fallopian tube

cervix

cervical canal

Plate 17   Uterus, tubes, and ovaries

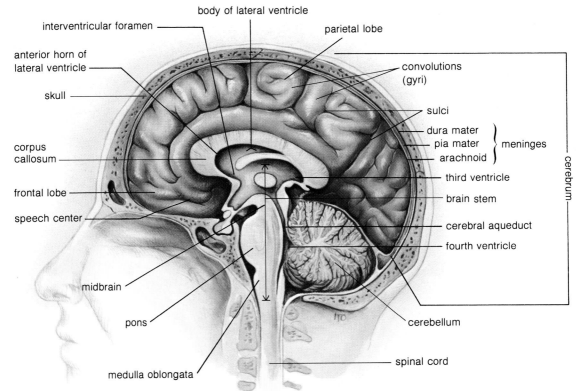

interventricular foramen

body of lateral ventricle

parietal lobe

anterior horn of
lateral ventricle

skull

corpus
callosum

frontal lobe

speech center

midbrain

pons

medulla oblongata

convolutions
(gyri)

sulci

dura mater
pia mater } meninges
arachnoid

third ventricle

brain stem

cerebral aqueduct

fourth ventricle

cerebellum

spinal cord

cerebrum

Plate 18 Cross section of the brain

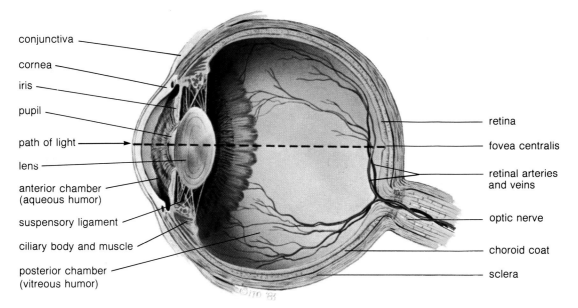

conjunctiva

cornea

iris

pupil

path of light

lens

anterior chamber
(aqueous humor)

suspensory ligament

ciliary body and muscle

posterior chamber
(vitreous humor)

retina

fovea centralis

retinal arteries
and veins

optic nerve

choroid coat

sclera

Plate 19   Internal view of the eye

THE LYMPHATIC SYSTEM AND IMMUNITY

KEY WORDS

acquired
  immunity
acquired
  immunodefi-
  ciency
  syndrome
  (AIDS)
active acquired
  immunity
adentis
allergen
anaphylactic
  shock
anaphylaxis
antigen
artificial acquired
  immunity
asymptomatic
  infection
autoimmune
  disorder
autoimmunity
axillary node

colostrum
cytomegalovirus
  (CMV)
hepatomegaly
histoplasmosis
HTLV-III
hypersensitive
hypersensitivity
immunity
immunization
immunoglobulin
immunosuppressed
incubation
  period
inguinal
intercellular
  (interstitial)
  fluid
Kaposi's sarcoma
leukopenia
lymph
lymphadenopathy
lymph nodes

lymph vessels
lymphatic system
lymphoma
metastasize
natural acquired
  immunity
natural immunity
opportunistic
  infection
passive acquired
  immunity
right lymphatic
  duct
spleen
splenomegaly
thoracic duct
  (left lymphatic
  duct)
thymus gland
toxoplasmosis

OBJECTIVES

- Describe the lymphatic system
- Define the components of the lymphatic system
- Outline the function of the lymph nodes
- Explain what is meant by immunity
- Identify the causative agent of AIDS
- List the symptoms of AIDS
- Describe the modes of AIDS transmission and measures used to prevent its transmission and acquisition
- Define the Key Words relating to this unit of study

The **lymphatic system** can be considered a supplement to the circulatory system. It is composed of lymph, lymph nodes, lymph vessels, the spleen, the thymus gland, lymphoid tissue in the intestinal tract, and the tonsils. Unlike the circulatory system, it has no muscular pump or heart.

LYMPH

Lymph is a straw-colored fluid, similar in composition to blood plasma. Plasma is what diffuses from the capillaries into the tissue spaces. Since lymph bathes the surrounding spaces between tissue cells, it is also referred to as **intercellular** or **interstitial fluid.** Lymph is composed of water, lymphocytes, some granulocytes, oxygen, digested nutrients, hormones, salts, carbon dioxide, and urea. It does not contain any red blood cells or protein molecules too large to diffuse through the capillaries.

Lymph acts as an intermediary between the blood in the capillaries and the tissues. It carries digested food, oxygen, and hormones to the cells. It also carries metabolic waste products (carbon dioxide, urea wastes) away from the cells and back into the capillaries for excretion.

Unlike the circulatory system, the lymphatic system has no pump; other factors operate to push lymph through the lymph vessels. The contractions of the skeletal muscles against the lymph vessels cause the lymph to surge forward into larger vessels. The breathing movements of the body also cause lymph to flow. Valves located along the lymph vessels prevent backward lymph flow.

LYMPH VESSELS

The lymph vessels accompany and closely parallel the veins. They form an extensive, branch-like system throughout the body which may be considered as an auxiliary to the circulatory system.

Lymph vessels are located in almost all the tissues and organs that have blood vessels. They are not found in the cuticle, nails, and hair. Lymphatic capillaries are not in the cartilage, central nervous system, epidermis, eyeball, the inner ear, or the spleen.

The lymph surrounding tissue cells enters small lymph vessels, figure 22–1. These, in turn, join to form larger lymph vessels called **lymphatics.** They continue to unite, forming larger and larger lymphatics, until the lymph flows into one of two large, main lymphatics. They are the **thoracic duct** and the **right lymphatic duct.**

The thoracic duct, also called the **left lymphatic duct,** receives lymph from the left side of the chest, head, neck, abdominal area and lower limbs. Lymph in the thoracic duct is carried to the left subclavian vein, and from there to the superior vena cava and the right atrium. In this manner, lymph carrying digested nutrients and other materials can return to the systemic circulation. Lymph from the right arm,

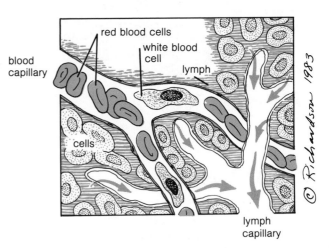

Figure 22-1   Lymph circulation

right side of the head and upper trunk enters the right lymphatic duct. From there, it enters the right subclavian vein at the right shoulder, then flows into the superior vena cava, figure 22–2.

Unlike the circulatory system, which travels in closed circuits through the blood vessels, lymph travels in only one direction: from the body organs to the heart. It does not flow continually through vessels forming a closed circular route.

LYMPH NODES

Lymph nodes are tiny, oval-shaped structures ranging from the size of a pinhead to that of an almond, figure 22–3. They are located alone or grouped in various places along the lymph vessels throughout the body, figure 22–4. Their function is to provide a site for lymphocyte production and to serve as a filter for screening out harmful substances (such as bacteria or cancer cells) from the lymph. If the harmful substances occur in such large quantities that they cannot be destroyed by the lymphocytes before the lymph node is injured, the

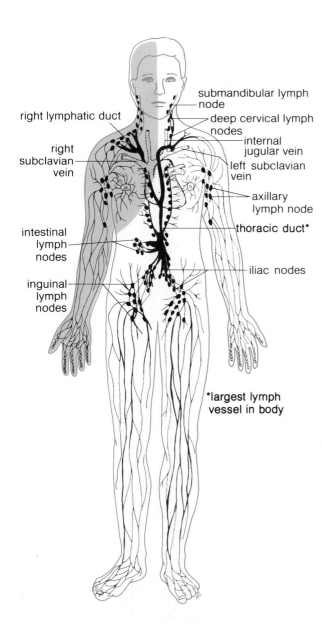

right lymphatic duct

right subclavian vein

submandibular lymph node

deep cervical lymph nodes

internal jugular vein

left subclavian vein

axillary lymph node

thoracic duct*

intestinal lymph nodes

iliac nodes

inguinal lymph nodes

*largest lymph vessel in body

Figure 22-2   Lymph drainage. Most of the lymph enters the circulation via the thoracic duct, but the right lymphatic ducts drain lymph from the right side of the head, right half of the thorax, and the right arm. (From *Human Anatomy and Physiology* **by Joan G. Creager. © 1983 by Wadsworth Inc. Reprinted by permission of Wadsworth Publishing Company, Belmont, California 94002)**

node becomes inflamed. This causes a swelling in the lymph glands, a condition known as **adenitis**.

Knowledge of the location of lymph nodes is important to any health care provider. For example, when giving care to patients with severe infections of the upper leg or thigh, the lymph nodes of the groin (**inguinal**) and the popliteal area are checked for tenderness and swelling.

Another example of care based on knowledge may be applied to patients with breast cancer. In such cases, lymph nodes under the arms (**axillary nodes**) and near the breasts may contain entrapped cancer cells. These cancer cells are filtered out of the lymph that comes from the breast area.

Early detection of unusual lumps in the breast is possible through monthly self-examination. Surgery, chemotherapy, and/or radiation may cure such conditions. But early detection and treatment are *vital*, because if discovered too late, the cancer cells can spread (**metastasize**) to other areas. It is the lymphatic vessels which spread them.

SPLEEN

The **spleen** is a sac-like mass of lymphatic tissue. It is located near the upper left area of the abdominal cavity, just beneath the diaphragm. The spleen forms lymphocytes and monocytes. Blood passing through the spleen is filtered, as in any lymph node.

The spleen stores large amounts of red blood cells. During excessive bleeding or vigorous exercise, the spleen contracts, forcing the stored red blood cells into circulation. It also destroys and removes old or fragile red blood cells, and forms erythrocytes in the embryo.

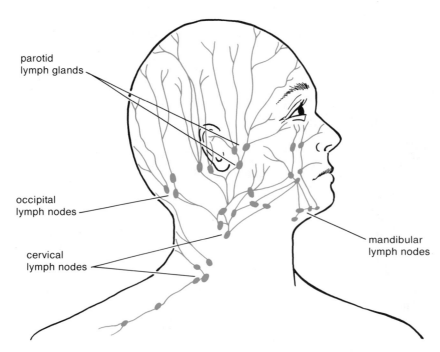

parotid
lymph glands

occipital
lymph nodes

cervical
lymph nodes

mandibular
lymph nodes

Figure 22-3   Lymph nodes and lymph vessels found in the head

THYMUS GLAND

The **thymus gland** is located in the upper anterior part of the thorax, above the heart. Its function is to produce lymphocytes. The thymus is often classified with the lymphatic organs because it is composed largely of lymphatic tissue. It is also considered an endocrine gland because it secretes a hormone which stimulates production of lymphoid cells (this is discussed further in unit 44).

Sometimes pathogens and foreign materials succeed in penetrating a person's first line of defense, the unbroken skin. The body's ability to resist these invaders and the diseases they cause is called **immunity**. Individuals differ in their ability to resist infection. In addition, an individual's resistance varies at different times.

NATURAL AND ACQUIRED IMMUNITIES

There are two general types of immunity: natural and acquired. **Natural immunity** is the immunity with which we are born. It is inherited and is permanent. This inborn immunity consists of anatomical barriers, such as the unbroken skin, and cellular secretions, such as mucus and tears. Blood phagocytes and local inflammation are also part of one's natural immunity.

When the body encounters an invader, it tries to kill the invader by creating a specific substance to combat it. The body also tries to make itself permanently resistant to these intruders. **Acquired immunity** is the reaction that occurs as a result of exposure to these invaders. This is the immunity developed during an

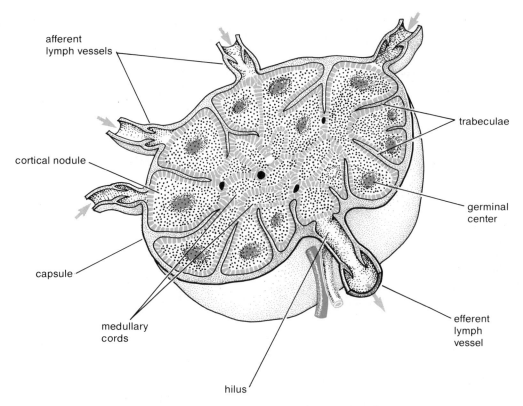

afferent
lymph vessels

trabeculae

cortical nodule

germinal
center

capsule

efferent
lymph
vessel

medullary
cords

hilus

Figure 22-4 Cross section of a lymph node

individual's lifetime. It may be passive or active.

Passive acquired immunity is borrowed immunity. It is acquired artificially by injecting antibodies from the blood of other individuals or animals into a person's body in order to protect him or her from a specific disease. The immunity produced is immediate in its effect. However, it lasts only from three to five weeks. After this period, the antibodies will be inactivated by the individual's own macrophages.

Because it is immediate, passive immunity is used when one has been exposed to a virulent disease, such as diptheria, measles, tetanus, and infectious hepatitus, and has not acquired active immunity to that disease. The borrowed antibodies will confer temporary protection.

A baby has temporary passive immunity from the mother's antibodies. These antibodies pass through the placenta to enter the baby's blood. In addition, the mother's milk, **colostrum**, also offers the baby some passive immunity. Thus a newborn infant may be protected against poliomyelitis, measles, and mumps. However, this passive immunity against poliomyelitis only lasts for about six weeks after birth. For measles and mumps it may last for nearly a year. Then the child must develop his or her own active immunity.

Active acquired immunity is preferable to passive immunity because it lasts longer. There are two types of active acquired immunity: natural acquired immunity and artificial acquired immunity. Here is how these two types of immunity are acquired:

- **Natural acquired immunity** is the result of having had and recovered from the disease. For example, a child who has had measles and has recovered will not ordinarily get it again because the child's body has manufactured antibodies. This form of immunity is also acquired by having a series of unnoticed or mild infections. For example, a person who has had a mild form of a disease one or more times and has fought it off, sometimes unnoticed, is later immune to the disease.

- **Artificial acquired immunity** comes from being inoculated with a suitable vaccine, antigen, or toxoid. For example, a child vaccinated for smallpox has been given a very mild form of the disease; the child's body will thus be stimulated to manufacture its own antibodies.

Immunization is the process of increasing an individual's resistance to a particular infection by artificial means. An **antigen** is a substance that is injected to stimulate production of antibodies. For example, toxins produced by bacteria, dead or weakened bacteria, viruses, and foreign proteins are examples of antigens. Toxin stimulates the body to produce antibodies, while the antitoxin weakens or neutralizes the effect of the toxin.

An **immunoglobulin** is a protein that functions specifically as an antibody. There are five classes of immunoglobulins; immunoglobulin G (IgG), and the others, IgM, IgA, IgD, and IgE.

Autoimmunity

Autoimmunity is when an individual's immune system goes awry. It forms antibodies to its own tissues, which destroy these tissues. This is also known as **an autoimmune disorder.**

A well-known example of this disorder is rheumatic fever. A person may get a streptococcal infection, as in a "strep" throat, that slightly alters heart tissue. Later streptococcal infections can cause further heart damage. This is because the antibodies formed against the streptococci will also attack the altered heart tissue. This type of heart damage is known as rheumatic heart disease.

Hypersensitivity

Hypersensitivity occurs when the body's immune system fails to protect itself against foreign material. Instead, the antibodies formed irritate certain body cells. A **hypersensitive** or allergic individual is generally more sensitive to certain allergens than most people.

An **allergen** is an antigen that causes allergic responses. Examples of allergens include grass, ragweed pollen, ingested food, penicillin and other antibiotics, and bee and wasp stings. Such allergens stimulate antibody formation, some of which are known as the IgE antibodies. Antibodies are found in individuals who are allergic, drug sensitive, or hypersensitive. The antibodies bind to certain cells in the body, causing a characteristic allergic reaction.

In asthma, the IgE antibodies bind to the bronchi and bronchioles; in hayfever they bind to the mucous membranes of the respiratory tract and eyes, causing runny nose and itchy eyes. In hives and rashes, they bind to the skin cells.

An even more severe and sometimes fatal allergic reaction is called **anaphylaxis** or **anaphylactic shock.** It is the result of an antigen-antibody reaction that stimulates a massive secretion of histamine. Anaphylaxis can be caused by insect stings and injected drugs like penicillin. A person suffering from anaphylaxis experiences breathing problems, headache, facial swelling, falling blood pressure, stomach cramps, and vomiting. The antidote is an injection of either adrenaline or antihistamine. If proper care is not given right away, death may occur in minutes.

Health care professionals should always ask patients whether they are sensitive to any allergens or drugs. This precaution is necessary to prevent negative and sometimes fatal allergic responses to injected drugs. People with such hypersensitivities should wear a Med-Alert tag about the neck or wrist. This will alert health professionals in the event of an emergency. Such tags have saved the lives of patients rendered unconscious or otherwise unable to communicate.

AIDS VIRUS

At this point, some very important and basic information about the virus that causes AIDS should be presented in a logical and forthright manner to the microbiology student and health care professional.

To date, much publicity and media hype has unfortunately created, at times, an air of controversy and emotionalism surrounding AIDS.

The following information is intended to answer the various questions that a health care professional may have about AIDS, such as: What causes AIDS? What are its symptoms? What is the mode of transmission of AIDS? How infectious is it? What are the preventive measures taken to avoid its transmission or acquisition?

Discovery of AIDS

Between October 1980 and May 1981, five young, previously healthy homosexual men were treated for a pneumonia caused by a parasite, *Pneumocystis carinii*. They were treated at three different hospitals in Los Angeles. Doctors and health care professionals took special note of this. Before this, P. carinii pneumonia occurred only in **immunosuppressed** (suppression of the immune system so there is a decreased ability to fight disease and infections) patients, especially those receiving cancer therapy. At the same time, a rare and unusual blood vessel malignancy called **Kaposi's sarcoma** was being diagnosed with increasing frequency in young homosexual males in California and New York. By July, 1981, 26 cases of Kaposi's sarcoma had been diagnosed in young homosexual males. Seven of these males also had serious infections, and four of them had P. carinii pneumonia.

These cases were an early indication of an epidemic of a previously unknown disease. Later, it was called the **Acquired Immunodeficiency Syndrome (AIDS)**. As of October 1983, 2500 cases had been reported in the United States, and AIDS is now reported in other countries. About 40% of the total number of diagnosed AIDS patients and 75% of those patients diagnosed in 1981 have died. Recent data show that as of October 1985, over 13,000 cases have been reported in the United States. For people who have contracted AIDS, it is usually fatal.

Causative Agent of AIDS

The causative agent of AIDS is called **HTLV-III.** HTLV-III stands for *h*uman *T-l*ymphotrophic *v*irus type *III.* The virus is called by other names, such as HTLV-III/LAV ("LAV" is the French name for it), AIDS-Related Virus (ARV), and the "AIDS Virus."

Symptoms of AIDS

First of all, AIDS is a disease that suppresses the body's natural immune system.

Thus, a patient with AIDS cannot fight off cancers and most infections. The term AIDS or Acquired Immunodeficiency Syndrome stands for:

- **A-Acquired**—The disease is not inherited or caused by any form of medication

- **I-Immuno**—Refers to the body's natural defenses against cancers, disease, and infections

- **D-Deficiency**—Lacking in cellular immunity

- **S-Syndrome**—The set of diseases or conditions that are present to signal the diagnosis.

There are three possible outcomes that can result from infection with the HTLV-III virus. One is the actual development of AIDS, the second is the development of a condition called AIDS-Related Complex (ARC), and the third condition is known as an asymptomatic infection.

Acquired Immunodeficiency Syndrome (AIDS)

AIDS is the most severe type of HTLV-III infection. When a patient has AIDS, the immune system is severely suppressed. Thus, the person becomes highly susceptible to certain cancers and **opportunistic infections.** (An opportunistic infection can normally be fought off by a healthy individual with a normal functioning immune system but infects a person with immune dysfunction.) The opportunistic conditions include:

- Cancers, especially Kaposi's sarcoma and at times primary **lymphoma** (tumors) of the brain.

- Parasitic infections such as *Pneumocystis carinii* pneumonia and *toxoplasmosis.**

- Fungal infections such as candidiasis and histoplasmosis.*

- Viral infections such as cytomegalovirus disease,* herpes simplex, hepatitis B, and non-A, non-B hepatitis.

The symptoms of AIDS are often nonspecific. These symptoms are often similar to illnesses like the common cold or the flu. Unfortunately, these symptoms usually do not go away. They include:

- Prolonged fatigue that is not due to physical exertion or other disorders

- Persistent fevers or night sweats

- A persistent, unexplained cough

---

*Toxoplasmosis is a disease caused by a sporozoan protozoa called *Toxoplasma gondii.* Human toxoplasmosis is acquired either orally or congenitally through the placenta from an infected mother. Oral transmission has a source either in cat feces or in inadequately prepared meat or infected animals. Orally acquired toxoplasmosis seldom causes illness and may often go undetected, marked only by fatigue and muscle pains. Acute toxoplasmosis is rare. Symptoms range from fever, **lymphadenopathy** (lymph node enlargement), muscle fatigue, and pain to cerebral infection. Its symptoms can mimic aseptic meningitis, hepatitis, myocarditis, or pneumonia, depending on the site of the parasite.

---

*Histoplasmosis is an infection caused by the fungus, *Histoplasma capsulatum.* The symptoms range from a mild respiratory infection to more severe ones such as fever, anemia, **hepatomegaly** (liver enlargement), **splenomegaly** (spleen enlargement), **leukopenia** (reduction of the number of white blood cells in the peripheral blood), pulmonary lesions, gastrointestinal ulcerations, and suprarenal necrosis.

---

*Cytomegalovirus (CMV) disease is a disease that is particularly severe in immunosuppressed persons, especially those with AIDS. Symptoms range from hepatitis and mononucleosis to pneumonia.

- A thick, whitish hairlike coating in the throat or on the tongue

- Easy bruising or unexplained bleeding

- Recent appearance of discolored or purplish lesions of the mucous membranes or skin that do not go away and slowly increase in size

- Chronic diarrhea

- Shortness of breath

- Unexplained lymphadenopathy (swollen glands) that has persisted over three months

- Unexplained weight loss of ten or more pounds in less than two months

Incubation Period. The **incubation period** (the period between becoming infected and the actual development of the disease symptoms) for AIDS is quite long, ranging from six months to as much as 12 years. However, only a minority of infected individuals develop symptoms, and only a fraction of these later develop AIDS. The persons who actually develop AIDS usually die within two years.

At present, there is no cure for AIDS. However, the opportunistic infections can be treated. Several experimental drugs are being developed and tested on AIDS patients in the United States and Europe, particularly at the Pasteur Institute in Paris. Other doctors and health care professionals are treating patients with only minimal symptoms early in the onset of their disease to see if more serious symptoms can be prevented. The development of various vaccines, such as AZT, have been reported, but these findings must be taken with precaution. It is unlikely that a vaccine will be available for a few years because of the complexity and newness of the HTLV-III virus.

AIDS-Related Complex (ARC)

An individual can contract the HTLV-III virus and develop other conditions, but not AIDS itself. These conditions are called AIDS-Related Complex (ARC). Symptoms range from chronic diarrhea, to chronic lymphadenopathy, to unexplained weight loss. Some individuals with ARC develop a life-threatening opportunistic infection; when this occurs, the person is then said to have AIDS.

Asymptomatic Infection

Most people who have been infected with the HTLV-III virus usually do not develop any symptoms. These are known as **asymptomatic infections** and occur with all viruses, and AIDS is no exception. It is estimated that the HTLV-III virus has probably infected over one million people in the United States. Only long-term follow-up studies of infected, asymptomatic people will show whether or not they will later develop AIDS or ARC.

High-Risk Groups for Aids

The individuals who are at the highest risk of contracting AIDS are:

- Homosexual and bisexual men with multiple sexual partners

- Male and female IV (intravenous) drug users who share needles and syringes

Other risk groups are:

- Female sexual partners of males in the high-risk group

- Infants born to parents who are at risk for AIDS

- Persons who have received blood or blood products, previously including hemophiliacs

Transmission of AIDS

The transmission of he HTLV-III virus occurs in three ways:

- Sexual intercourse where semen enters the body (about 75% of the adults in the United States who have AIDS contracted it through sexual intercourse)

- Sharing of hypodermic needles among IV drug users where infected blood is injected into the body (accounts for 17–25% of the AIDS cases in the United States)

- In utero or at birth from an infected mother to her unborn or newborn infant

Transmission of the HTLV-III virus through transfusion of blood or blood products has been almost eliminated. This is possible because blood banks test all blood donors to determine whether or not they have been exposed to the HTLV-III virus. Also, federal guidelines recommend that individuals in the high-risk group do not donate blood or blood products.

So far, it seems unlikely that AIDS can be contracted through casual contact. The virus cannot be contracted through air, feces, food, urine, or water. Even close nonsexual contact such as coughing, sneezing, embracing, shaking hands, and sharing eating utensils cannot spread the virus.

Measures to Prevent Transmission and Acquisition

Persons in the risk groups having AIDS must take precautions to reduce the chances of giving the virus to others. At the same time, those in the risk groups must take measures to reduce their chances of contracting AIDS. Thus, these measures should be followed by the above persons.

- Limit the number of sexual contacts, as each new sexual partner increases the chance of infection.

- Do not donate blood, blood products, sperm, or any other parts of the body if you are in the high-risk group.

- Abstain from sexual acts where blood or semen are exchanged, as in anal, oral, and vaginal intercourse.

- Do not share hypodermic needles or syringes.

- Make sure that soiled articles, materials, and surfaces are thoroughly cleaned with soap and hot water after incidents involving bleeding.

- Cover an open cut, sore, or wound with a bandage.

- Discuss with your doctor the possible delay of a pregnancy until more is known about the risk of transmitting HTLV-III to the baby.

Some recommendations for health care personnel to prevent the acquisition of AIDS are:

- Use the same precautions when caring for AIDS patients as for those patients with hepatitis B virus.

• Avoid direct contact of skin and mucous membranes with blood, blood products, excretions, secretions, and tissues of people with AIDS or who are likely to have it.

For more specific recommendations consult the Morbidity and Mortality Weekly Report, *Acquired Immune Deficiency Syndrome (AIDS): Precautions for Clinical and Laboratory Staffs,* Vol. 31, No. 43, November 5, 1982.

The HTLV-III Antibody Test

Recently the HTLV-III antibody test was developed to detect the presence of antibodies in a person's blood. This test has proved quite useful in the testing and screening of potential blood donors. Thus, the nation's blood supply is kept free of the HTLV-III virus.

Basically, the HTLV-III antibody test detects the presence of antibodies in the bloodstream of a person who has been exposed to the virus. What does this possibly mean for the person with a positive antibody test? The person may have fought off the infection, in which case the person may be immune to HTLV-III; the person may be carrying the infection but is not sick; or the person may be developing or may have AIDS. It is still not known what a positive test means for a person's future health. Due to the limited experience with the test, it is wise to remember that the HTLV-III antibody test:

• CANNOT test for AIDS

• CANNOT accurately test for the presence of the HTLV-III virus

• CANNOT measure immunity to, or protection from, the virus

• CANNOT determine the ability to transmit the virus to others

• CANNOT predict future illness with AIDS or a related condition

As of this moment, because no one knows just what the presence of antibodies in a person's blood means, this test is used for limited purposes only.

The HTLV-III antibody test — because it is *not* a test for AIDS — should not be used to diagnose AIDS.

Further Study and Discussion

• Discuss the diagram in figure 22–1. Explain how the materials that the cells need are transported.

Assignment

Briefly answer the following questions.

1. From what substance is lymph formed?

2. What name is given to the enlarged portion of the lymph vessel?

3. The lymph allows exchange of digested food, oxygen, and waste products between two mediums of the body. Name them.

4. What body mechanism forces lymph to move through the lymphatic vessels?

5. Through which vessel does the lymph re-enter the general circulation?

6. Name the two veins which receive lymph drainage at the shoulder.

7. Name two functions of the lymph nodes.

8. Name the inflammatory disorder that produces swelling of the lymph nodes.

9. Identify three body areas where lymph nodes are located.

10. Which of the three major types of blood cells may enter the lymph?

11. What is immunity?

12. What is natural immunity?

13. Name four sources of natural immunity.

14. What is acquired immunity?

15. Identify the two types of acquired immunity.

16. How is an individual's health related to immunity?

17. How is active acquired immunity obtained?

18. How long does active acquired immunity last?

19. How is passive acquired immunity attained?

20. How does an infant obtain passive acquired immunity?

21. How long does passive acquired immunity last?

22. What is the main difference between active and passive immunity?

23. When is passive immunization used?

24. What is an antigen?

25.   What are antibodies?

26.   What is hypersensitivity?

27.   What are the common forms of hypersensitivity in humans?

28.   What is anaphylaxis?

29.   What are the symptoms of anaphylaxis?

30.   How can anaphylaxis be effectively treated?

31.   To what diseases may humans become immune?

32.   What is an allergy?

33. Give two common examples of allergies.

34. Name some common substances that cause people to be allergic.

35. What causes AIDS?

36. What do the initials A-I-D-S signify?

37. What are the three possible outcomes from infection by the causative agent for AIDS?

38. Describe three of the possible opportunistic infections that can trouble an AIDS patient.

39. What are the symptoms of AIDS, and what is its incubation period?

40.   Who are the people at risk of contracting AIDS?

41.   What are the three ways of transmitting the causative agent of AIDS?

42.   What are some preventive measures a health care professional should use to avoid the acquisition of AIDS?

43.   What is the one useful benefit of the HTLV-III antibody test?

REPRESENTATIVE DISORDERS OF THE CIRCULATORY SYSTEM

KEY WORDS

acute rheumatic
  heart disease
anemia
aneurysm
angina pectoris
arrhythmia
arteriosclerosis
ascites
atrial fibrillation
bradycardia
cerebral
  hemorrhage
congenital heart
  disease
congestive heart
  failure
Cooley's anemia
coronary
  occlusion

dyspnea
embolism
endocarditis
familial
  hemolytic
  jaundice
gangrene
heart block
heart failure
heart murmur
hematoma
hemophilia
hemorrhoid
hyperemia
hypertension
hypotension
iron-deficiency
  anemia
leukemia

myocardial
  infarction
myocarditis
pericarditis
pernicious
  anemia
phlebitis
phlegmasia Alba
  dolens
polycythemia
precordial
sickle cell
  anemia
sickling trait
tachycardia
thrombosis
thrombus
varicose vein

OBJECTIVES

- List disorders of the circulatory system
- Describe some disorders of the heart and blood vessels
- Define the Key Words related to this unit of study

One of the leading causes of death is cardiovascular disease. Some of the disorders of the heart and blood vessels are defined and briefly discussed in this unit.

DISORDERS OF THE HEART

Acute rheumatic heart disease is an infection of the membrane lining of the heart, usually caused by a streptococcus organism. A streptococcal infection (like a strep throat) may slightly alter heart tissue (e.g., affect heart valves). Subsequent streptococcal infections can cause further heart damage. This is be-

cause the antibodies formed against the streptococci also attack the altered heart tissue.

Arrhythmia is a term used to describe any change or deviation from the normal orderly rhythm of the heart action.

Atrial fibrillation is a condition in which the atria are never completely emptied of blood. Their walls quiver instead of giving the usual contraction of a normal heartbeat. This occurs when irregular and weak nerve impulses arrive at the S-A node, or pacemaker. The pacemaker is stimulated irregularly, and ventricular contraction can occur when it is filled with less than the normal quantity of blood. This causes a highly irregular wrist pulse and abnormal heart rate.

Congenital heart disease is a condition in which the heart did not develop properly during fetal life. Various factors may cause improper heart development during fetal life. For instance, a woman in her second month of pregnancy, who contracts a contagious disease like chickenpox, measles, mumps, or rubella (German measles) can pass the pathogenic microorganisms through her placenta into the fetus. The second month is critical, because that is when heart malformations are likely to develop in the fetus. Also, the ingestion of large quantities of aspirin during pregnancy may cause an abnormal heart to develop in the fetus.[1]

Endocarditis is an inflammation of the membrane that lines the heart. This causes the formation of rough spots in the endocardium, which may lead to a potentially fatal thrombosis or blood clot.

Heart block is the loss of ability of the A-V node to carry nerve impulses. This happens when the A-V node is damaged, possibly due to blockage of a coronary artery leading to the septum. The heart block causes the ventricles to contract at a highly irregular rate, often as slowly as 40 to 50 beats per minute. Heart block is treated by the implantation of a battery-powered pacemaker. This artificial pacemaker stimulates the heart electrically, causing ventricular contractions. Such contractions occur at a sufficiently rapid rate to maintain normal blood circulation.

Heart failure is the inability of the heart muscles to beat efficiently due to high blood pressure or other pathological conditions. Different symptoms can arise depending upon

which ventricle fails to beat properly. If the left ventricle fails, **dyspnea** (difficulty or rapid breathing) occurs. Engorgement of organs with venous blood, edema and **ascites** (abnormal accumulation of serous fluid in the abdominal cavity) takes place when the right ventricle fails. Other symptoms include lung congestion and coughing.

Congestive heart failure is similar to heart failure, but in addition there is edema (swelling) of the lower extremities. Blood backs up into the lung vessels, and fluid extends into the air passages. The patient actually drowns in his or her own fluid.

Myocarditis is an inflammation of the heart muscle. An area of the heart muscle may become damaged because of a lack of blood supply, usually due to an occluded artery or a **myocardial infarction.** The symptoms are **hyperemia** (accumulation of blood, leading to distention of blood vessels), cloudy swelling, fatty degeneration, and necrosis. The necrotic (dead) myocardial tissue causes a mild inflammation, resulting in the formation of fibrous tissue.

Pericarditis is an inflammation of the membrane covering the heart. The symptoms are **precordial** (chest area overlying the heart) pain and tenderness, cough, dyspnea, rapid pulse and slight fever. It is caused by rheumatic fever, septicemia (poisoning of the blood by the toxic products of invading bacteria), nephritis (kidney inflammation), or the extension of infection from an adjacent area.

Angina pectoris is the severe chest pain which arises when the heart does not receive enough oxygen. It is not a disease in itself, but a symptom of an underlying problem with coronary circulation.

The chest pain radiates from the precordial area to the left shoulder, down the arm along the ulnar nerve. Victims often expe-

---

1. Sherman and Sherman, *Biology* (New York: Oxford University Press, 1980).

rience an apprehension of impending death. Angina pectoris occurs quite suddenly, brought on by emotional stress or physical exertion. It commonly affects men over 40 years old, but rarely women.

Murmurs can indicate some defect in the valves of the heart. They may take the form of "gurgling" and "hissing" sounds as the valves fail to close properly. Cardiac murmurs are designated as bicuspid (mitral), tricuspid, pulmonary or aortic, depending on which valve is damaged. They are also classified according to the period of the heart's cycle during which they occur. A systolic murmur occurs during systole; the diastolic murmur happens during diastole. A presystolic murmur occurs just before systole.

Coronary occlusion is a condition in which the heart does not receive enough blood because a coronary artery is blocked. This heart disease is also known as coronary thrombosis, and may result from a myocardial infarction.

Bradycardia is an abnormally slow heartbeat rate less than 60 beats per minute.

Tachycardia is an abnormally rapid heartbeat rate. In paroxysmal tachycardia, the heart suddenly begins to beat as fast as 100 or more beats per minute.

DISORDERS OF THE BLOOD VESSELS

Arteriosclerosis is a thickening of the walls of the arteries. This is caused by fibrous connective tissue, fat deposition, and calcification, causing loss of contractility and elasticity.

Gangrene is death of body tissue due to an insufficient blood supply caused by disease or injury.

Phlebitis is an inflammation of the lining of a vein, accompanied by clotting of blood in the vein. Symptoms include *edema* (swelling) of the affected area, pain and redness along the length of the vein.

Varicose veins are the swollen inelastic veins which result from the slowing up of blood flow back to the heart. Blood backs up in the veins if the muscles do not massage them. The weight of the stagnant blood distends the valves; the continued pooling of blood then causes distention and inelasticity of the vein walls. This condition develops due to hereditary weakness in vein structure. In addition, the human bipedal posture, prolonged periods of standing, and physical exertion can cause valves in the superficial leg veins to enlarge and weaken. Age and pregnancy are other factors responsible for varicose veins.

Hemorrhoids are varicose veins in the walls of the lower rectum and the tissues around the anus.

Cerebral hemorrhage refers to bleeding from blood vessels within the brain. It can be caused by arteriosclerosis, disease, or an injury like a blow to the head.

Aneurysm is a sac caused by enlargement of the blood vessel, accompanied by thinning of the vessel wall. The aneurysm also forms a blood-containing tumor, which pulsates with each systole, causing a murmur. The symptoms are pain and pressure. The most common aneurysm occurs in the aorta.

DISORDERS OF THE BLOOD

Anemia is a deficiency in the number of red blood cells and/or in the percentage of hemoglobin in the blood. Anemia results from a large or chronic loss of blood (hemorrhage) which decreases the number of erythrocytes. Extreme erythrocyte destruction and malformation of the hemoglobin of red blood cells also causes this condition. Since there is always some hemoglobin deficiency, there is never enough oxygen transported to the cells for cellular oxidation. Consequently, not enough energy is being released. Anemia is characterized by varying degrees of dyspnea, pallor, palpitation, and fatigue.

Iron-deficiency anemia is a condition that often exists in children and adolescents. It is caused by a deficiency of adequate amounts of iron in the diet. This leads to insufficient hemoglobin synthesis in the red blood cells. The condition is easily alleviated by ingestion of iron supplements and green, leafy vegetables that contain the mineral.

Pernicious anemia is a condition affecting erythrocyte development due to vitamin B_{12} deficiency. It leads to both inadequate and abnormally large, misshapen red blood cells. If pernicious anemia is not diagnosed early and continues to progress, death usually occurs. Pernicious anemia is commonly caused by poor absorption of vitamin B_{12} into the blood due to a missing factor (intrinsic factor) in the stomach.

Polycythemia is a condition in which too many red blood cells are formed. Blood viscosity increases due to friction between the erythrocytes, and also between them and the blood vessel walls. Consequently, there is an increase in blood pressure.

Embolism is a condition where an embolus is carried by the bloodstream until it reaches an artery too small for passage. An embolus is a substance foreign to the bloodstream. It may be air, a blood clot, cancer cells, fat, bacterial clumps, a needle, or even a bullet (that was lodged in tissue and breaks free).

Thrombosis is a blood clot which forms in a blood vessel – or in the heart – and stays in the same place in which it was formed. The blood clot formed is called a **thrombus.** It is caused by unusually slow blood circulation, or changes in the blood or blood vessel walls.

Hemophilia is a hereditary disease in which the blood clots slowly or abnormally. This causes prolonged bleeding with even minor cuts and bumps. Although sex-linked hemophilia occurs only in males, it is transmitted genetically by females to their sons.

Leukemia is a condition in which there is a great increase in the number of white blood cells. The overabundant immature leukocytes replace the erythrocytes, thus interfering with the transport of oxygen to the tissues. They can also hinder the synthesis of new red blood cells from bone marrow. Leukemia is usually fatal. Acute leukemia, which develops quickly and runs its course rapidly, occurs most often in children and young adults.

Sickle cell anemia is a chronic blood disease inherited from both parents. The disease causes red blood cells to form in the abnormal crescent shape. These cells carry less oxygen and break easily, causing anemia. The **sickling trait,** a less serious disease, occurs with inheritance from only one parent. Sickle cell anemia occurs almost exclusively among Blacks.

Cooley's anemia is a blood disease similar to sickle cell anemia, affecting people of Mediterranean descent.

Familial hemolytic jaundice occurs when the spleen functions abnormally, rendering the erythrocytes extremely fragile; they break down quite readily and release their hemoglobin into the blood. This condition can generally be cured by removal of the spleen.

Hematoma is a localized clotted mass of blood found in an organ, tissue, or space. It is caused by an injury, like a blow, that can cause a blood vessel to rupture.

Phlegmasia Alba dolens ("milk leg") is an acute edema that starts in the ankle. It is caused by an obstruction of venous blood return. It usually occurs as a result of septic infection following childbirth or surgery.

DISORDERS OF BLOOD PRESSURE _____

Hypertension is high blood pressure in which the systolic reading stays above 140 millimeters of mercury. The average adult reading depends on weight, age, and build.

Hypotension is low blood pressure; usually systolic reading is under 100 millimeters of mercury.

Further Study and Discussion

• Refer to reading references and other outside sources to find out why phlebitis is dangerous.

• Discuss why patients with damaged hearts must restrict physical activity to limits recommended by their doctor.

Assignment

A. Select the correct item which completes each statement.

1. Myocarditis is an inflammation of the
   a. lining of the heart   c. arteries of the heart
   b. covering of the heart   d. muscle of the heart

2. Leukemia is a condition in which there is a great increase in
   a. erythrocytes   c. fibrinogen
   b. neurocytes   d. leukocytes

3. Hypertension or high blood pressure is a condition in which the systolic reading stays above
   a. 190 mm of mercury   c. 140 mm of mercury
   b. 160 mm of mercury   d. 120 mm of mercury

4. Hemophilia is a condition in which the blood clots slowly and is acquired by
   a. environmental contracts and poor nutrition
   b. being inherited by the male but transmitted by the female
   c. close contact with persons who have the disorder
   d. contact with animals in the home and yard

5. A clot which is carried by the blood until it blocks a blood vessel too small for passage is called
   a. an embolism   c. an aneurysm
   b. a thrombus   d. a stenosis

B. Briefly answer the following questions:

1. What is bradycardia?

2. What can cause a hematoma?

3. What is "milk leg"?

4 TRANSPORT OF BLOOD AND OXYGEN

A. Match each term in column I with its correct description in column II.

Column I	Column II
_____ 1. aorta	a. lower chambers of the heart
_____ 2. atria	b. white blood cells which absorb and destroy harmful bacteria
_____ 3. cardiac	c. referring to the lungs
_____ 4. coronary	d. largest artery in body
_____ 5. endocardium	e. liquid part of blood
_____ 6. hemoglobin	f. upper chambers of heart
_____ 7. lymphatic	g. vessel transporting lymph
_____ 8. phagocytes	h. circulation through kidneys
_____ 9. pericardium	i. lining of heart
_____ 10. portal circulation	j. arteries which nourish heart
_____ 11. pulmonary	k. largest vein in body; returns to right atrium
_____ 12. plasma	l. oxygen-carrying part of the blood
_____ 13. renal	m. pertaining to the heart
_____ 14. valves	n. goes to liver from small intestine
_____ 15. vena cava (superior and inferior)	o. covering of heart
_____ 16. ventricles	p. structures in heart and veins, permit blood flow in one direction only
	q. membrane that lines the chest cavity

B. Select the letter which precedes the correct answer.

1. An infection of the membrane lining the heart, usually caused by the streptococcus organism is
   a. acute pericarditis
   b. acute myocarditis
   c. acute rheumatic heart disease
   d. acute atrial fibrillation

2. Hypotension is a condition in which the systolic reading usually continues below
   a. 75 millimeters of mercury
   b. 100 millimeters of mercury
   c. 110 millimeters of mercury
   d. 120 millimeters of mercury

3. A condition in which there are too many red blood cells is
   a. pernicious anemia
   b. leukemia
   c. polycythemia
   d. simple or primary anemia

4. A condition in which a blood clot may be carried by the bloodstream until it reaches a blood vessel too small for passage is a (an)
   a. embolism
   b. thrombus
   c. aneurysm
   d. stenosis

5. A condition in which there is an inability to absorb vitamin B_{12} is known as
   a. simple anemia
   b. pernicious anemia
   c. leukemia
   d. polycythemia

C. Match each term in column I with its description in column II.

Column I	Column II
_____ 1. adenitis	a. varicose veins in walls of rectum
_____ 2. anemia	b. blood clot in artery which leads to the heart
_____ 3. angina pectoris	c. inflammation of a vein
_____ 4. arteriosclerosis	d. moving blood clot in bloodstream
_____ 5. coronary thrombosis	e. inflammation of membrane which lines the heart
_____ 6. embolism	f. hardening of the arteries
_____ 7. endocarditis	g. severe chest pain
_____ 8. hemorrhoids	h. deficiency of red blood cells
_____ 9. myocarditis	i. inflammation of heart muscle
_____ 10. phlebitis	j. inflammation of lymph glands
	k. inflammation of membrane that covers the heart
	l. crescent-shaped red blood cells

D. Briefly answer the following questions.

1. Summarize the five functions of blood.

2. Why are immunosuppressants administered to heart transplant patients?

3. What is hemolysis?

4. What are the characteristic symptoms of inflammation?

5. What is natural immunity? Name four sources of natural immunity.

6. What causes AIDS? What do the initials A-I-D-S stand for?

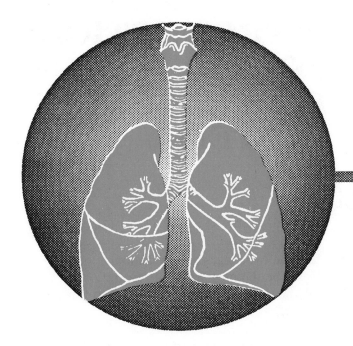

CHAPTER 5

BREATHING PROCESSES

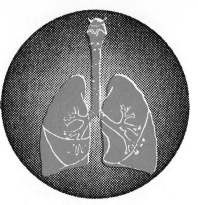

INTRODUCTION TO THE RESPIRATORY SYSTEM

KEY WORDS

bicarbonate ions
(HCO$_3^-$)
cellular respiration
(oxidation)

external
respiration

internal
respiration

The countless millions of cells which make up the human body require a constant supply of energy. This energy is needed to help cells perform their many chemical activities in maintaining the body's homeostasis. For this to occur, energy-rich nutrient (fuel) molecules must be transported to the cells. Oxygen also facilitates the release of energy stored in nutrient molecules. So it must be in constant supply to the body; without oxygen, a human being can live no more than a few minutes at best.

The respiratory system is composed of organs which bring oxygen into the body and remove carbon dioxide. Human respiration is subdivided into three stages: external respiration, internal respiration, and cellular respiration (oxidation).

External respiration is also known as breathing, or ventilation. This is the exchange of oxygen and carbon dioxide between the body and the outside environment. The breathing process consists of inhalation and exhalation. As one inhales, the air is warmed, moistened, and filtered on its passage into the air sacs of the lungs (alveoli). The concentration of oxygen in the alveoli is greater than in the bloodstream. Thus oxygen diffuses from the area of greater concentration (the alveoli) to an area of lesser concentration (the bloodstream), then into the red blood cells. Consequently, the concentration of carbon dioxide in the bloodstream becomes greater, and it diffuses into the alveoli. Exhalation expels much of the carbon dioxide in the blood through the alveoli of the lungs. Some water vapor is also given off in the process.

Internal respiration includes the exchange of carbon dioxide and oxygen between the cells and the lymph surrounding them, plus the oxidative process of energy in the cells. The differences in concentration of carbon dioxide and oxygen govern the exchange which occurs among the air in the alveoli, the blood, and the tissue cells. After inhalation, the alveoli are rich with oxygen and transfer the oxygen into the blood. The resulting greater concentration of oxygen in the blood moves the oxygen into the tissue cells. Through respiration, the tissue cells use up the oxygen. At the same time, the cells build up a higher carbon dioxide concentration. The concentration increases to a point which exceeds the level in the blood. This causes the carbon dioxide to diffuse out of the cells and into the blood where it is then carried away to be eliminated, figure 24–1.

Deoxygenated blood, produced during internal respiration, carries carbon dioxide in the form of **bicarbonate ions (HCO_3^-).** These ions are transported by both blood plasma and red blood cells. Exhalation expels carbon dioxide from the red blood cells and the plasma; it

is released from the body in the following manner:

$$H_2CO_3 \longrightarrow H_2O + CO_2$$

(Bicarbonate ions decompose to form water and carbon dioxide)

Cellular respiration, or **oxidation,** involves the use of oxygen to release energy stored in nutrient molecules like glucose. This chemical reaction occurs within the cells. Just as wood, when burned (oxidized), gives off energy in the form of heat and light, so does food give off energy when it is burned, or oxidized, in the cells. Much of this energy is released in the form of heat to maintain body temperature. Some of it, however, is used directly by the cells for such work as contraction of muscle cells. It is also used to carry on other vital processes.

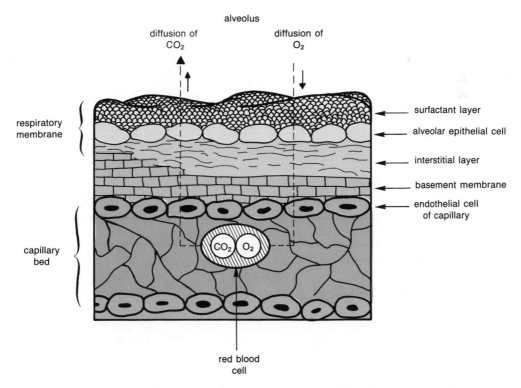

Figure 24-1 Mechanics of internal respiration

As wood burns, the carbon and hydrogen combine with oxygen to form carbon dioxide (CO_2) and water vapor (H_2O). Similarly, food, when oxidized, gives off waste products including carbon dioxide and water vapor. These are transported from the cells through the circulatory system to the lungs where they are exhaled.

Further Study and Discussion

- Breathe on a mirror. Note the moisture which appears from the exhaled air. Discuss the fact that carbon dioxide, heat, and water vapor are given off in exhalation.

- Jog in place. Note the effect of body activity on the rate of breathing. How does exercise change breathing? Why?

- Why does a young child breathe more rapidly than an aged person?

Assignment

A. Briefly answer the following questions.

1. Name and describe the three stages of respiration.

2. Describe the oxidation process. What happens to the energy and waste products released?

B. Match each term in column I with its description in column II.

Column I	Column II
_____ 1. external respiration	a. exchange of gases between the cells and lymph surrounding them
_____ 2. oxidation	b. carbon dioxide and water vapor
_____ 3. waste products of oxidation	c. air sacs in lungs
	d. filtering of air
_____ 4. alveoli	e. combining of food and oxygen in tissues
_____ 5. internal respiration	f. the inhalation of oxygen and exhalation of carbon dioxide
	g. water vapor only

RESPIRATORY ORGANS AND STRUCTURES

KEY WORDS

adenoid
alveoli
anterior nares
apex of the lung
base of the lung
bifurcate
bronchi
bronchial tubes
bronchiole
cardiac
  impression
cilia
fissure of the lung

interpleural space
laryngopharynx
larynx
mediastinum
nasal conchae
nasal septum
nasopharynx
olfactory nerve
oropharynx
parietal pleura
pharyngeal arch
pharynx
pleural cavity

pleural fluid
pleurisy
pneumothorax
pulmones
sinus
surfactant
thoracentesis
tonsil
trachea
turbinate
visceral pleura
  (pulmonary)

OBJECTIVES

- List the organs used in breathing
- Define the structures within the lungs
- Describe functions of parts of the respiratory system
- Define the Key Words that relate to this unit of study

Color plate 14 illustrates how air moves into the lungs through several passageways. The following structures are included: nasal cavity, pharynx, larynx, trachea, bronchi, bronchioles, alveoli, lungs, pleura, and mediastinum.

THE NASAL CAVITY

In humans, air enters the respiratory system through two oval openings in the nose. They are called the nostrils, or **anterior nares.** From here, air enters the nasal cavity, which is divided into a right and left chamber, or smaller cavity, by a partition known as the **nasal septum.** Both cavities are lined with mucous membranes.

Protruding into the nasal cavity are three **turbinate,** or **nasal conchae** bones. These three scroll-like bones (superior, middle and inferior concha), divide the large nasal cavity into

three narrow passageways. The turbinates increase the surface area of the nasal cavity, causing turbulence in the flowing air. This causes the air to move in various directions before exiting the nasal cavity. As it moves through the nasal cavity, air is being filtered of dust and dirt particles by the mucous membranes lining the conchal and nasal cavity. The air is also moistened by the mucus and warmed by blood vessels which supply the nasal cavity. At the front of the nares are small hairs or **cilia** which entrap and prevent the entry of larger dirt particles. By the time the air reaches the lungs, it has been warmed, moistened, and filtered. Nerve endings providing the sense of smell **(olfactory nerves)** are located in the mucous membrane, in the upper part of the nasal cavity.

The **sinuses,** named frontal, maxillary, sphenoid, and ethmoid, are cavities of the skull in and around the nasal region, figures

25–1 and 25–2. Short ducts connect the sinuses with the nasal cavity. Mucous membrane lines the sinuses and helps to warm and moisten air passing through them. The sinuses also give resonance to the voice. The unpleasant voice sound of a nasal cold results from the blockage of sinuses.

THE PHARYNX

After air leaves the nasal cavity it enters the **pharynx,** commonly know as the throat. The pharynx serves as a common passageway for air and food. It is about 5 inches long can be subdivided into three sections. The uppermost section, just after the nasal cavity, is the **nasopharynx.** The **oropharynx** lies behind the mouth. The lowest portion is known as the **laryngopharynx.** Air travels down the pharynx on its way to the lungs; food travels this route on its way to the stomach. **Adenoids** and **tonsils** are lymphatic tissue, located in the nasopharynx and oropharynx respectively. An upper respiratory infection or cold may cause them to enlarge. Enlargement of the adenoids makes it difficult to breathe. When this happens, breathing is performed through the mouth instead of the nose. The affected individual is said to be "adenoidal."

The left and right eustachian tubes open directly into the nasopharynx, connecting each middle ear with the nasopharynx. Because of this connection, nasopharyngeal inflammation can lead to middle ear infections.

THE LARYNX

The **larynx,** or voice box, is a triangular chamber found below the pharynx. The laryngeal walls are composed of nine fibrocartilagi-

nous plates. These plates are derived from embryonic structures called **pharyngeal arches.** Of these nine fibrocartilaginous plates, the largest is the thyroid cartilage, commonly known as the "Adam's apple."

The larynx is lined with a mucous membrane, continuous from the pharyngeal lining above to the tracheal lining below. Within the larynx are the characteristic vocal cords. Muscles attached to the laryngeal cartilages can exert tension upon the vocal cords, lengthening and relaxing them, or making them short and tense. The voice is low-pitched in the former case when the vocal cords are long and relaxed, and high-pitched when they are short and tense.

THE TRACHEA

The **trachea,** or windpipe, is a tube-like passageway some 11.2 centimeters (about 4.5 inches) in length. It extends from the larynx, passes in front of the esophagus, and continues to form the two bronchi (one for each lung). The walls of the trachea are composed of alternate bands of membranes, and 15 to 20 C-shaped rings of hyaline cartilage. These C-shaped rings are virtually noncollapsible, keeping the trachea open for the passage of oxygen into the lungs. However, the trachea can be obstructed by large pieces of food, tumorous growths, or the swelling of inflamed lymph nodes in the neck.

The walls of the trachea are lined with both mucous membrane and ciliated epithelium. The function of the mucus is to entrap inhaled dust particles, whereupon the cilia sweep such dust-laden mucus upward to the pharynx. Coughing or regurgitation then dislodges and eliminates the dust-laden mucus from the pharynx, figure 25–3.

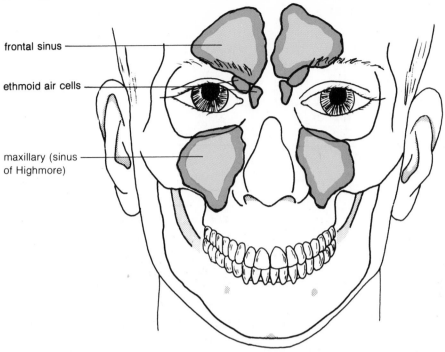

Figure 25-1   Paranasal sinuses, front cross-section view (From P. Anderson. *The Dental Assistant*. Albany: Delmar Publishers Inc.)

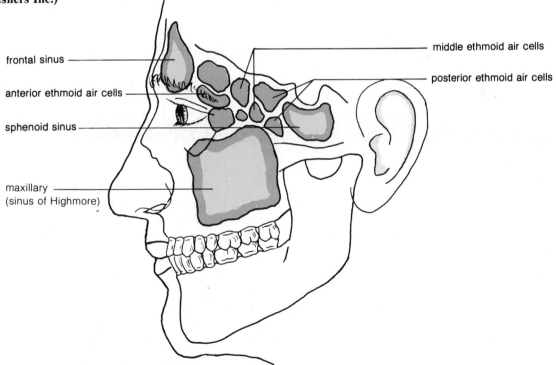

Figure 25-2   Paranasal sinuses, side cross-section view (From P. Anderson. *The Dental Assistant*. Albany: Delmar Publishers Inc.)

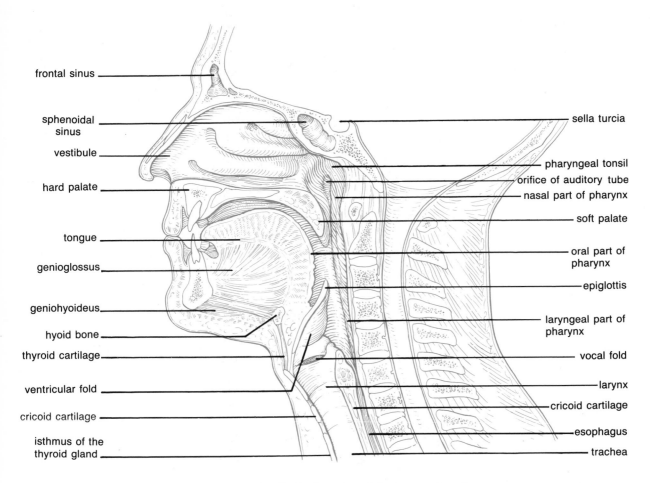

Figure 25-3   Sagittal section of the face and neck

THE BRONCHI AND THE BRONCHIOLES

The lower end of the trachea **bifurcates** (divides in two) into the **right bronchus** and the **left bronchus.** There is a slight difference between the two bronchi, the right bronchus being somewhat shorter, wider and more vertical in position.

As the bronchi enter the lung, they subdivide into **bronchial tubes** and smaller **bronchioles.** The divisions are Y-shaped in form. The two bronchi are similar in structure to the trachea, because their walls are lined with ciliated epithelium and ringed with hyaline cartilage. However, the bronchial tubes and smaller bronchi are ringed with cartilaginous plates instead of incomplete C-shaped rings. The bronchioles lose their cartilaginous plates and fibrous tissue. Their thinner walls are made from smooth muscle and elastic tissue lined with ciliated epithelium. At the end of each bronchiole, there is an alveolar duct which ends in a sac-like cluster called **alveolar sacs (alveoli).**

THE ALVEOLI

The alveolar sacs consist of many alveoli and are composed of a single layer of epithelial tissue. There about 300 million alveoli in the adult lung.[1] Each alveolus forming a part of the alveolar sac possesses a globular shape. Their inner surfaces are covered with a lipid material known as **surfactant.** The surfactant helps to stabilize the alveoli, preventing their collapse. Each alveolus is encased by a network of blood capillaries.

It is through the moist walls of both the alveoli and the capillaries that rapid exchange of carbon dioxide and oxygen occurs. In the blood capillaries, carbon dioxide diffuses from the erythrocytes, through the capillary walls, into the alveoli.

Carbon dioxide leaves the alveoli, exhaled through the mouth and nose. The opposite process occurs with oxygen, which diffuses from the alveoli into the capillaries, and from there into the erythrocytes.

If one were to spread out the internal lung surface to form a single sheet of tissue, the entire area would cover an estimated 90 square meters (or 3543.30 square inches.)[2] This is more than 100 times the skin surface of the adult human body!

THE LUNGS

The lungs, or **pulmones,** are fairly large, cone-shaped organs filling up the two lateral chambers of the thoracic cavity, see plate 14. They are separated from each other by the mediastinum and the heart. The upper part of the lung, underneath the collarbone, is the **apex;**

the broad lower part is the **base.** Each base is concave, allowing it to fit snugly over the convex part of the diaphragm.

Lung tissue is porous and spongy, due to the tremendous amount of air it contains. If you were to place a specimen of a cow lung into a tankful of water, for example, it would float quite easily.

The right lung is larger and broader than the left. This is because the heart inclines to the left side. The right lung is also shorter due to the diaphragm's upward displacement on the right in order to accommodate the liver. The right lung is divided by **fissures** (clefts) into three lobes: superior, middle and inferior.

The left lung is smaller, narrower, and longer than its counterpart. It is subdivided into two lobes: superior and inferior. The concave area occupied by the heart, on the left side of the lung, is called the **cardiac impression.**

THE PLEURA

The lungs are covered with a thin, moist, slippery membrane made up of tough endothelial cells, or **pleura.** There are two pleural membranes. The one lining the lungs and dipping between the lobes is the *pulmonary,* or **visceral pleura.** Lining the thoracic cavity and the upper surface of the diaphragm is the **parietal pleura.** Consequently, each lung is enclosed in a double-walled sac.

The space between the two pleural membranes is the **pleural cavity,** filled with serous fluid called **pleural fluid.** This fluid is necessary to prevent friction as the two pleural membranes rub against each other during each breath.

Unfortunately, the pleural cavity may, on occasion, fill up with an enormous quantity of serous fluid. This occurs when there is an inflammation of the pleura (called **pleurisy**). The

---

[1] Morrison, Cornett, Tether, and Gratz, *Human Physiology* (New York: Holt, Rinehart, and Winston, 1977).

[2] See note 1 above.

increased pleural fluid compresses and sometimes even causes parts of the lung to collapse. This obviously makes breathing extremely difficult. To alleviate such pressure, a **thoracentesis** may be performed. This procedure entails the insertion of a hollow, tubelike instrument through the thoracic cavity and into the pleural cavity, so as to drain the excess fluid.

Another disorder which can affect the pleural cavity is **pneumothorax.** This condition occurs if there is a buildup of air within the pleural cavity on one side of the chest. The excess air increases pressure on the lung, causing it to collapse. Breathing is not possible with a collapsed lung, but the unaffected lung can still continue the breathing process.

THE MEDIASTINUM

The **mediastinum,** also called the **interpleural space,** is situated between the lungs along the median plane of the thorax. It extends from the sternum to the vertebrae. The mediastinum contains the thoracic viscera: the thymus gland, heart, aorta and its branches, pulmonary arteries and veins, superior and inferior vena cava, esophagus, trachea, thoracic duct, lymph nodes and vessels.

Further Study and Discussion

- Using a plastic model or charts, trace the air passage from the nostrils to the air sacs of the lungs.

- If laboratory facilities are available, examine beef lungs and trace the trachea and bronchi into the tissues of the lung. Blow into the trachea with a glass tube and inflate the lungs. Observe the action.

- Discuss the effect that lung congestion has on breathing (e.g., during a severe chest cold).

Assignment

A. Explain how the air sacs are particularly adapted to permit a rapid exchange of oxygen and carbon dioxide.

B. Match each term in column I with its correct description in column II.

Column I	Column II
_____ 1. alveoli	a. help give resonance to voice
_____ 2. ciliated epithelium	b. air sacs
_____ 3. intercostal muscles	c. lines nasal passage
_____ 4. larynx	d. voice box
_____ 5. lobes	e. divisions of lungs
_____ 6. mucous membrane	f. double lining of the thoracic cavity
_____ 7. nasal septum	g. chest
_____ 8. pleura	h. collects dust particles
_____ 9. sinuses	i. made of cartilage
_____ 10. thoracic cavity	j. support and aid the breathing process
	k. respiratory center

C. Briefly answer the following questions.

1. What tissue makes up the alveolar sac?

2. What structure forms a tight network around the alveolar sac?

3. What structure, found in the nasal passage and sinuses, will warm, moisten and filter air passing through it?

4. Name the four sinuses in the nasal area.

5. Name the two muscles primarily responsible for the breathing movements.

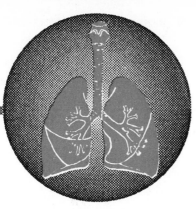

UNIT 26

MECHANICS OF BREATHING

KEY WORDS

apnea	inspiration	polypnea
barometer	inspiratory	pulmonary
compliance	reserve volume	ventilation
dyspnea	(IRV)	residual volume
eupnea	intercostal	(RV)
expiration	muscle	respiratory
expiratory	(external and	movement
reserve volume	internal)	tachypnea
(ERV)	medulla	tidal volume (TV)
Hering-Brewer	oblongata	vagus nerve
reflex	orthopnea	vital capacity
hyperpnea	phrenic nerves	

OBJECTIVES

- Explain how breathing movements are controlled
- Describe the action of the diaphragm and the ribs in breathing
- Define the various lung capacities
- Describe the various factors that can alter the rate of respiration
- Identify the various types and conditions of respiration
- Define the Key Words relating to this unit of study

Pulmonary ventilation (breathing) of the lungs is due to changes in pressure which occur within the chest cavity. This variation in pressure is brought about by cellular respiration and mechanical breathing movements.

THE BREATHING PROCESS

Pulmonary ventilation allows the exchange of oxygen between the alveoli and erythrocyte, and eventually between the erythrocyte and cells.

Inhalation

There are two groups of intercostal muscles: **external intercostals** and **internal intercos-**

tals. Their muscle fibers cross each other at an angle of 90°. During inhalation, or **inspiration,** the external intercostals lift the ribs upward and outward, figure 26–1. This increases the volume of the thoracic cavity. Simultaneously, the sternum rises along with the ribs and the dome-shaped diaphragm contracts and becomes flattened, moving downward. As the diaphragm moves downward, pressure is exerted on the abdominal viscera. This causes the anterior muscles to protrude slightly, increasing the space within the chest cavity in a vertical direction. As a result, there is a decrease in pressure. Since atmospheric pressure is now greater, air rushes in all the way down to the alveoli, resulting in inhalation.

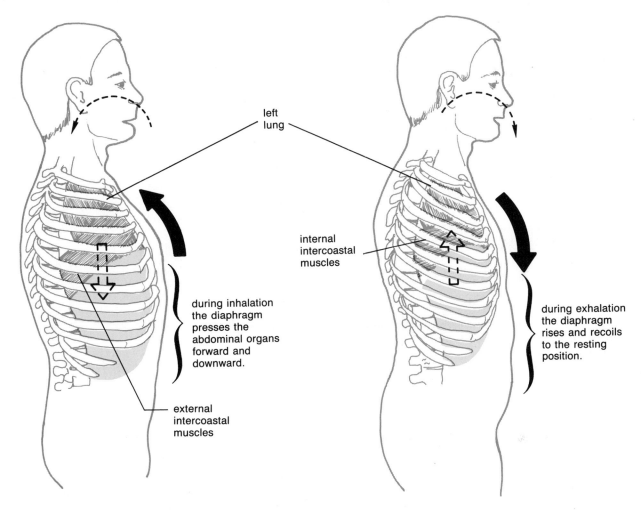

left
lung

internal
intercoastal
muscles

during inhalation
the diaphragm
presses the
abdominal organs
forward and
downward.

during exhalation
the diaphragm
rises and recoils
to the resting
position.

external
intercoastal
muscles

Figure 26-1   Mechanics of breathing—inhalation and exhalation

Exhalation

In exhalation, or **expiration,** just the op-posite takes place. Expiration is a passive pro-cess; all the contracted intercostal muscles and diaphragm relax. The ribs move down, the dia-phragm moves up. In addition, the surface ten-sion of the fluid lining the alveoli reduces the elasticity of the lung tissue and causes the alve-oli to collapse. This action, coupled with the relaxation of contracted, respiratory muscles,

relaxes the lungs; the space within the thoracic cavity decreases, thus increasing the internal pressure. Increased pressure forces air from the lungs, resulting in exhalation. Figure 26–2 illustrates this concept. Two glass bell jars, equipped with a rubber stopper and balloons, are used to demonstrate the mechanics of breathing.

The lungs are extremely elastic. They are able to change capacity as the size of the tho-racic cavity is altered. This ability is known as

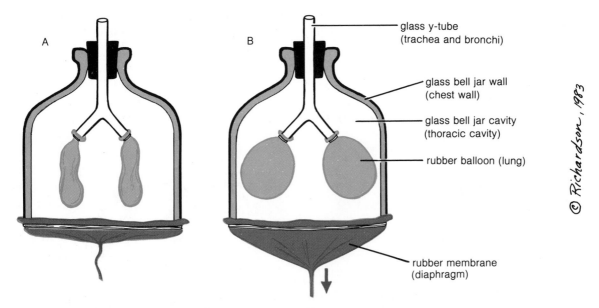

A

B

glass y-tube
(trachea and bronchi)

glass bell jar wall
(chest wall)

glass bell jar cavity
(thoracic cavity)

rubber balloon (lung)

rubber membrane
(diaphragm)

© Richardson, 1983

Figure 26-2   Glass bell jar models to demonstrate the process of inhalation and exhalation. Model A represents exhalation—the rubber diaphragm is relaxed, deflating the two rubber balloons (lungs). Model B represents inhalation—the rubber diaphragm is pulled downward, inflating the two rubber balloons. This occurs because the volume of the bell jar cavity has been increased.

compliance. When lung tissue becomes diseased and fibrotic, the lung's compliance decreases and ventilation decreases.

Pressure Changes During Respiration

During inhalation, as the thoracic cavity expands so do the lungs. Lung expansion lowers the air pressure in the alveoli and air sacs, resulting in a pressure gradient which, in turn, allows air to rush into the alveoli. This helps to equalize the air pressure between the outside and the alveoli, decreasing pressure in the pleural cavity.

In order to understand the concept of gaseous pressure, a brief discussion of atmospheric pressure will prove helpful. The pressure of a gas is measured by the height of a column of mercury which the gas is able to support. Imagine that a glass cylinder, sealed at

one end, is filled with mercury; it is then inverted into a shallow receptacle containing mercury. Eventually the mercury in the cylinder drops to where its weight is balanced by the atmospheric pressure exerted on the surface of the mercury in the shallow container. At sea level, the mercury in the cylinder will rise to a height of 760 millimeters, or 30 inches. This figure (760mm) is known as 1 atmosphere of pressure of air at sea level at zero degree Celsius (0°C or 32°F). At higher elevations, the column of mercury will decrease due to the decrease in atmospheric pressure, and vice-versa. The instrument that measures atmospheric pressure is called a **barometer.**

During inhalation, alveoli pressure decreases in proportion to pressure in the pleural cavity, by about 2–3 millimeters of mercury 757–758 millimeters of mercury (mm Hg). This slight change in air pressure is enough to push air into the lungs and alveoli. Exhalation causes the alveoli pressure to rise about $+3$ mm Hg to 763 mm Hg. Consequently air rushes out of the alveoli and lungs.

Respiratory Movements and Frequency of Respiration

The rhythmic movements of the rib cage where air is drawn in and expelled from the lungs makes up the respiratory movements. Inspiration and expiration combined is counted as one **respiratory movement.** Thus, the normal rate in quiet breathing for an adult is about 14 to 20 breaths per minute. This rate is changeable. The respiratory rate can be increased by muscular activity, increased body temperatures (as in fever), and in certain pathological disorders like hyperthyroidism. (See unit 47 on *Disorders of the Endocrine System* for further information on hyperthyroidism.) It changes with **sex,** females having the higher rate at 16 to 20 breaths per minute. *Age* will also change the respiratory rate. For example, at birth the rate is 40 to 60 breaths per minute; at 5 years, 24 to 26 breaths; at 15 years, 20 to 22 breaths; at 25 years and above, 14 to 20 breaths per minute. The *body's position* also affects the respiration rate. When the body is asleep or prone, the rate is 12 to 14 breaths per minute; if the body is in a sitting position, it is 18; and in a standing position, it is 20 to 22 breaths per minute. *Emotions* play a role in decreasing or increasing the respiratory rate, probably through the hypothalamus and pons. (See unit 49 on *The Central Nervous System: Brain and Spinal Chord* for further information on the hypothalamus and pons.)

CONTROL OF BREATHING

The rate of breathing is controlled by neural (nervous) and chemical factors. Although both have the same goal – that of respiratory control – they function independently of one another.

Neural Factors. The respiratory center is located in the **medulla oblongata** in the brain. It is subdivided into two centers: one to regulate inspiration, the other for expiratory control, see figure 26–3.

The upper part of the medulla contains a grouping of cells that is the seat of the respiratory center. This has been experimentally proven by applying electrical and thermal stimulation to the medulla of research animals. Application of stimuli to this respiratory center causes the rate of respiration to increase or decrease.

Two neuronal pathways are involved in the breathing process. One group of motor nerves, called the **phrenic nerves,** leads to the diaphragm and the intercostal muscles. The other nerve pathway carries sensory impulses from the nose, larynx, lungs, skin, and abdominal organs via **vagus nerve** in the medulla. As you can see, various stimuli from different parts of the body help to control breathing.

The rhythm of breathing can be changed by stimuli originating within the body's surface membranes. For example, a sudden drenching with cold water can make us gasp, while irritation to the nose or larynx can make us sneeze or cough.

Although the medulla's respiratory center is primarily responsible for respiratory control, it is not the only part of the brain that controls breathing. A lung reflex, called the **Hering-Brewer reflex,**[1] is involved in preventing the overstretching of the lungs. When the lungs are inflated, the nerve endings in the walls are stimulated. A nerve message is sent

---

1. Karl Hering (1834-1918), German physiologist and Josef Brewer (1842-1925), Austrian psychiatrist.

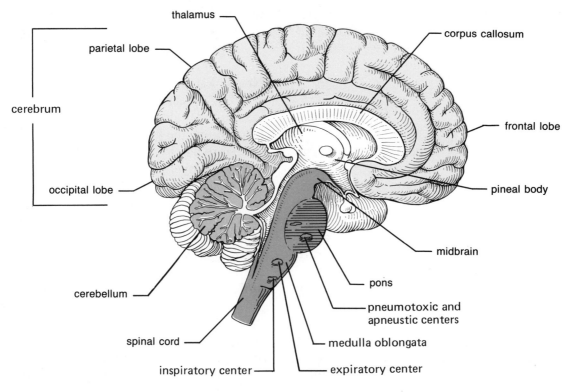

Figure 26-3 Cross section of the brain. Note the expiratory and inspiratory centers.

from the lungs to the medulla by way of the vagus nerve, inhibiting inspiration and stimulating expiration. This mechanism prevents overinflation of the lungs, keeping them from being ripped apart like an over-inflated balloon. Also it prevents the lungs from taking up too much blood, and so depriving the left side of the heart of its blood supply.

Chemical Factors. The respiratory center can be inactivated by sleep-inducing drugs, or other central nervous system depressants such as excessive and toxic amounts of barbiturates, chloroform, ether, and morphine. These drugs interfere with oxygen utilization by the cells of the respiratory center. They also damage nerve impulse transmissions and decrease the blood flow into the respiratory center. If

such damage to the respiratory center is not avoided, death will occur. Currently, there are few chemical substances which can reactivate the respiratory center. Therefore, a "chemical antidote" for overdose of sleep-inducing drugs is not available. In many cases, artificial respiration is used to reactivate the respiratory center.

Chemical control of respiration is dependent upon the level of carbon dioxide in the blood. When blood circulates through an active tissue, it receives carbon dioxide and other metabolic waste products of cellular respiration. As blood circulates through the respiratory center, it becomes sensitive to the increased carbon dioxide in the blood. Consequently, a person performing vigorous exercise or physical labor breathes more deeply and quickly.

LUNG CAPACITY AND VOLUME

Vital capacity refers to the amount of air one can forcibly expire after a maximum inhalation; in other words, it is a measure of the ability to inspire and expire air. Disease processes that weaken the respiratory muscles (such as polio) or decrease the ability of the lungs to expand (such as emphysema) can decrease the vital capacity. The vital capacity of an average person is about 4500 milliliters. See figure 26–4.

Tidal volume (TV) is the amount of air that is inhaled and exhaled during rest. Normal tidal volume is about 500 milliliters.

Inspiratory reserve volume (IRV) is the extra volume of air that can be inhaled over and beyond the tidal volume. It is usually about 3000 milliliters.

The **expiratory reserve volume (ERV)** is the amount of air that can be forced by expiration after the end of a normal exhalation. This is about 1100 milliliters.

The **residual volume (RV)** is what remains in the lungs even after a forced expiration; this is about 1200 milliliters.

TYPES OF RESPIRATION

The health care professional should be aware of the various changes to the respiratory rate and sounds of human respiration. These changes can alert a health professional to an abnormal respiratory condition in a patient they are caring for or treating. The following conditions describe various kinds and conditions of respiration.

Apnea is the temporary stoppage of breathing movements.

Dyspnea is difficult, labored, or painful breathing, usually accompanied by discomfort and breathlessness.

Eupnea is normal or easy breathing with the usual quiet inhalations and exhalations.

Hyperpnea is an increase in the depth and rate of breathing accompanied by abnormal exaggeration of respiratory movements.

Orthopnea is difficult or labored breathing when the body is in a horizontal position. It is usually corrected upon taking a sitting or standing position.

Polypnea is very rapid respiration or panting due to increased muscular activity or from emotional trauma.

Tachypnea is an abnormally rapid and shallow rate of breathing.

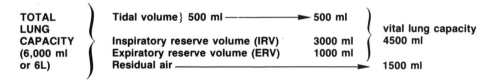

Figure 26-4   Lung capacity and volume

Further Study and Discussion

- Demonstrate breathing movements by placing the hands near the base of the ribs on both sides of the chest. Note how the ribs rise and fall during breathing. Then place the hands horizontally across the stomach (at the base of the diaphragm) as inhalation and exhalation take place.

- Discuss the effects of the following on healthful breathing: posture, exercise, deep breathing, mouth breathing, enlarged tonsils and adenoids.

- Using library sources, look up the "iron lung." How does its action compare with natural breathing movements?

- Discuss why a "respirator" machine is properly called a ventiltor.

Assignment

A. Explain the function of:

   a. The diaphragm

   b. The intercostal muscles

B. Match each term in column I with its function or description in column II.

Column I	Column II
_____ 1. respiratory control center	a. opposite of inhalation
_____ 2. inspiration and expiration	b. measure of the ability to inspire and expire air
_____ 3. vital capacity	c. complemental air
_____ 4. exhalation	d. located in the medulla
_____ 5. increases respiratory rate	e. occur from 16 to 24 times a minute
_____ 6. diaphragm	f. result of increase in carbon dioxide content of the blood
_____ 7. intercostal muscles	g. becomes flattened and moves downward during inhalation
_____ 8. tidal air	h. air which cannot be forcibly expelled from the lungs
_____ 9. residual air	i. corresponds with atmospheric pressure
_____ 10. chest cavity space	j. air inhaled and exhaled during rest
	k. muscles in between the ribs which contract during inhalation
	l. moves upward during inhalation

C. Briefly answer the following questions.

   1. List three factors that can increase the human respiratory rate.

   2. What is dyspnea, hyperpnea, and polypnea?

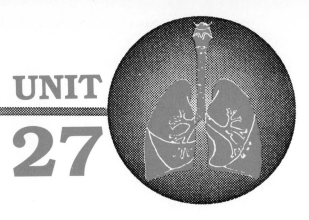

UNIT 27

REPRESENTATIVE DISORDERS OF THE RESPIRATORY SYSTEM

KEY WORDS

asthma
atelectasis
bronchiectasis
bronchitis
cancer of the
   larynx
cancer of the
   lungs
causative agent
complication
consolidation
crepitation
diphtheria
dysphagia

emphysema
inflammatory
   exudate
influenza
laryngitis
mucopurulent
   discharge
pharyngitis
pleurisy
pneumonia
rales
respiratory
   distress
   syndrome

rhinitis
rhinorrhea
silicosis
sinusitis
tonsillitis
tuberculosis
viral or atypical
   pneumonia
whooping cough
   (pertussis)

OBJECTIVES

- Describe some common respiratory diseases caused by a virus or a bacterium
- Describe some respiratory disorders unrelated to infectious causes
- Suggest proper health professional care for respiratory ailments
- Define the Key Words related to this unit of study

The greatest loss in production hours each year is caused by the common cold. This respiratory infection spreads quickly through the classroom, factory, or business office. It is often the basis for more serious respiratory disease. It lowers body resistance, making it subject to infection. The direct cause of a cold is usually a virus. Indirect causes include: chilling, fatigue, lack of proper food, and not enough sleep. A person who has a cold should stay in bed, drink warm liquids and fruit juice, and eat wholesome, nourishing foods.

INFECTIOUS CAUSES

The respiratory system is subject to various infections and inflammations caused by bacteria, viruses, and irritants.

Pharyngitis is a red, inflamed throat which may be caused by one of several bacteria or viruses. It also occurs as a result of irritants such as too much smoking or speaking. It is characterized by painful swallowing and extreme dryness of the throat.

Laryngitis is an inflammation of the larynx, or voice box. It is often secondary to other respiratory infections. It can be recognized by the incidence of hoarseness or loss of voice. The most common form is chronic catarrhal laryngitis. This is characterized by dryness, hoarseness, sore throat, coughing and **dysphagia** (difficulty in swallowing).

Tonsillitis is an infection of the tonsils caused by one of several bacteria. Frequent occurrence of this infection, which is accompanied by severe sore throat, difficulty in swallowing, elevation of temperature, chills and aching muscles, may require surgical removal of the tonsils.

Sinusitis is an infection of the mucous membrane which lines the sinus cavities. One or several of the cavities may be infected. Pain and nasal discharge are symptoms of this infection which, if severe, may lead to more serious complications. The sinuses affected can be the ethmoid, frontal, sphenoid, and maxillary sinuses.

Pleurisy is the result of inflammation of the pleura, the delicate membrane that lines the thorax and folds back over the lung surface. Pleurisy is often a **complication** (a disease that occurs at the same time as another disease) of a more severe illness such as pneumonia or tuberculosis. One type is acute pleurisy, which can originate from a lung infection such as pneumonia, or an inflammation in the mediastinum or adjacent structures. **Acute pleurisy** is characterized by fever, painful breathing, and **crepitation** (production of sounds from the lungs). Another type is **chronic pleurisy.** Here, fibrinous attachments grow between the parietal and visceral pleural surfaces. Chronic pleurisy may be a complication of tuberculosis.

Bronchitis is an inflammation of the mucous membrane of the trachea and the bronchial tubes. It may be acute or chronic and often follows infections of the upper respiratory tract. **Acute bronchitis** can be caused by the spreading of an inflammation from the nasopharynx, or by inhalation of irritating vapors. This condition is characterized by a cough, fever, substernal pain and by **rales.**

Chronic bronchitis occurs in middle or old age, characterized by a cough and dry rales. It can result from repeated bouts with acute bronchitis, gout, rheumatism or tuberculosis; it is sometimes a secondary symptom to cardiac or renal disorders.

Influenza is an infectious disease characterized by inflammation of the mucous membrane of the respiratory system. The infection is accompanied by fever, a **mucopurulent discharge,** muscular pain, and extreme exhaustion. An influenza virus is the **causative agent** responsible for the disease, various strains being labelled as strain A, B, etc. Complications such as bronchopneumonia, neuritis, otitis media (middle ear infection), and pleurisy often follow influenza.

Pneumonia is an infection of the lung. The alveoli fill up with an **inflammatory exudate** (intercellular fluid mixed with pieces of injured cells which results from an inflammation). Pneumonia is usually caused by bacteria although there may be other causes. Onset is often sudden and is marked by chills and chest pain. When caused by a virus, it is called **viral** or **atypical** pneumonia.

Tuberculosis is an infectious disease of the lungs, caused by the tubercle bacillus *Mycobacterium tuberculosis.* The bacterium can affect any organ or tissue of the body. Most related deaths, however, result from tuberculosis of the lungs. Since there are no obvious early signs of this infection, yearly check-ups and chest X rays are highly recommended. If the tuberculosis bacterium is present in the lungs, lesions occur containing lymphocytes and epithelioid cells.

Diphtheria is a very infectious disease caused by the *Corynebacterium diphtheriae.* The disease affects the upper respiratory tract. It can be recognized by the formation of a false, grayish-white or yellow membrane on the pharynx, larynx, trachea, and tonsils. Locally, diphtheria causes pain, swelling and obstruction. If the diphtheria toxin is circulated through the bloodstream, it leads to cardiac damage, fever, extreme fatigue, occasional paralysis, and all too often — death.

Whooping cough (pertussis) is an infectious disease. It is characterized by repeated coughing attacks that end in a "whooping" sound. It is caused by the Bordet Gengou bacillus. Pertussis is often fatal to very young infants.

NONINFECTIOUS CAUSES

Respiratory ailments which are unrelated to infectious causes sometimes develop in the respiratory system.

Rhinitis is the inflammation of the nasal mucous membrane causing swelling and increased secretions. Various forms include **acute rhinitis** (the common cold); **allergic rhinitis,** caused by any allergen (more commonly known as hay fever); **atrophic rhinitis,** which is an atrophy of the mucous membrane of the nose, and **chronic rhinitis,** caused by repeated attacks of acute rhinitis and characterized by the presence of dark, putrid crusts.

Asthma is a respiratory disorder with symptoms of difficult breathing, wheezing, coughing, the presence of a mucoid sputum, and a feeling of tightness in the chest. Serious episodes of wheezing may occur from emotional stress or from breathing irritants. Emergency care may be needed.

Atelectasis is a condition in which the lungs fail to expand normally, due to bronchial occlusion.

Bronchiectasis is the dilation of a bronchus caused by an inflammation, accompanied by heavy pus secretion.

Silicosis is caused by breathing dust containing silicon dioxide over a long period of time. The lungs become fibrosed which results in a reduced capacity for expansion. Silicosis is also called *chalicosis, lithosis, miner's asthma, miner's disease,* or *grinder's rot.*

Emphysema is a noninfectious condition in which the alveoli become overextended, with resulting overinflation of the lungs. Breathing becomes increasingly difficult. Treatment is aimed at relieving the discomfort of the symptoms. At present, there is no cure, only treatment.

Cancer of the lungs is a malignant tumor which often forms in the bronchial epithelium. The incidence of this condition is high in middle-aged men, especially those who are regular smokers. Early diagnosis is difficult, depending on examinations rather than apparent symptoms. Surgery is often indicated. If done soon enough, it is often successful.

Cancer of the larynx is curable if early detection is made of the disorder. It is found most frequently in men over fifty.

Consolidation is the accumulation of matter in the air spaces of the lungs.

Respiratory Distress Syndrome (RDS; Hyaline Membrane Disease) is a condition generally affecting premature babies. It is characterized by the formation of a hyaline-like false membrane within the alveoli. This causes the alveoli to collapse.

Rhinorrhea is the discharge of thin, watery fluid from the nose.

Professional health care in many of these respiratory ailments is directed toward maintaining external respiration while making the patient as comfortable as possible. In addition, sufficient rest and proper nourishment are essential.

Further Study and Discussion

- Explain why sinusitis is more common among people who live at sea level. Explain why the climate in Arizona is usually beneficial to people who have sinusitis.

- Discuss how a minor infection can lower the body's resistance to other infections.

- Discuss how public health measures could help reduce the incidence of emphysema and lung cancer.

Assignment

1. Describe what should be done for a person who is developing the symptoms of a cold.

2. Name five common respiratory disorders caused by a virus or bacterium.

3. Name three respiratory disorders of a noninfectious nature.

4. Why is pertussis also called "whooping cough"? What causes pertussis?

5. What is respiratory distress syndrome?

5

BREATHING PROCESSES

A. Describe the process of external and internal respiration.
   (1) External respiration

   (2) Internal respiration

B. Explain the function of the hemoglobin in internal respiration.

C. Label figure SE5–A by inserting the name of the structure to which the line is pointing (e.g., esophagus).

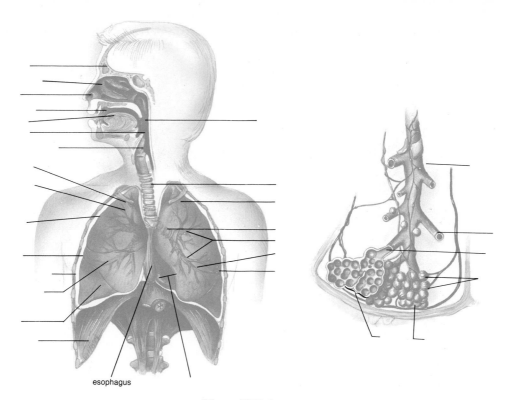

esophagus

Figure SE5-A

D. Complete the following statements.

1. During inhalation, the ribs are _____ by contraction of the rib muscles.

2. The microscopic air sacs in the lungs are called_____ .

3. Laryngitis is an inflammation of the_____ .

4. When the diaphragm moves_____ , inhalation takes place.

5. Energy and waste products are given off when food unites with _____ .

6. The principal waste product of exhalation is _____ .

7. The respiratory system is dependent upon the _____ system for transporting oxygen to the body cells and carbon dioxide away from the body cells.

8. The lining of the thoracic cavity is called_____ .

9. The most common respiratory ailment is _____ .

10. The sinuses are lined with_____ .

E. Explain how the action of the respiratory center affects the breathing rate.

F. Briefly answer the following questions.
   1. Describe the following kinds of breathing.
      a. Apnea

      b. Eupnea

      c. Orthopnea

      d. Polyphea

   2. What causes whooping cough? What are the symptoms of whooping cough?

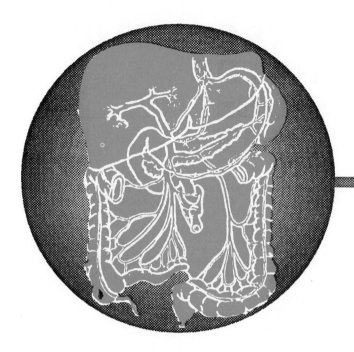

CHAPTER 6

DIGESTION OF FOOD

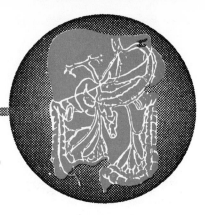

UNIT 28

INTRODUCTION TO THE DIGESTIVE SYSTEM

KEY WORDS

accessory
  digestive
  organs
alimentary canal
bicuspids
bolus
buccal cavity
canines
circular muscle
crypts
cusps
deciduous
deglutition
dentition
  formula
digestion
duct of Bartholin
ducts of Rivinus
enzymes

enzymatic
  hydrolysis
feces
gingivae
hard palate
hydrolytic juices
  (digestive)
incisors
longitudinal
  muscle
masticate
molars
mucosa
muscle tonus
papillae
  • filiform
  • fungiform
  • circumvallate
    (vallate)

parotid papilla
peristalsis
permanent
premolar
ptyalin
salivary glands
  • parotid
  • sublingual
  • submandibular
soft palate
submucosa
taste buds
tonsillitus
tonsils
  • lingual
  • palatine
uvula
wisdom teeth

OBJECTIVES

- Describe the general function of the digestive system
- List the structures of the digestive system
- Relate the function of the mouth and teeth to digestion
- Define the Key Words that relate to this unit of study

All food which is eaten must be changed into a soluble, absorbable form within the body before it can be used by the cells. This means that certain physical and chemical changes must take place to *change the insoluble complex food molecules into simpler soluble ones.* These can then be transported by the blood to the cells and be *absorbed through the cell membranes.* The process of changing complex solid foods into simpler soluble forms which can be absorbed by the body cells is called **digestion,** or **enzymatic hydrolysis.** It is accomplished by the action of various digestive juices containing enzymes. **Enzymes** are chemical substances that promote chemical re-

actions in living things although they themselves are unaffected by the chemical reactions.

Digestion is performed by the digestive system, which includes the alimentary canal and accessory digestive organs. The **alimentary canal** is also know as the digestive tract, gastrointestinal tract (GI tract), or gut. Its organs are found in the head, thorax, abdomen, and pelvis. Most are concentrated within the abdominal cavity. The alimentary canal consists of the mouth (oral cavity), pharynx (throat), esophagus (gullet), stomach, small intestine, large intestine (colon), and the anus, see color plate 15. It is a continuous tube some 30 feet (9 meters) in length, from the mouth to anus. However, during life, the length of the alimentary canal is much shorter (12–15 feet) due to **muscle tonus** (a continual state of partial contraction).

The walls of the alimentary canal are composed of four layers: (1) the innermost lining, called the **mucosa,** is made of epithelial cells, (2) the **submucosa,** consists of connective tissue with fibers, blood vessels, and nerve endings, (3) the third layer is comprised of **circular muscle,** (4) the fourth has **longitudinal muscle.** The mucosa secretes slimy mucus. In some areas, it also produces **hydrolytic (digestive) juices.** This slimy mucus lubricates the alimentary canal, aiding in the passage of food. It also insulates the digestive tract from the effects of powerful hydrolytic enzymes while protecting the delicate epithelial cells from abrasive substances within the food.

A very important concept must be stressed here regarding the relationship of the alimentary canal to the human body. The body has a "tube-within-a-tube" body plan. The digestive tract can be viewed as the inner tube, the body wall as the outer tube surrounding the digestive tract. In a very real sense, food within the alimentary canal is not yet part of the body and its cells. Thoroughly *digested* food molecules must first pass through the small intestine into the bloodstream, then into the blood capillaries. Here the food molecules diffuse into the interstitial fluid, and finally into the body's tissue cells.

The **accessory organs** are the teeth, tongue, salivary glands, pancreas, liver and gallbladder.

GENERAL OVERVIEW OF DIGESTION

Food enters the gastrointestinal tract via the mouth. In the oral cavity, the food is mechanically digested by the cutting, ripping, and grinding action of the teeth. Chemical digestion of carbohydrates is initiated by the secretion of saliva containing a hydrolytic enzyme. Then, the action of the saliva and rolling motion of the tongue turn the food into a soft, pliable ball called a **bolus.** The bolus slides down to the throat (pharynx) to be swallowed. Next it travels through the esophagus into the stomach. Food is pushed along the esophagus by rhythmic, muscular contractions called **peristalsis.** From the stomach, peristaltic contractions continue to push the food into the small intestine.

Each part of the alimentary canal contributes to the overall digestive process. Protein digestion, for instance, is initiated by the stomach. Then the small intestine starts and finishes fat digestion, as well as completes the digestion of carbohydrates and proteins. Numerous digestive glands are located in the stomach and small intestine, which secrete hydrolytic juices containing powerful enzymes to chemically digest the food. Due to digestion, insoluble food becomes a soluble fluid substance. This substance is then transported across the small intestinal wall into the bloodstream.

Circulated and absorbed through the blood capillaries into the interstitial fluid and finally into the body cells, the soluble food molecules are utilized for energy, repair, and production of new cells. The remaining undigested substances **(feces)** pass into the large intestine and leave the alimentary canal via the anus.

Mouth and Digestion

Food enters the digestive tract through the mouth (oral or **buccal cavity).** The inside of the mouth is covered with a mucous membrane. Its roof consists of a hard and soft palate. The **hard palate** is hard because it is formed from the maxillary and palatine bones, which are covered by mucous membrane. Behind the hard plate is the **soft palate** made from a movable mucous membrane fold. It encloses blood vessels, muscle fibers, nerves, lymphatic tissue and mucous glands. The soft palate is an arch-shaped structure, separating the mouth from the nasopharynx. Hanging from the middle of the soft palate is a conical flap of tissue called the **uvula.** This prevents food from entering the nasal cavity when swallowing, figure 28–1.

Tonsils

Located on either side of the pharyngeal opening are soft masses of lymph tissue known as the **palatine tonsils.** There are also masses of lymph tissue under the tongue called the **lingual tonsils.** Usually, however, the word **tonsils** refers to the palatine tonsils. The tonsils

have little openings called **crypts.** Tonsils act like lymph nodes by producing lymphocytes and filtering out microbes that might enter the body and cause infection. Occasionally bacteria may grow inside the crypts, causing an infection which can spread into the lymph and eventually into the blood. This type of infection is known as **tonsillitis.**

Tongue

The tongue and its muscles are attached to the floor of the mouth, helping in both chewing and **deglutition** (swallowing). The tongue is made from skeletal muscles that lie in many different planes. Because of this, the tongue can be moved in various directions. It is attached to four bones: the hyoid, the mandible, and two temporal bones. On the tongue's epithelial surface are projections called **papillae,** figure 28–2. There are nerve endings located in

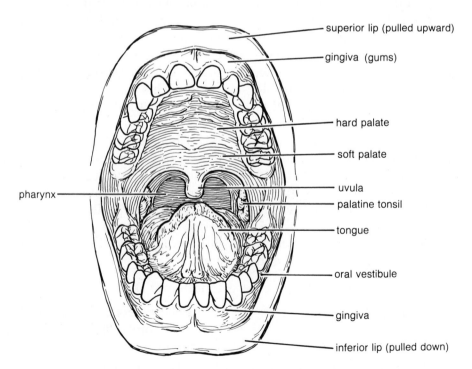

superior lip (pulled upward)
gingiva (gums)
hard palate
soft palate
uvula
palatine tonsil
tongue
oral vestibule
gingiva
inferior lip (pulled down)
pharynx

© Richardson 1983

Figure 28-1 The mouth and its structures

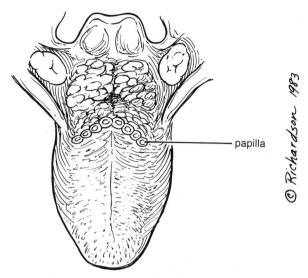

Figure 28-2 There are about 9000 taste buds on the tongue, contained in knoblike elevations called papillae.

many of these papillae forming the sense organs of taste, or **taste buds.** These taste buds respond to bitterness, saltiness, sweetness, and sourness in foods, figure 28–3(A). They are also sensitive to cold, heat, and pressure. The tongue is made up of three kinds of papillae:

fungiform on the tip of the tongue, **filiform** near the center and sides, and **vallate,** or **circumvallate,** near the back, forming a wide "V."

In order for food to be tasted, it must be in solution. The solution passes through the taste bud openings, stimulating the nerve endings in the taste cells. A nerve impulse is created and carried to the brain via nerve fibers at the base of the taste buds, figure 28–3(B).

The sensation of taste is coupled with the sense of smell. When we experience an odor, it stimulates the olfactory nerve endings in the upper part of the nasal cavity. Thus we may confuse the odor of a food with its flavor when it is simultaneously present in the mouth. A bad cold, with nasal congestion, frequently impedes the ability to taste the flavor of foods. This is because increased mucous secretions cover the olfactory nerve endings.

Salivary Glands

The **salivary glands** produce a watery secretion called saliva. Saliva has many functions. It softens and lubricates food, making it

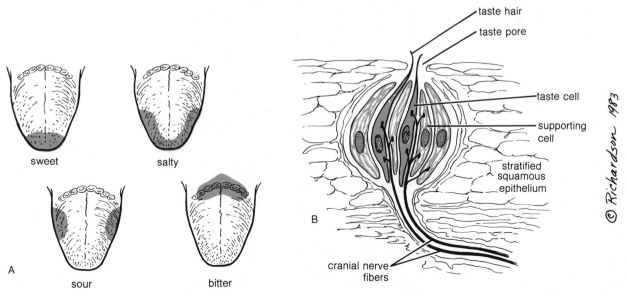

Figure 28-3 Taste buds are sensitive to four basic tastes as shown in (A). Sketch of a taste bud with its nerve fibers is shown in (B).

easier to chew and swallow. At the same time, the saliva dissolves a portion of the food so it can be tasted. Saliva contains the enzyme **ptyalin** (salivary amylase), which partially digests starches to simpler substances (dextrose). Since food stays in the mouth only for a short time, ptyalin continues its digestion of the dextrose in the stomach.

Food is swallowed in the form of a bolus, which doesn't break up immediately upon reaching the stomach. Therefore the ptyalin's digestive action can continue as long as thirty minutes more. Eventually the stomach's gastric juice, containing hydrochloric acid, will stop the digestive action of the ptyalin. By that point, as much as 75% of the starches in foods like bread, pasta, potatoes, and rice have been broken down.

Saliva also neutralizes mouth acids, washes the teeth, and keeps the mouth cavity flexible and moist. A moist mouth helps in the speech process.

Saliva is a watery mixture of different chemical compounds. It consists of 99% water and contains dissolved traces of salts like calcium, potassium, and sodium, as well as mucin and the enzyme ptyalin.

Saliva is secreted into the oral cavity by three pairs of salivary glands: the parotid, the submandibular, and the sublingual, figure 28–4. The **parotid salivary glands** are found on both sides of the face, in front and below the ears. They are the largest salivary glands, the ones that become inflamed during an attack of mumps. Chewing, at such times, is painful, because the motion squeezes these tender, inflamed glands. A parotid duct, also called Stenson's duct,[1] carries its secretion (almost entirely ptyalin) into the mouth. It opens upon the inner surface of the cheeks, opposite the second molar of the upper jaw. This area is

_____

1. Nicholas Stenson (1638–1686), Danish anatomist

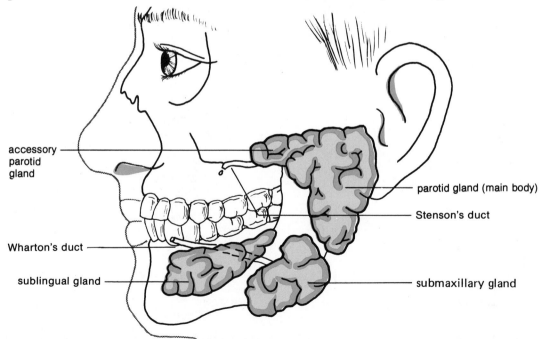

accessory parotid gland

Wharton's duct

sublingual gland

parotid gland (main body)

Stenson's duct

submaxillary gland

Figure 28-4   Salivary glands (From P. Anderson, *The Dental Assistant.* Albany: Delmar Publishers Inc.)

marked by a flap of tissue called the **parotid papilla.**

Below the parotid salivary gland and near the angle of the lower jaw is a **submaxillary gland.** This gland is about the size of a walnut, and its secretions contain both mucin and ptyalin. The secretions enter the buccal cavity via the submandibular duct, or Wharton's duct,[2] at the anterior base of the tongue.

The final pair of salivary glands are the **sublingual glands,** the smallest of the three. They are found under the sides of the tongue. Their secretion consists mainly of mucus and contains no ptyalin. There are some 8–20 small ducts **(ducts of Rivinus),** and a larger one **(duct of Bartholin),** which either join the submandibular duct or open directly onto the mouth floor. An infected sublingual gland causes swelling of the floor of the mouth, resulting in pain during any motion of the tongue, such as in chewing and talking.

Gingivae and Teeth

The **gingivae,** or gums, support and protect the teeth. They are made up of fleshy tis-

---

2. Thomas Wharton (1610–1673), English anatomist

sue covered with mucous membrane. This membrane surrounds the narrow portions of the teeth (also called cervix or neck), and covers the structures in the upper and lower jaws.

Food ingested by the mouth must be thoroughly chewed, or **masticated,** by the teeth. Teeth help break food down into very small morsels, increasing the food's surface area. This activity enables the digestive enzymes to digest the food more efficiently and quickly than if it were swallowed without being chewed. During normal growth and development, the human mouth develops two sets of teeth: (1) the deciduous or milk teeth, which are later replaced by (2) the permanent teeth.

Deciduous teeth start to erupt at about 6 months and continue until around two years of age. In total, 20 deciduous teeth are cut during the first two years — 10 in the upper and 10 in the lower jaw. They are: 4 incisors, 2 canines, and 4 molars. This relationship is expressed in the **dentition formula** as shown in figure 28–5(A). The **incisors** have sharp edges for biting, the **canines** are pointed for tearing, and the **molars** have ridges, or **cusps,** designed for crushing and grinding. There are no **premolars** among the deciduous teeth. Deciduous teeth last only up to the age of six.

A. The dentition formula for deciduous teeth is:

	Molars		Canine		Incisors		Canine		Molars
Upper jaw	2	:	1	:	4	:	1	:	2
Lower jaw	2	:	1	:	4	:	1	:	2

B. The dentition formula for permanent teeth is:

	Molars		Premolars		Canine		Incisors		Canine		Premolars		Molars
Upper jaw	3	:	2	:	1	:	4	:	1	:	2	:	3
Lower jaw	3	:	2	:	1	:	4	:	1	:	2	:	3

Figure 28-5   Dentition formulas for deciduous and permanent teeth

Permanent teeth begin developing at this point, pushing out their deciduous predecessors. The first molars lead the way between the fifth and seventh years. The last to emerge are the third molars, or **"wisdom teeth,"** which may appear anywhere from 17 to 25 years of age. In total, the adult mouth develops 32 teeth, 16 in each jaw, figure 28–5(B).

Based on the dentition formula, the adult mouth has 8 premolars, or **bicuspids:** 4 in the upper and 4 in the lower jaw. Bicuspids are broad, with two cusps on each crown, and have only one root. Their design is ideal for grinding food. Figure 28–6 shows the arrangement of the deciduous and permanent teeth, and the years during which they normally erupt.

Further Study and Discussion

- Discuss what measures are necessary for the proper care of teeth.

- Make a list of foods which are rich in calcium and phosphorus.

- Discuss other nutrients important in maintaining the health of the mouth.

Assignment

A. Briefly answer the following questions.

　1. What is the purpose of the salivary glands?

　2. Name four kinds of permanent teeth, and give the uses of each.

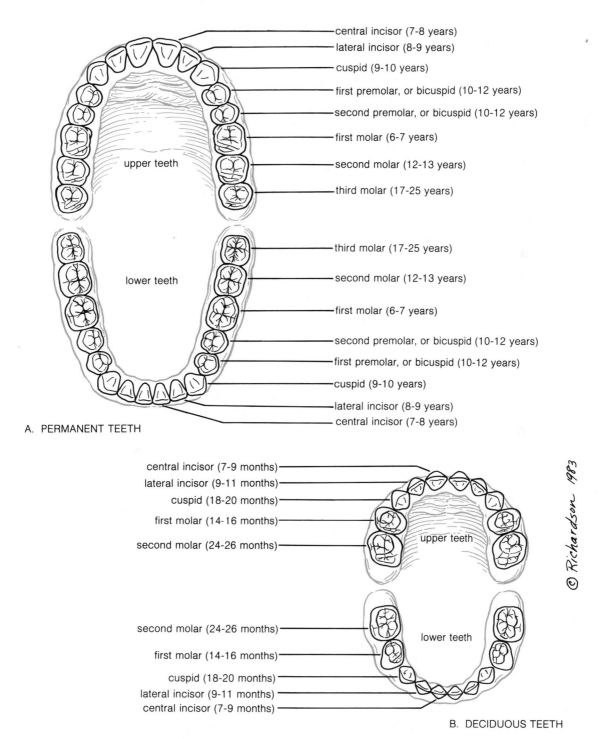

A. PERMANENT TEETH

central incisor (7-8 years)
lateral incisor (8-9 years)
cuspid (9-10 years)
first premolar, or bicuspid (10-12 years)
second premolar, or bicuspid (10-12 years)
first molar (6-7 years)
second molar (12-13 years)
third molar (17-25 years)

third molar (17-25 years)
second molar (12-13 years)
first molar (6-7 years)
second premolar, or bicuspid (10-12 years)
first premolar, or bicuspid (10-12 years)
cuspid (9-10 years)
lateral incisor (8-9 years)
central incisor (7-8 years)

upper teeth
lower teeth

central incisor (7-9 months)
lateral incisor (9-11 months)
cuspid (18-20 months)
first molar (14-16 months)
second molar (24-26 months)

second molar (24-26 months)
first molar (14-16 months)
cuspid (18-20 months)
lateral incisor (9-11 months)
central incisor (7-9 months)

upper teeth
lower teeth

B. DECIDUOUS TEETH

© Richardson 1983

Figure 28-6   Teeth and their eruption times

B. Match each of the terms in column I with its correct statement in column II.

Column I	Column II
_____ 1. papillae	a. substances that promote chemical reactions in living things
_____ 2. calcium and phosphorus	b. bleeding gums
_____ 3. digestion	c. a small soft structure suspended from the soft palate
_____ 4. the teeth	d. gums which protect the teeth
_____ 5. enzymes	e. tract consisting of the mouth, stomach and intestines
_____ 6. gingivae	f. minerals contained in teeth
_____ 7. accessory organs and structures of digestion	g. teeth, tongue, salivary glands, pancreas, liver, gallbladder, and appendix
_____ 8. ptyalin	h. hardest structure in the body
_____ 9. uvula	i. projections on the surface of the tongue containing the taste buds
_____ 10. alimentary canal	j. the process of changing complex solid foods into soluble forms to be absorbed by cells
	k. the enzyme manufactured by the salivary glands

C. Label the teeth indicated on figure 28–7. (The teeth on the left are the deciduous ones; those on the right are permanent teeth.)

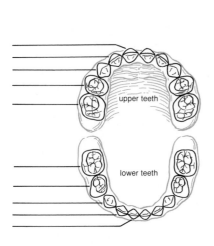

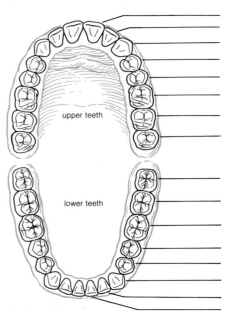

Figure 28-7

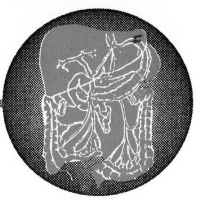

UNIT 29

DIGESTION IN THE STOMACH

KEY WORDS

cardiac sphincter
casein
chief cells
chyme
curdling
deglutition
duodenum
epiglottis
fundus
gastric glands
greater curvature
  (body of
  stomach)
greater omentum
intrinsic factor

laryngeal
  pharynx
mucin
mucous coat
mucous neck cells
mucus
muscular coat
nasopharynx
oropharynx
parietal cells
pepsin
pepsinogen
peptone
peristalsis

peritoneum
pharynx
protease
proteose
pyloric sphincter
pyloric stenosis
pylorospasm
pylorus
rennin
rugae
stomach or
  gastric
  serosa
submucosa coat

After having been chewed and moistened with saliva in the mouth, food is swallowed by the action of the **pharynx.** The walls of the pharynx consist of skeletal muscle layers lined with mucous membrane. The pharynx is subdivided into three parts: the upper, or **nasopharynx;** the middle, or **oropharynx;** and the **laryngeal pharynx** which reaches from the hyoid bone to the esophagus. The pharyngeal passageway communicates with the ears, nose, mouth, and larynx. In addition, the mucous membrane lining the pharynx is continuous with the mucous membranes of the ears, nasal cavities, mouth, and larynx. The pharyngeal walls are well-lined with mucous glands.

DEGLUTITION

Swallowing, or **deglutition,** is a complex process involving the constrictor muscles of the pharynx. It begins as a voluntary process, changing to an involuntary process as the food enter the esophagus. When we swallow, the tip of the tongue arches slightly and moves backward and upward. This action forces the food against the hard palate; simultaneously, the soft palate and the uvula shut off the opening to the nasopharynx. Food is thus prevented from entering the nasopharynx.

In swallowing, the constrictor muscles of the pharynx contract, pushing food into the upper part of the esophagus. At the same time, other pharyngeal muscles raise the pharynx, causing the **epiglottis** to cover the larynx (windpipe) to prevent food from entering it. As a further precaution, the nerve impulses causing breathing stop so that breathing and swallowing cannot occur simultaneously. For these reasons, food can only travel in one direction — towards and down the esophagus.

The act of swallowing is voluntary. But, as a bolus of food passes over the posterior part of the tongue and stimulates receptors in the walls of the pharynx, swallowing becomes an involuntary reflex action. With the contraction of the pharyngeal muscles, followed by the contraction of the muscles lining the esophagus, food passes down into the stomach.

THE ESOPHAGUS

When food is swallowed it enters the upper portion of the esophagus. The esophagus is a muscular tube about 25 centimeters (10 inches) long. It begins at the lower end of the pharynx, behind the trachea. It continues downward through the mediastinum, in front of the vertebral column, and passes through the diaphragm. From there the esophagus enters the upper part, or cardiac portion, of the stomach. This point can be located at the end of the sternum, near the level of the xiphoid process.

The esophageal walls consist of four coats or layers. From the innermost layer to the outermost, they are:

1. the *internal mucous layer*
2. the *submucous* or *areolar layer*
3. a *muscular layer*
4. an *external serous layer* of tough, fibrous connective tissue.

The muscular layer is composed of external longitudinal muscle and internal circular muscle. The muscles in the upper third of the esophagus are striated, and the lower portion consists exclusively of smooth muscle.

After food is swallowed, a series of wavelike involuntary muscular contractions, called **peristalsis,** moves a bolus of food down the esophagus to the stomach. From the time it is swallowed, it takes food five to six seconds to travel the length of the esophagus. When the peristaltic wave reaches the stomach, the **cardiac sphincter** muscle near the entrance to the stomach (cardiac portion) relaxes. This allows food to pass from the esophagus into the stomach. Once the food is in the stomach the cardiac sphincter contracts, preventing reflux, or backflow of food into the esophagus.

THE STOMACH

The stomach is found in the upper part of the abdominal cavity, just to the left of and below the diaphragm. It is an elastic bag generally shaped like the letter *J*. The shape and position are determined by several factors. These include the amount of food contained within the stomach, the stage of digestion, the position of a person's body, and the pressure exerted upon the stomach from the intestines below.

The stomach is divided into three portions: the upper part or **fundus;** the middle section, called the **body** or **greater curvature;** and the lower portion called the **pylorus.** At the opening into the stomach is found a circular layer of muscle **(cardiac sphincter)** which controls passage of food into the stomach. It is called the cardiac sphincter because of its proximity to the heart. Toward the other end of the stomach lies the **pyloric sphincter** valve which regulates entrance of food into the **duodenum** (the first part of the small intestine). Sometimes the pyloric sphincter valve fails to relax in infants. In such cases, food remaining in the stomach does not get completely digested and eventually is vomited. This condition is called **pylorospasm.** Another abnormal condition is **pyloric stenosis,** a narrowing of the pyloric sphincter which may occur at any age.

The stomach wall consists of four layers: mucous, submucous, muscular, and serous layers.

1. The **mucous coat** is the innermost layer. It is an extremely thick layer made up of small **gastric glands** embedded in areolar connective tissue. When the stomach is not distended with food, the gastric mucosa is thrown into folds called **rugae,** figure 29–1.

2. The **submucosa coat** is made of loose areolar connective tissue. It connects the mucous coat to the muscular coat.

3. The **muscular coat** consists of three layers of smooth muscle: the outer, longitudinal layer; a middle, circular layer; and an inner, oblique layer, figure 29–1. These muscles help the stomach to undergo peristalsis which helps in digestion and in pushing food into the small intestine. The muscular coat is closely connected to the serosa.

4. The **serosa** is the thick outer layer covering the stomach. It is continuous with the **peritoneum** (the membrane lining the entire inner abdominal cavity). The serosa and peritoneum meet at certain points, surrounding the organs around the stomach and holding them in a kind of sling. From the left, or greater curvature of the stomach, the peritoneum extends downward, forming the apron-like **greater omentum** which hangs in front of the intestines. The greater omentum contains large amounts of fat.

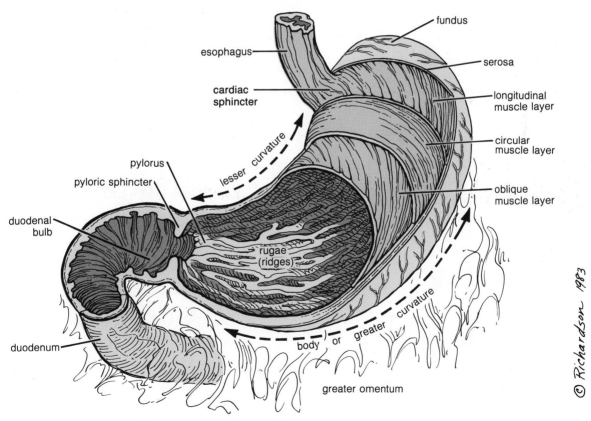

Figure 29-1   Parts of the stomach

The Gastric Glands

The gastric mucosa is estimated to have approximately 35 million gastric glands lining its surface. These glands secrete gastric juice, which is used in digestion.

The gastric glands are comprised of three types of cells: **chief cells, mucous neck cells,** and **parietal cells,** figure 29–2. The chief cells secrete **pepsinogen,** an inactive form of the enzyme **pepsin.** Mucus cells secrete **mucus** and **mucin,** a protein-like substance. The parietal cells secrete hydrochloric acid and the **intrinsic factor.** This is a glycoprotein that helps the body absorb vitamin B_{12}. If insufficient intrinsic factor is secreted, a condition known as pernicious anemia results (see unit 23).

Gastric Juice

The millions of gastric glands which line the stomach secrete a gastric juice. This gastric juice consists of water, hydrochloric acid, mucus, and the **protease** pepsin (an enzyme that specifically digests proteins).

Hydrochloric acid gives gastric juice a very acidic pH (about 1.5). The functions of hydrochloric acid are:

- It helps to convert the inactive enzyme, pepsinogen, into its active form, pepsin.

- It provides the necessary acidic environment so that the pepsin can begin to digest protein.

- It helps to dissolve certain mineral salts found in the foods we consume.

- It destroys the bacteria and microorganisms that enter the stomach in our foods. This action is so efficient that partially digested food leaving the stomach is virtually sterile under normal conditions.

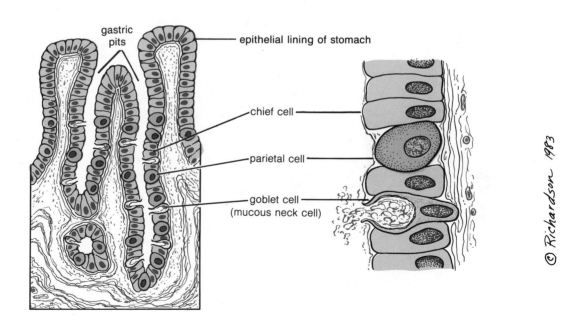

Figure 29-2   Three types of gastric gland cells make up the gastric glands that line the stomach.

The enzyme **pepsin** acts only on proteins in the stomach. The optimum conditions for the functioning of pepsin are an acidic pH of 1.5 and a temperature of 37°C (body temperature of 98.6°F). Pepsin breaks down large protein molecules into intermediate-sized protein molecules called **proteoses** and **peptones.** As the proteose and peptone molecules are still too large for absorption into the bloodstream, they must pass into the small intestine for final digestion. It was once believed that human gastric juice contained a second protein-splitting enzyme called **rennin.** This was thought to act on the milk protein, **casein.** It has since been proven that rennin does not exist in the adult stomach, and that pepsin can curdle milk. Rennin is, however, found in the stomach of infants and certain young mammals (such as calves). **Curdling** is the changing of the liquid casein into a solid form, or curd. It prepares milk for eventual digestion by other enzymes. It is of interest to note that rennin, obtained from calves' stomachs, is used commercially to curdle milk for cheeses and various milk desserts.

The action of the gastric juice is helped by the churning of the stomach walls. The semi-liquid food which results is called **chyme.** When the chyme is ready to leave the stomach, a valve (the **pyloric sphincter)** at the lower end of the stomach opens from time to time. This allows the food to spurt on into the duodenum. The contraction and relaxation of smooth muscles in the walls of the alimentary tract move the food along the entire alimentary canal.

Further Study and Discussion

- Identify each organ of the digestive system on a wall chart or a torso model.

- Add 5 mL of 0.5% hydrochloric acid to an equal volume of warm milk; note the reaction. Can this action be related to digestion?

- Explain why the stomach may change its shape before and after a meal.

- If laboratory facilities are available, place a small quantity of finely chopped, hard-boiled egg white into each of four test tubes. To test tube #1, add 5 mL water; to test tube #2, add 5 mL 0.5% hydrochloric acid; to test tube #3, add a tiny amount of pepsin in 5 mL water; to test tube #4, add both a little pepsin and 5 mL of 0.5% hydrochloric acid. Place all the test tubes in an incubator overnight. Observe the results and complete the following table.

TEST TUBE	CONTENTS	OBSERVATION	CONCLUSION
1	White of egg plus water	No change	Water alone does not dissolve protein
2	White of egg plus 0.5% hydrochloric acid		
3	White of egg plus pepsin and water		
4	White of egg plus pepsin plus 0.5% hydrochloric acid		

Assignment

A. Briefly answer the following questions.

1. List the organs of the alimentary canal and the accessory organs of digestion (as discussed in the preceding unit).

      Alimentary Canal   *Accessory Organs*

2. Explain the importance of hydrochloric acid in the stomach.

3. Name the main enzyme found in gastric juice and explain its function.

B. Match each term in column I with its correct description in column II.

Column I	Column II
_____ 1. chyme	a. semiliquid condition of food found in the stomach
_____ 2. esophagus	
_____ 3. hydrochloric acid	b. acts upon protein in the stomach
_____ 4. pepsin	c. oversecretion may cause peptic ulcer
_____ 5. peristalsis	d. involuntary muscle action of alimentary canal
_____ 6. pharynx	e. passageway to the stomach
_____ 7. ptyalin	f. storage place for food
_____ 8. pylorus	g. lower section of stomach
_____ 9. stomach	h. passage where swallowing action takes place
_____ 10. fundus	i. enzyme which changes starch to sugar
	j. upper portion of stomach
	k. sphincter muscle at entrance to stomach

C. List the parts of the stomach and the organs through which food enters and leaves the stomach. (Study figure 29–1 before answering.)

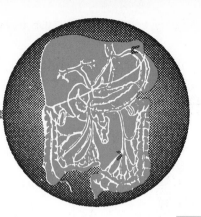

DIGESTION IN THE SMALL INTESTINE

KEY WORDS

absorption	chymotrypsinogen	liver
ampulla of Vater	dextrins	mucilaginous
bile	emulsified	nucleoalbumin
bilirubin	enterokinase	pancreatic juice
biliverdin	gallbladder	secretin
carboxypoly-	glycogen	steapsin
peptidase	ileum	trypsin
cholecystokinin	intestinal juice	trysinogen
chymotrypsin	jejunum	villi

OBJECTIVES

■ Describe how the small intestine prepares food for absorption
■ Describe the digestive function of the liver
■ Explain the digestive function of the gall-bladder
■ Define the Key Words relating to this unit of study

The small intestine is a coiled portion of the alimentary canal and is about twenty-five feet long and one inch in diameter, figures 30–1 and 30–2. It contains thousands of small intestinal glands which produce intestinal juice. In addition to intestinal juice, bile from the liver and pancreatic juice from the pancreas are poured into the duodenum, the first part of the small intestine, see color plate 15.

Liver bile is needed for the digestion of fat. It breaks up the fat into small droplets upon which the digestive juices can act. Pancreatic juice contains enzymes that: (a) continue the digestion of protein started in the stomach, (b) act on starch, and (c) digest fat. The enzymes of the intestinal juice complete the digestion of proteins and carbohydrates. Therefore, the combined action of bile, pancreatic juice, and intestinal juice completes the process of breaking down food mass into sub-stances which can be absorbed into the bloodstream.

Absorption is possible because the lining of the small intestine is not smooth. It is covered with millions of tiny projections called **villi.** Each microscopic villus contains a network of blood and lymph capillaries, figures 30–3 and 30–4. The digested portion of the food passes through the villi into the bloodstream and on to the body cells. The undigestible portion passes on to the large intestine.

CHANGES THAT OCCUR IN THE SMALL INTESTINE

There are three juices that are of importance in small intestinal digestion. They are **pancreatic juice, intestinal juice,** and **bile.**

Secretion of Pancreatic Juice. The secretion of pancreatic juice is started by nerve stimulation

loop of small intestine

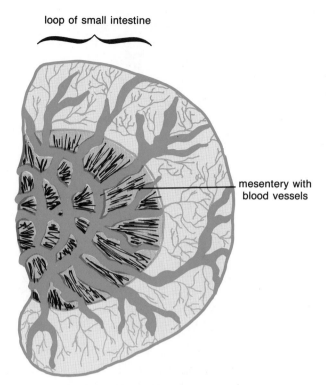

mesentery with
blood vessels

Figure 30-1   Showing mesentery

and chemical stimulation. The nerve stimulation is caused by the vagus and splanchnic nerves. A chemically controlled secretion is caused by the dual action of the hormones **secretin** and **cholecystokinin.** These two hormones are produced by the duodenum and **jejunum.*** They are stimulated by the acidic gastric juice and the partially digested proteins from the stomach. After these two hormones are secreted by the small intestine, they are circulated to the pancreas via the bloodstream. In the pancreas, they cause the secretion of a large quantity of fluid rich in pancreatic digestive enzymes.

The hormonally stimulated pancreatic juice secretion is rich in sodium bicarbonate but poor in enzymes. However, the neurally stimulated pancreatic secretion is small in quantity but rich in enzymes. It is believed

*Jejunum is the part of the small intestine between the duodenum and the ileum.

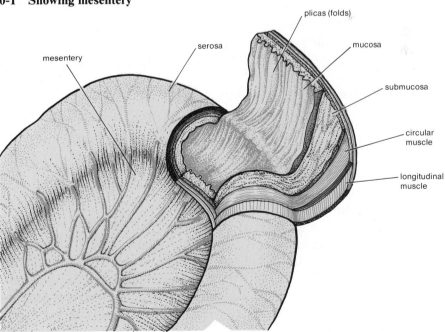

plicas (folds)

serosa

mucosa

mesentery

submucosa

circular
muscle

longitudinal
muscle

Figure 30-2   Portion of the jejunum showing the inner structure

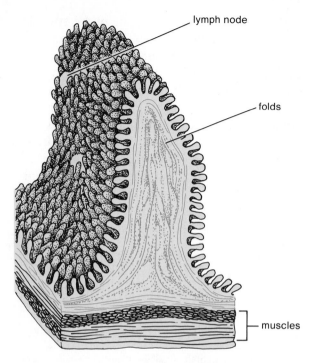

Figure 30-3   Diagram of the wall of a portion of the small intestine showing the villi arrangement

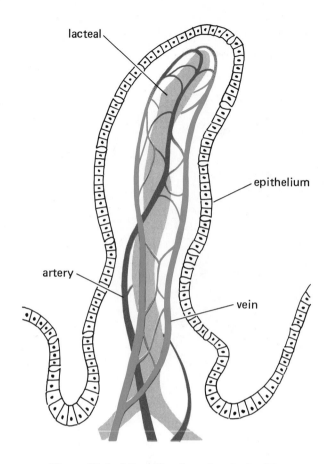

Figure 30-4   Magnification of a single villus

that the neurally stimulated secretion supplies pancreatic juice during the early stages of intestinal digestion. The chemically induced secretion maintains the flow until the entire food contents of the stomach reaches the duodenum.

Pancreatic Juice. The neurally induced secretion of pancreatic juice is very thick and rich in enzymes and proteins. The chemically stimulated secretion is thin and watery, but it is also rich in enzymes. Pancreatic juice is alkaline or basic in pH. It becomes more so with increasing rates of secretion. This is due to the effect of secretin. Secretin increases the flow of bicarbonate ions as well as decreases the flow of gastric juice.

    Pancreatic juice contains four different types of enzymes:
1. Pancreatic proteases
    a. carboxypolypeptidase
    b. chymotrypsin
    c. trypsin
2. Pancreatic amylase
3. Pancreatic lipase
    a. steapsin
4. Pancreatic ribonuclease

    The amount of pancreatic juice secreted daily ranges from 500 to 800 milliliters. There are three proteolytic enzymes. One of these enzymes is **carboxypolypeptidase,** which breaks down polypeptides into their component amino acids. Another enzyme is **trypsin.** It is secreted in an inactive form called **trypsino-**

gen. In the small intestine, trypsinogen is converted to trypsin by the influence of **enterokinase,** an intestinal enzyme that is secreted by glands lining the small intestine. In turn trypsin will turn inactive **chymotrypsinogen** into **chymotrypsin.** Both chymotrypsin and trypsin will digest proteins or incompletely digested proteins turning them into peptones, proteoses, polypeptides, peptides, and finally into amino acids.

Pancreatic amylase continues the digestion of starches which started in the mouth by ptyalin in saliva. In the small intestine, the starches are digested to **dextrins** that are in turn hydrolyzed to maltose. Maltose is digested further into glucose by maltase.

Steapsin is a pancreatic lipase that will digest fats. However, before fats can be digested, they must be **emulsified.** Large fat globules will be physically broken down into smaller fat globules by the action of bile. Bile is secreted into the duodenum from the liver. Bile emulsification of fats helps to increase the surface area of fat globules. This way steapsin can digest the smaller fat globules more efficiently. Once the fats are emulsified, steapsin will digest them into diglycerides, monoglycerides, fatty acids, and glycerol.

Finally, there is pancreatic ribonuclease. It is a nucleic acid-splitting enzyme. It will split DNA and RNA into their component nucleotides.

INTESTINAL SECRETIONS

The small intestine, itself, secretes a fluid that contains various enzymes. This intestinal secretion is a clear, yellowish liquid. Its composition is changeable. In the duodenum and the jejunum of the small intestine, it is slightly acidic. In the **ileum,** the lower portion of the small intestine, the intestinal secretion is almost neutral. In the duodenal bulb and in the

ampulla of Vater* it is almost entirely mucous. The intestinal secretion has been analyzed and has been found to contain many enzymes. The enzymes are enterokinase, aminopeptidase, carboxypeptidase, and dipeptidase. The latter three will digest peptides into amino acids. Thus, it will finish the digestion started by gastric pepsin and intestinal trypsin.

Maltase, lactase, and sucrase are also enzymes found in intestinal fluid. Maltase converts maltose into two glucose molecules. Lactase will digest the disaccharide lactose into two simple sugars, galactose and glucose. While sucrase will hydrolyze sucrose (common table sugar) into fructose and glucose.

Finally nucleases are also found in intestinal fluid.

THE LIVER AND GALLBLADDER

During the process of digestion, the **liver,** a large organ located just below the diaphragm on the right side, mainly acts on fat metabolism. It manufactures **bile** and passes it along to its storehouse, the **gallbladder.** When bile is needed for the digestion of fats, the gallbladder releases it through a duct into the duodenum of the small intestine.

In addition to manufacturing bile, the liver produces and stores **glycogen** (animal starch) from unused digested sugars. The liver also aids in removing certain waste products from the bloodstream, changing them into a form that can be excreted by the kidneys.

The bile contains mineral salts. If stored too long, these salts may crystallize and form gallstones either in the gallbladder or in the ducts through which the bile passes. Gall-

---

Ampulla of Vater is a junction or common passageway formed from the common bile duct of the liver and the pancreatic duct. It helps to empty bile into the duodenum. It is named after the German anatomist who discovered it.

stones may keep the bile from reaching the small intestine.

Figure 30–5 shows how starch, fat, and protein are broken into simple forms and made ready for absorption.

Bile

Bile is secreted continuously from the liver at the rate of about 800 to 1,000 ml daily. It is alkaline, pH 6.8 to 7.7, and usually yellow, brown-yellow, or olive green in color. The color of bile is determined by the varying amounts of two bile pigments, **bilirubin** and **biliverdin**. Bilirubin is reddish in color, and biliverdin is greenish in color. These two bile pigments come from the breakdown of hemoglobin in the bone marrow, liver, and spleen by phagocytosis. Bile collectively contains water, bile pigments, bile acids, bile salts, cholesterol, lecithin, and neutral fats. The mucous membranes of the bile ducts and gallbladder add a mucus-like protein called **nucleoalbumin** to the bile. This along with mucin gives bile its **mucilaginous** (gum-like) consistency.

At this point, a summary of all the digestive enzymes involved in the process of human digestion from the mouth to the small intestine is included in Table 30–1.

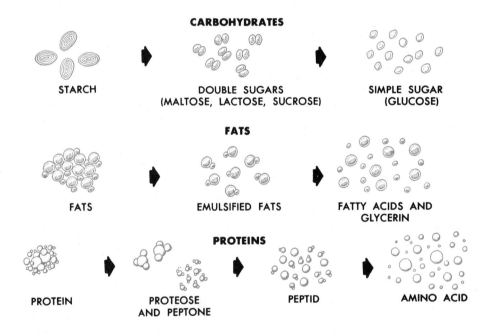

CARBOHYDRATES

STARCH → DOUBLE SUGARS (MALTOSE, LACTOSE, SUCROSE) → SIMPLE SUGAR (GLUCOSE)

FATS

FATS → EMULSIFIED FATS → FATTY ACIDS AND GLYCERIN

PROTEINS

PROTEIN → PROTEOSE AND PEPTONE → PEPTID → AMINO ACID

Figure 30-5   Phases in the digestion of starch, fat, and protein

Table 30–1 Summary of Digestive Enzymes Involved in Human Digestion

ORGAN	JUICE	GLAND	ENZYME(S)	ACTION	ADDITIONAL FACTS
Mouth	Saliva	Salivary	Amylase found in ptyalin	Starch ⟶ Maltose	Physical as well as chemical hydrolysis Mucus flow starts here and continues throughout digestive tract
Esophagus	Mucus	Mucous	None	Lubrication of food	Peristalsis begins here
Stomach	Gastric juice along with HCL acid	Gastric	Protease, pepsin	Proteins ⟶ peptones and proteoses	Gastrin activates the gastric glands HCL supplies an acidic medium and kills bacteria Temporary food storage
Small intestine	Intestinal	Intestinal	Peptiadases	Peptones and proteoses amino acids	Absorption of end products occurs in small intestine
			Maltase	Maltose ⟶ glucose	Villi facilitates absorption
			Lactase	Lactose ⟶ glucose and galactose	
			Sucrase	Sucrose ⟶ glucose and fructose	
			Lipase	Fats ⟶ fatty acids and glycerol	
	Bile	Liver	None	Emulsifies fat	Neutralizes stomach acid
	Pancreatic	Pancreas	Protease (trypsin)	Proteins ⟶ peptones, and amino acids	Secretin stimulates the flow of pancreatic juice
			Amylase (amylopsin)	Starch ⟶ maltose	
			Lipase (steapsin)	Fats ⟶ fatty acids and glycerol	
			Nucleases	Nucleic acids (DNA/RNA) nucleotides	

Further Study and Discussion

- Discuss reasons for giving hospital patients dilute glucose solution through their veins instead of a regular diet by mouth.

Assignment

A. Match each term in column I with its description in column II.

Column I	Column II
_____ 1. small intestine	a. substances which contain enzymes capable of acting on the digestion of proteins, starch and fats
_____ 2. end result of protein digestion	
_____ 3. villi	b. tiny projections in the small intestines which greatly increase absorption area
_____ 4. pancreatic juice	
_____ 5. enzymes of intestinal juice	c. receives the undigested portion of food at the end of the alimentary canal
_____ 6. duodenum	
_____ 7. liver bile	d. region into which bile from the liver and pancreatic juice are poured
_____ 8. large intestine	
_____ 9. glucose	e. amino acids
_____ 10. usable products of fat metabolism	f. fatty acids and glycerin
	g. sucrose
	h. is about 25 feet long and one inch wide
	i. emulsifies fat
	j. digestive juice for fat metabolism
	k. substance which may result from the breakdown of starch
	l. enzymes which complete digestion of proteins and carbohydrates

B. Briefly answer the following questions:

1. What are the three juices that are of importance in small intestinal digestion?

2. Name the four different types of enzymes contained in pancreatic juice.

3. Why must fat be emulsified before fat digestion can occur?

4. What will lactase and sucrase digest?

5. What are the names of the two bile pigments? How are they formed?

THE LARGE INTESTINE

KEY WORDS

anal sphincter	colonic stasis	laxative
anus	defecation	mass peristalsis
appendicitis	descending colon	nonpathogenic
ascending colon	feces	rectal columns
bowel	hemorrhoids	rectum
cathartic	(piles)	sigmoid colon
cecum	ileocecal (colic)	transverse colon
cellulose	valve	vermiform
colon		appendix

OBJECTIVES

- Locate the large intestine
- Describe the functions of the large intestine
- List foods which aid the function of the colon
- Define the Key Words related to this unit of study

The large intestine, or **colon,** is 1.5 meters long (about 5 feet) and 2 inches in diameter (twice as wide as the small intestine). It is called the large intestine because of its larger lumen. The colon forms three sides of a square starting at the lower right hand corner of the abdominal cavity (up, across, and down).

CECUM AND APPENDIX

The ileum empties its intestinal chyme into the side wall of the colon through an opening called the **colic** or **ileocecal valve,** figure 31–1. This valve permits passage of the intestinal chyme toward the colon, while preventing backsliding into the ileum. Located slightly below this valve, in the lower right portion of the abdomen, is a blind pouch which we call the **cecum.**

Just below the ileocecal valve, to the lower left of the cecum, is the **vermiform appendix.** The appendix is a finger-like projection protruding into the abdominal cavity. It has no

digestive function. Because the appendix is a blind sac, it fills up easily, but drains quite slowly; substances can remain within the appendix for prolonged periods. Irritation of the lining of the appendix, which may be caused by hard or rough materials, can make it a suitable area for bacterial growth. This often leads to the painful inflammatory condition known as **appendicitis.**

COLON

The colon continues upward, along the right side of the abdominal cavity, to the underside of the liver, forming the **ascending colon.** Then it veers abruptly to the left of the abdominal cavity, near the level of the third lumbar vertebra, forming the **transverse colon.** The **descending colon** travels down the left side of the abdominal cavity. As the descending colon reaches the left iliac region, it enters the pelvis in an S-shaped bend. This section is known as the **sigmoid colon,** which extends

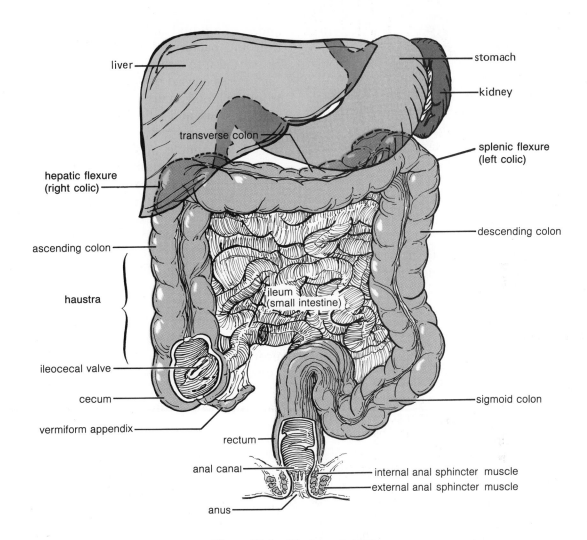

liver

stomach

kidney

transverse colon

splenic flexure
(left colic)

hepatic flexure
(right colic)

descending colon

ascending colon

haustra

ileum
(small intestine)

ileocecal valve

cecum

sigmoid colon

vermiform appendix

rectum

anal canal

internal anal sphincter muscle

external anal sphincter muscle

anus

Figure 31-1   The large intestine

some 7 or 8 inches as the **rectum.** The rectum opens exteriorly into the anus.

ANAL CANAL

The anal canal is the last portion of the large intestine; its external opening is the anus. The anus is guarded by two **anal sphincter muscles.** One is an internal sphincter of smooth, involuntary muscle, the other an external sphincter of striated, voluntary muscle. Both of these remain contracted to close the anal opening until defecation takes place. The mucous membrane lining the anal canal is folded into vertical folds called **rectal columns.** Within each rectal column is an artery and a vein. The condition leading to inflammation or enlargement of the rectal column veins is known as **hemorrhoids,** or **piles.**

FUNCTIONS OF THE LARGE INTESTINE

The large intestine is concerned with water absorption, bacterial action, fecal formation, and defecation. The purpose of these functions is to regulate the body's water balance while storing and excreting waste products of digestion.

Water Absorption

The large intestine aids in the regulation of the body's water balance by absorbing large quantities of water back into the bloodstream. The water is drawn from the undigested food and indigestible material (like cellulose) that pass through the colon.

Bacterial Action

A few hours following the birth of an infant, the lining of the colon starts to accumulate bacteria. These bacteria enter the body via ingested food and persist throughout the person's lifetime. A proportion of the bacteria are destroyed by the action of hydrochloric acid contained in gastric juice in the stomach. Those bacteria that survive are passed along to the colon, where they multiply rapidly, to form the bacterial population or flora, of the colon. The intestinal bacteria are harmless (**nonpathogenic**) to their host. They act upon the undigested food remains, turning them into acids, amines, gases, and other waste products. Some of these decomposed products are eventually excreted through the colon. Another benefit of the bacterial action is the synthesis (formation) of moderate amounts of B-complex vitamins and vitamin K (needed for blood clotting).

Fecal Formation

Initially, the undigested or indigestible material in the colon contains a lot of water and is in a liquid state. Due to water absorption and bacterial action, it is subsequently converted into a semisolid form, called feces.

Feces consist of bacteria, waste products from the blood, acids, amines, inorganic salts, gases, mucus, and cellulose. The acids are acetic, butyric, and lactic. Amines that are produced are indole and skatole. Amines are waste products of amino acids. The gases are ammonia, carbon dioxide, hydrogen, hydrogen sulfide, and methane. The characteristically foul odor of feces derives from these substances — especially indole, skatole, and hydrogen sulfide.

Cellulose is the fibrous part of plants that humans are unable to digest. It contributes to the bulk of the feces. This bulk stimulates the muscular activity of the colon, resulting in defecation. Regular **defecation** (regularity) can be promoted by exercising daily and eating foods containing bulk, like whole-grain cereals, fruits and vegetables. These foods supply the necessary roughage to initiate bowel movements.

Defecation

Once approximately every 12 hours, the fecal material moves into the lower **bowel** (lower colon and rectum) by means of a series of long contractions called **mass peristalsis.** When the rectum becomes distended with the accumulation of feces, a defecation reflex is triggered. Nerve endings in the rectum are stimulated, and a nerve impulse is transmitted to the spinal cord. From the spinal cord, nerve impulses are sent to the colon, rectum, and internal anal sphincter. This causes the colon and rectal muscles to contract and the internal sphincter to relax, resulting in emptying of the bowels.

For defecation to occur, the external anal sphincter must also be relaxed. The external anal sphincter surrounds and guards the outer opening of the anus and is under conscious control. Due to this control, defecation can be prevented when inconvenient, despite the defecation reflex. However, if this urge is continually ignored, it lessens or disappears totally, resulting in constipation, or **colonic stasis.** Temporary relief from constipation may be obtained with the use of **laxatives** and **cathartics.** (A laxative is a substance that induces gentle bowel movement; a cathartic stimulates more vigorous movement, which may eventually reduce the bowel's muscle tone.)

Further Study and Discussion

- Discuss what effect waste products could have on the general health were they not removed from the intestines.

- Discuss the special care needs of a person on bedrest based upon the information in this unit.

- Prepare a list of foods commonly recommended for persons suffering from constipation.

Assignment

A. Briefly answer the following questions.

  1. What causes constipation?

  2. What is the function of the large intestine other than storage and elimination of wastes?

B. Read each statement carefully and determine if it is true or false. Encircle the letter *T* for true or *F* for false.

T   F   1. The large intestine is called the colon.

T   F   2. The large intestine is 20 feet long and 2 inches wide.

T   F   3. The cecum is located where the small intestine joins the large intestine.

T   F   4. The function of the appendix is unknown.

T   F   5. The large intestine stores and eliminates the waste products of digestion.

T   F   6. Regulation of water balance occurs in the large intestine because its lining absorbs water.

T   F   7. Constipation may be overcome by intensive and long periods of work and exercise.

T   F   8. Bulk foods such as whole-grain cereals, fruits and vegetables may help avoid constipation.

T   F   9. The rectum is an extension of the descending colon.

T   F   10. The transverse colon lies between the ascending and the descending colon.

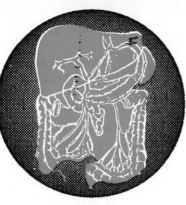

UNIT 32

ROLE OF NUTRIENTS, VITAMINS, AND MINERALS IN HEALTH CARE

KEY WORDS

anorexia nervosa
bulimia
calorie
cholesterol
complete proteins
essential amino
  acids

incomplete
  proteins
kilocalorie
microgram
milligram
mineral
nutrient

nutritionist
obesity
osteoporosis
roughage
RDA
trace element
vitamin

OBJECTIVES

■ Define the term nutrient
■ Identify the different types of nutrients
■ Describe the function(s) of the different types of nutrients
■ Differentiate between the fat-soluble and water-soluble vitamins
■ Describe the concept of "Recommended Daily Dietary Allowances"
■ List the Dietary Guidelines for Americans
■ Define the Key Words relating to this unit of study

The pace of an active daily life can at times be hectic and stress-filled. This can occasionally cause one to eat "on the run," to "grab a bite" at a fast-food restaurant, or to forget to eat nutritiously.

The food one eats and drinks may or may not be nutritious. For food to be nutritious, it must contain the materials needed by the individual cells for proper cell functioning. These materials or **nutrients** are:

- water
- carbohydrates
- lipids
- proteins
- minerals
- vitamins

WATER

Water is an essential component of all body tissues. It has several important functions in the human body:

- Acts as a solvent for all biochemical reactions
- Serves as a transport medium for substances

Portions of this unit were contributed by Loretta Chiarenza, M.A., M.S., Associate Professor of Biology and Associate Dean, State University of New York at Farmingdale, Farmingdale, NY 11735.

- Functions as a lubricant for joint movement and the digestive tract

- Controls body temperature by evaporation from the pores of the skin

- Serves as a cushion for body organs, such as the lungs and brain

Water makes up between 55 percent and 65 percent of our total body weight. The body is continually losing water through evaporation, excretion, and respiration. This water loss must be replaced. We supply some of this need by drinking plain water. However, most of the body's water comes from the food we eat (including liquids). Practically all the foods we eat contain water, even those that seem to be dry.

Water is the only nutrient we can sense a need for. When the body needs water, we experience thirst.

CARBOHYDRATES

Carbohydrates include simple sugars, such as monosaccharides like glucose ($C_6H_{12}O_6$), and some longer molecules that contain a number of monosaccharides joined together. Depending upon the number of simple sugars found in the carbohydrate, they are classified as monosaccharides, disaccharides, or polysaccharides. Only the monosaccharides are small enough to be absorbed and eventually taken into the cells. The other carbohydrates are broken down by digestion in the digestive tract into the smallest possible molecular subunits prior to absorption.

Carbohydrates are the main source of energy for the body. Excess carbohydrates are converted into fat and stored in fat tissue. **Nutritionists** recommend that carbohydrates comprise between 50 percent and 60 percent of the daily intake of calories.

A **calorie** is a unit that measures the amount of energy contained within the chemical bonds of different foods. The small calorie is defined as the amount of heat required to raise the temperature of one gram of water by one degree Celsius. A **kilocalorie** or large calorie is equal to 1000 small calories. The calorie content of food is determined by measuring the amount of heat released when food is burned. The energy content of fat (9 kilocalories per gram) is slightly more than twice that of carbohydrate (4 kilocalories per gram) or protein (4 kilocalories per gram).

A normal adult usually requires between 1600 and 3000 kilocalories a day depending on age, sex, body weight, and degree of physical activity. Newborn infants and young children have higher energy requirements per unit of body weight than adults because of the high energy expenditure of growth. See Table 32–1 for daily recommended energy intakes.

An excess of the wrong foods can cause an overweight condition called **obesity**. Obesity usually results when we take in more calories than we use. There are carbohydrates that should be avoided or minimized in the daily diet. These foods are candies, cakes, cookies, jams, sugar-coated cereals, and sugary soft drinks. All of these foods contain large amounts of highly refined carbohydrates as sugar. They supply calories, but little else. Energy obtained from such foods is commonly referred to as "empty calories." Intake of these foods can also contribute to tooth decay. Foods containing starches and cellulose are a healthier source of carbohydrates. These foods, besides providing energy, can also provide needed minerals, roughage, and vitamins. **Roughage** is the undigestible part of food. Examples are whole grain breads and cereals, fruits, vegetables, macaroni, rice, and potatoes.

LIPIDS

Lipids are a group of compounds containing fatty acids combined with an alcohol. They

Table 32–1 Mean Heights and Weights and Recommended Energy Intake*

Category	Age, years	Weight		Height		Energy needs (with range)	
		kg	lb	cm	in.	kcal	
Infants	0.0-0.5	6	13	60	24	kg × 115	(95-145)
	0.5-1.0	9	20	71	28	kg × 105	(80-135)
Children	1-3	13	29	90	35	1300	(900-1800)
	4-6	20	44	112	44	1700	(1300-2300)
	7-10	28	62	132	52	2400	(1650-3300)
Males	11-14	45	99	157	62	2700	(2000-3700)
	15-18	66	145	176	69	2800	(2100-3900)
	19-22	70	154	177	70	2900	(2500-3300)
	23-50	70	154	178	70	2700	(2300-3100)
	51-75	70	154	178	70	2400	(2000-2800)
	76 +	70	154	178	70	2050	(1650-2450)
Females	11-14	46	101	157	62	2200	(1500-3000)
	15-18	55	120	163	64	2100	(1200-3000)
	19-22	55	120	163	64	2100	(1700-2500)
	23-50	55	120	163	64	2000	(1600-2400)
	51-75	55	120	163	64	1800	(1400-2200)
	76 +	55	120	163	64	1600	(1200-2000)
Pregnancy						+ 300	
Lactation						+ 500	

*The data in this table have been assembled from the observed median heights and weights of children, together with desirable weights for adults for the mean heights of men (70 inches) and women (64 inches) between the ages of 18 and 34 years as surveyed in the U.S. population.

The energy allowances for the young adults are for men and women doing light work. The allowances for the two older age groups represent mean energy needs over these age spans, allowing for a 2-percent decrease in basal (resting) metabolic rate per decade and a reduction in activity of 200 kcal/day for men and women between 51 and 75 years, 500 kcal for men over 75 years, and 400 kcal for women over 73 years. The customary range of daily energy output is shown in parentheses for adults and is based on a variation in energy needs of ±400 kcal at any one age, emphasizing the wide range of energy intakes appropriate for any group of people.

Energy allowances for children through age 18 are based on median energy intakes of children of these ages followed in longitudinal growth studies. The values in parentheses are 10th and 90th percentiles of energy intake, to indicate the range of energy consumption among children of these ages.

Source: Recommended Dietary Allowances, Revised 1980, Food and Nutrition Board, National Academy of Sciences—National Research Council.

can be subdivided into two groups: simple lipids (fats, oils, waxes) and compound lipids (phospholipids, glycolipids, sterols). Like carbohydrates, fats are a source of energy. The same amount of fats can release more than twice as many calories as the same amount of carbohydrate or protein. The human body stores reserves of energy as fat in fat cells. Likewise, any excess carbohydrate and protein in the diet is transformed into fat and stored along with any excess fat.

Fats are an essential nutrient to the maintenance of the human body. Stored fats provide a supply of energy during emergencies such as sickness or during deficient caloric intakes. Fats also cushion the internal organs and serve as an insulation against the cold. Fats are components of the cell membrane, and contribute to the formation of bile and steroid hormones, such as the sex hormones. Fats also contain certain kinds of vitamins called fat-soluble vitamins which are an important part of our daily diet. It is therefore essential to have a diet containing fats without exceeding the body's calorie needs. Total daily dietary fat intake should not exceed 25 percent to 30 percent of the daily caloric intake.

A common animal fat is **cholesterol**. Cholesterol is found in the cell membranes of animal cells; it is the fat necessary for the formation of bile and for the steroid hormones. In addition, cholesterol in our skin is activated by sunlight to become vitamin D. Unfortunately, in certain people, cholesterol is also involved in the formation of arterial plaques which contribute to heart disease by blocking the passage of blood through the blood vessels.

PROTEINS

Proteins are structurally more complex than carbohydrates and lipids and contain an amino (NH_2) group. They are synthesized in the cell cytoplasm from constituent molecules called **amino acids**.

Proteins serve many different functions in the body. Some are enzymes and regulate the rate of chemical reactions; others are important in growth and repair of tissues. When necessary, proteins can also be used as a source of energy. In addition, contractile systems (muscles), hormonal systems, plasma transport systems, clotting and defense systems (antibodies) are all dependent upon proteins.

The body can synthesize some amino acids, but not all. The amino acids that cannot be made in the body are **"essential" amino acids**. Proteins that contain all the essential amino acids are known as **complete proteins**. Sources of such complete proteins are eggs, meat, milk, and milk products. Proteins that do not contain all the essential amino acids are called **incomplete proteins**. Vegetables contain incomplete proteins. However, a varied diet including vegetables will supply all the necessary complete proteins. For example, beans and wheat eaten alone will not provide all of

the necessary complete proteins. However, when eaten together, they will complement each other and supply the necessary complete proteins.

Unlike fats, the human body is unable to store excess amino acids. Any unused amino acids are broken down by the body, and the amino group is excreted as a nitrogenous waste product called **urea**. The remainder of the amino acid may be burned for immediate energy or stored as fat or glycogen, a polysaccharide.

Protein synthesis cannot occur without all of the essential amino acids present at the same time. Therefore, it is important to include some source of complete protein throughout the various foods we eat during the day. The daily intake of calories from proteins should be no more than 15 percent to 20 percent.

Most adults in the United States eat a daily intake of protein in excess of the recommended dietary allowance. This practice puts an extra burden on the liver, which produces urea during the degradation of proteins, and on the kidney, which must eliminate the urea from the body.

MINERALS AND TRACE ELEMENTS

A **mineral** is a chemical element that is obtained from inorganic compounds in food. Our knowledge of the role of the essential minerals and trace elements is incomplete. Many are notably necessary for normal human growth and maintenance.

Among the most important of these nutrients are sodium, potassium, calcium, iron, phosphorous, and zinc.

Trace elements are present in the body in very small amounts. These include zinc, copper, iodine, cobalt, manganese, selenium, chromium, molybdenum, and fluorine.

The toxic limits of some trace elements are extremely close to the required dosages. This means that there is a critical difference between toxicity, health, and deficiency. Most of the essential minerals and trace elements are already present in the average normal American diet in sufficient concentrations, and supplementation is only indicated for special conditions of disease, during pregnancy, and old age. However, governmental surveys indicate that females in the United States might be consuming less than optimal daily intakes of calcium and iron.

Age-related **osteoporosis** is one of the most severely debilitating diseases in the United States and the most prevalent bone disease in the world. It is characterized by a decreased mass of bone which increases the risk of fractures. While the question of whether osteoporosis is a nutritional disorder remains unanswered, there is much convincing evidence that calcium deficiency accelerates the age-related loss of bone. The hormonal consequences of female menopause result in diminished calcium absorption in the intestines. This physiological consequence of reduced estrogen output, along with lower bone density in females than in males during young adulthood, requires that proper attention be paid to calcium intake throughout the life cycle to maximize peak bone density prior to menopause.

Women of child-bearing age have a tendency to be in low iron status because of blood loss during the menstrual flow. Fatigue and iron deficiency anemia in these women can usually be ameliorated by iron supplementation. Table 32–2 summarizes the most important minerals and trace elements in the human diet.

VITAMINS

A **vitamin** is defined as a biologically active organic compound, often functioning as a coenzyme, that is necessary for normal health and growth. Most enzymatic activity relies on the presence of coenzymes. A dietary deficiency of a vitamin results in a subclinical or obvious specific disorder. The term vitamin usually implies that the substance is not synthesized within the organism and, as a result, must be obtained from the diet. Vitamins are transported by the circulatory system to all the tissues of the body.

Recent evidence indicates that certain vitamins actually behave like hormones physiologically. For instance, both vitamin D and niacin are synthesized in the human (in inadequate amounts) conferring on them hormonal qualities, since hormones are produced in the body. The fat-soluble vitamins A, D, E, and K) are readily stored in the body, and within the cell they demonstrate many similarities to the steroid hormones (estrogen, testosterone, cortisol). The water-soluble vitamins are B_1, B_2, B_3, B_6, B_{12}, pantothenic acid, folic acid, biotin, and vitamin C. An excessive intake of these vitamins results in increased excretion rather than additional storage.

Certain conditions such as pregnancy, disease, emotional stress, old-age, and vitamin destruction caused by methods of processing, storage, and preparing of foods must be considered when determining daily individual vitamin requirements. Table 32–3 summarizes the major vitamins needed in the human diet.

BIOCHEMICAL INDIVIDUALITY AND RECOMMENDED DAILY DIETARY ALLOWANCES

Developing universal "minimum daily requirements" that can apply to everyone is an extremely difficult task. Nutritional requirements among individuals might vary for several reasons. Malabsorption disorders sometimes require that an individual needs greater than the average daily dosage of certain nutri-

Table 32–2 Summary of Essential Minerals and Trace Elements Needed for Health

MINERAL	FOOD SOURCES	FUNCTION	DEFICIENCY DISEASES
Calcium	Milk, cheese, dark green vegetables, dried legumes, sardines, shellfish	Bone and tooth formation Blood clotting Nerve transmission	Stunted growth Rickets Osteoporosis Convulsions
Chlorine	Common table salt, seafood, milk, meat, eggs	Formation of gastric juices Acid-base balance	Muscle cramps Mental apathy Poor appetite
Chromium	Fats, vegetable oils, meats, clams, whole-grain cereals	Involved in energy and glucose metabolism	Impaired ability to metabolize glucose
Copper	Drinking water, liver, shellfish, whole grains, cherries, legumes, kidney, poultry, oysters, nuts, chocolate	Constituent of enzymes Involved with iron transport	Anemia
Fluorine	Drinking water, tea, coffee, seafood, rice, spinach, onions, lettuce	Maintenance of bone and tooth structure	Higher frequency of tooth decay
Iodine	Marine fish and shellfish, dairy products, many vegetables, iodized salt	Constituent of thyroid hormones	Goiter (enlarged thyroid)
Iron	Liver, lean meats, legumes, whole grains, dark green vegetables, eggs, dark molasses, shrimp, oysters	Constituent of hemoglobin Involved in energy metabolism	Iron-deficiency anemia
Magnesium	Whole grains, green leafy vegetables, nuts, meats, milk, legumes	Involved in energy conversions and enzyme function	Growth failure Behavioral disturbances Weakness Spasms
Phosphorus	Milk, cheese, meat, fish, poultry, whole grains, legumes, nuts	Bone and tooth formation Acid-base balance Involved in energy metabolism	Weakness Demineralization of bone
Potassium	Meats, milk, fruits, legumes, vegetables	Acid-base balance Body water balance Nerve transmission	Muscular weakness Paralysis
Selenium	Fish, poultry, meats, grains, milk, vegetables (depending on amount in soil)	Necessary for vitamin E function	Anemia Increased mortality?
Sodium	Common table salt, seafood, most other foods except fruit	Acid-base balance Body water balance Nerve transmission	Muscle cramps Mental apathy
Sulfur	Meat, fish, poultry, eggs, milk, cheese, legumes, nuts	Constituent of certain tissue proteins	Related to deficiencies of sulfur-containing amino acids
Zinc	Milk, liver, shellfish, herring, wheat bran	Involved in many enzyme systems Necessary for vitamin A metabolism	Growth failure Lack of sexual maturity Impaired wound healing Poor appetite

Table 32–3 Summary of Major Vitamins Needed in the Human Diet

VITAMIN	FOOD SOURCES	FUNCTION	DEFICIENCY DISEASES
A (Fat soluble)	Butter, fortified margarine, green and yellow vegetables, milk, eggs, liver	Night vision Healthy skin Proper growth and repair of body tissues	Night blindness Dry skin Slow growth Poor gums and teeth
B_1 (thiamine) (Water-soluble)	Chicken, fish, meat, eggs, enriched bread, whole grain cereals	Promotes normal appetite and digestion Needed by nervous system	Loss of appetite Nervous disorders Fatigue Severe deficiency causes beriberi
B_2 (riboflavin) (Water-soluble)	Cheese, eggs, fish, meat, liver, milk, cereals, enriched bread	Needed in cellular respiration	Eye problems Sores on skin and lips General fatigue
B_3 (niacin) (Water-soluble)	Eggs, fish, liver, meat, milk, potatoes, enriched bread	Needed for normal metabolism Growth Proper skin health	Indigestion Diarrhea Headaches Mental disturbances Skin disorders
B_{12} (Cyanocobalamin) (Water-soluble)	Milk, liver, brain, beef, egg yolk, clams, oysters, sardines, salmon	Red blood cell synthesis Nucleic acid synthesis Nerve cell maintenance	Pernicious anemia Nerve cell malfunction
Folic Acid (Water-soluble)	Liver, yeast, green vegetables, peanuts, mushrooms, beef, veal, egg yolk	Nucleic acid synthesis Needed for normal metabolism and growth	Anemia Growth retardation
C (ascorbic acid) (Water-soluble)	Citrus fruits, cabbage, green vegetables, tomatoes, potatoes	Needed for maintenance of normal bones, gums, teeth, and blood vessels	Weak bones Sore and bleeding gums Poor teeth Bleeding in skin Painful joints Severe deficiency results in scurvy
D (Fat-soluble)	Beef, butter, eggs, milk	Needed for normal bone and teeth development Controls calcium and phosphorus metabolism	Poor bone and teeth structure Soft bones Rickets
E (tocopherol) (Fat-soluble)	Margarine, nuts, leafy vegetables, vegetable oils, whole wheat	Used in cell respiration Protects red blood cells from destruction	Anemia in premature infants No known deficiency in adults
K (Fat-soluble)	Synthesized by colon bacteria Green leafy vegetables, cereal	Essential for normal blood clotting	Slow blood clotting

ents. Differences in the microbial environment of the intestine, and genetic factors influencing biochemical reactions must also be considered. People experiencing psychological or physical stress often require a greater amount of certain nutrients to help the body maintain homeostasis or a relatively constant internal environment.

In recognition of individual variations in nutritional requirements, a table of **Recommended Dietary Allowances (RDA)** (see Table 32–4) has been approved by the Food and Nutrition Board, National Academy of Sciences. It contains the daily recommendations for protein, fat-soluble vitamins, water-soluble vitamins, and minerals. The allowances are intended to provide for individual variations among most normal persons as they live in the United States under usual environmental stresses.

DIETARY GUIDELINES FOR AMERICANS

Recently, a Scientific Advisory Committee was appointed by the United States Government to develop Dietary Guidelines for the American public. The importance of consuming a diet of a variety of foods to provide the essential nutrients at a caloric level to maintain desirable body weight is emphasized. The following specific guidelines are advocated by the Committee to help prevent the most prevalent and devastating diseases in our society: diabetes, cancer, hypertension, and heart disease.

1. Eat a variety of foods
2. Maintain desirable weight
3. Avoid too much fat, saturated fat (mostly animal fat), and cholesterol
4. Eat foods with adequate starch and fiber (roughage)
5. Avoid too much sugar
6. Avoid too much sodium
7. If you drink alcoholic beverages, do so in moderation.

EATING DISORDERS

Obesity is one of the most common "nutritional diseases" in our society. An obese person is one who contains excess body fat and who weighs fifteen percent more than the optimum body weight for gender, height, and bone structure.

Being obese can affect physical and mental health. Heart disease, high blood pressure, and non-insulin dependent diabetes mellitus are more common in significantly overweight people than in those closer to ideal body weight.

Since most cases of obesity are due to an excessive intake of calories in proportion to expenditure, a daily reduction of caloric intake along with an increase in exercise are recommended for most overweight individuals.

Unfortunately, the desire to be thin has resulted in a complex disorder, mostly seen in young women, called **anorexia nervosa.** In true anorexia nervosa, there is no real loss of appetite, but rather a refusal to eat because of a distorted body image and a fear of weight gain.

The criteria for diagnoisis of anorexia nervosa are identified by the American Psychiatric Association as follows:

1. Intense fear of becoming obese that does not diminish as weight loss progresses
2. Disturbance of body image, such as claiming to feel fat even when emaciated
3. Weight loss of at least twenty-five percent of the original body weight
4. Refusal to maintain body weight over

Table 32–4 1980 Recommended Dietary Allowances

Age and Sex Group	Weight		Height		Protein	Fat-soluble Vitamins			Water-soluble Vitamins		
						Vitamin A *μg R.E.**	Vitamin D *μg†*	Vitamin E *mgᵅ T.E.‡*	Vitamin C *mg*	Thiamin *mg*	Riboflavin *mg*
	kg	lb	cm	in							
Infants											
0.0-0.5 yr	6	13	60	24	kg × 2.2	420	10	3	35	0.3	0.4
0.5-1.0 yr	9	20	71	28	kg × 2.0	400	10	4	35	0.5	0.6
Children											
1-3 yr	13	29	90	35	23	400	10	5	45	0.7	0.8
4-6 yr	20	44	112	44	30	500	10	6	45	0.9	1.0
7-10 yr	28	62	132	52	34	700	10	7	45	1.2	1.4
Males											
11-14 yr	45	99	157	62	45	1,000	10	8	50	1.4	1.6
15-18 yr	66	145	176	69	56	1,000	10	10	60	1.4	1.7
19-22 yr	70	154	177	70	56	1,000	7.5	10	60	1.5	1.7
23-50 yr	70	154	178	70	56	1,000	5	10	60	1.4	1.6
51 + yr	70	154	178	70	56	1,000	5	10	60	1.2	1.4
Females											
11-14 yr	46	101	157	62	46	800	10	8	50	1.1	1.3
15-18 yr	55	120	163	64	46	800	10	8	60	1.1	1.3
19-22 yr	55	120	163	64	44	800	7.5	8	60	1.1	1.3
23-50 yr	55	120	163	64	44	800	5	8	60	1.0	1.2
51 + yr	55	120	163	64	44	800	5	8	60	1.0	1.2
Pregnancy					+ 30	+ 200	+ 5	+ 2	+ 20	+ 0.4	+ 0.3
Lactation					+ 20	+ 400	+ 5	+ 3	+ 40	+ 0.5	+ 0.5

1μg = 0.000,001 g
mg = 0.001 g
IU = International Unit

* Retinol equivalents; 1 retinol equivalent = 1μg retinol or 6μg β-carotene.
† As cholecalciferol: 10 μg cholecalciferol = 400 IU Vitamin D.

a minimal normal weight for age and height

5. No known physical illness that would account for the weight loss

6. Amenorrhea, or the cessation of menstruation

Another eating disorder associated with a fear of weight gain is **bulimia.** It is characterized by episodic binge eating followed by purging behavior such as self-induced vomiting and laxative abuse. Bulimic patients are most often women somewhat older than those with anorexia nervosa. In some instances, a young woman alternates between the two disorders.

The treatment of anorexia nervosa and bulimia is difficult and lengthy. The goals are restitution of normal nutrition and resolution of the underlying psychological problems. Early intervention is essential; the starvation associated with anorexia can cause irreversible tissue damage and the purging associated with bulimia can cause homeostatic imbalances that lead to cardiac irregularities and, in extreme cases, to death.

Further Study and Discussion

- Explain why a fat-free diet can result in a vitamin deficiency disorder.

- Explain why age-related bone loss is more of a problem in females than in males.

- Explain why some individuals might need more of a particular nutrient than the general population.

Assignment

1. What is a nutrient?

2. List the different nutrients.

3. What is the physiological function of carbohydrates? List some common food sources.

4. What physiological functions do proteins contribute to in the human body?

5. What physiological functions do fats contribute to in the human body?

6. List the fat-soluble vitamins and their physiological functions.

7. List the water-soluble vitamins and their physiological functions.

8. List the food sources of dietary iron.

9. List the Dietary Guidelines.

10. What is the most common cause of obesity?

REPRESENTATIVE DISORDERS OF THE DIGESTIVE SYSTEM

KEY WORDS

appendicitis
benign
carcinoma
chemotherapy
cholecystitis
cirrhosis
colitis
constipation
diarrhea
enteritis

gallstones
gastritis
gastroenteritis
"heartburn"
hiatal hernia
icterus
infectious
    hepatitis
jaundice

malignant
metastasize
mucus colitis
pancreatitis
peptic ulcer
peritonitis
pyloric stenosis
serum hepatitis
stomatitis

OBJECTIVES

- Identify common disorders which interfere with digestion
- Relate general treatment to these common disorders
- Define the Key Words relating to this unit of study

It is well to know the common disorders of the digestive system and the general treatment of them. Some of these are briefly described in this unit.

Stomatitis

Stomatitis is an inflammation of the soft tissues of the mouth cavity. Pain and salivation may occur also.

Hiatal Hernia

Hiatal hernia, or rupture, occurs when the stomach protrudes above the diaphragm through the esophagus opening. Changes in the diet may relieve the heartburn; surgery is not usually required.

Heartburn

So-called **"heartburn"** results from a backflow of the highly acidic gastric juice into the lower end of the esophagus. This irritates the lining of the esophagus, causing a burning sensation. Some individuals suffer chronic heartburn, occasioned by improper closure of the cardiac constrictor muscle at the junction of the esophagus and stomach. Temporary relief from this condition can usually be obtained by ingesting a solution of bicarbonate of soda. This is an alkaline, or basic substance that will neutralize the stomach's gastric juices.

Gastritis

Gastritis is an acute or chronic inflammation of the mucous membrane lining the stomach. It may be caused by irritants such as highly spiced foods or some drugs. There are many forms of gastritis, including:

- Atrophic gastritis — a chronic form in which the mucous membrane of the stomach has atrophied.

- Corrosive gastritis — this is an acute form of gastritis caused by corrosive poisons.

- Infectious gastritis — acute gastritis, associated with infectious diseases such as measles and scarlet fever.

Peptic Ulcers

Peptic ulcers are lesions which occur in either the stomach (gastric ulcers) or small intestine (duodenal ulcers). This condition affects approximately 1 of 10 adults in the United States, usually affecting 4 times as many men as women.

Increased psychological stress contributes to the development of peptic ulcers. The ulcers result from insufficient mucus secretion, and from oversecretion of gastric juice containing hydrochloric acid in the stomach. This process wears away the stomach's mucosal wall; it may even perforate the stomach or duodenum, leading to peritonitis and hemorrhage.

Most peptic ulcers are of the duodenal types. The pain accompanying a duodenal ulcer comes from the irritation of exposed nerves and muscle cells near the ulcer. Temporary relief from pain can be obtained by ingesting alkaline substances to neutralize stomach acid. These substances can neutralize the hydrochloric acid in the gastric juice and delay emptying of the stomach.

The characteristic burning pain associated with a peptic ulcer appears 2–3 hours after eating. By then, the food within the stomach has passed along into the small intestine; only the acid from the stomach is entering the duodenum.

Pyloric Stenosis

Pyloric stenosis is a narrowing of the pyloric sphincter at the lower end of the stomach. It is often found in infants. Projectile vomiting may result; surgery is often necessary.

Gastroenteritis

Gastroenteritis is the inflammation of the mucous membrane lining of the stomach and intestinal tract. This is a common disorder of infants and may lead to severe diarrhea and dehydration.

Enteritis

Enteritis is the inflammation of the intestine that may be caused by a bacterial, viral, or protozoan infection. For example, cholera and typhoid fever are caused by bacteria, the intestinal "flu" by a virus, and amebic dysentery by a protozoan. Enteritis can also be caused by an allergic reaction to certain foods or food poisoning.

Colitis

Colitis is a condition where the colon becomes inflamed. Colitis is often accompanied by excessive mucus secretion ("mucus colitis").

Appendicitis

Appendicitis occurs when the veriform appendix becomes inflamed. If it ruptures, the bacteria from the appendix can spread to the peritoneal cavity causing **peritonitis**.

Infectious Hepatitis

Infectious hepatitis is a viral infection of the liver, often spread through contaminated water or food. Symptoms include chills, fever, malaise, gastrointestinal disturbances, and jaundice. The skin takes on a yellowish tinge due to the excess bile in the bloodstream.

Serum Hepatitis

Serum hepatitis is an inflammation of the liver caused by a virus found only in the blood.

It is transmitted by a blood transfusion contaminated with the virus or through the use of inadequately sterilized syringes, needles, or surgical equipment. It is prevalent in drug addicts who use dirty hypodermic needles.

Cirrhosis

Cirrhosis is a chronic, progressive inflammatory disease of the liver, characterized by replacement of normal tissue with fibrous connective tissue. It is commonly caused by excessive alcohol consumption.

Jaundice

Jaundice or **icterus** is a disorder where bile pigments are deposited in the skin and mucous membranes giving a yellowish cast to an individual's skin. It can be caused by increased red blood cell phagocytosis by the spleen; blockage of the bile duct, which causes bile to be absorbed into the bloodstream; or infectious or toxic conditions where there is liver tissue damage.

Gallstones

Bile is normally stored in the gallbladder and secreted into the small intestine where fat is emulsified.

Sometimes collections of crystallized cholesterol form in the gallbladder. These are combined with bile salts and bile pigments to form **gallstones.** Gallstones can block the bile duct, causing pain and digestive disorders. In such cases, bile cannot flow into the small intestine to help in fat emulsification, digestion, and absorption. Most gallstones are small and may pass with undigested food. However, the larger and obstructive ones must be surgically removed.

Pancreatitis

Pancreatitis is the inflammation of the pancreas. The pancreas can become edema-

tous, hemorrhagic, or necrotic. Pancreatitis is often associated with alcoholism and obesity. It may be severe or chronic.

Cholecystitis

Cholecystitis is the inflammation of the lining of the gallbladder. The disorder may cause blockage of the cystic duct.

Peritonitis

Peritonitis is a condition in which the serous membrane lining of the abdominal cavity is inflamed. Vomiting and pain are symptoms of this condition.

Diarrhea

If the feces are passed along the colon too rapidly, insufficient water is reabsorbed, and the feces become watery. **Diarrhea** is characterized by loose, watery, and frequent bowel movements. It may result from irritation of the colon's lining by dysentery bacteria, poor diet, nervousness, toxic substances, or from irritants in food (as in prunes, which stimulate intestinal peristalsis).

Excessive water loss from chronic or severe diarrhea may lead to ulcerative colitis. This situation is caused by the rapid flow of digestive juices from the small intestine into the colon. Eventually the action of the digestive juices can lead to ulcers in the colon wall.

Chronic Constipation

Feces eliminated through the rectum are normally in a semisolid state,. When defecation is delayed, however, the colon absorbs excessive water from the feces rendering them dry and hard. When this occurs, defecation (or evacuation) becomes difficult.

For this reason, suppressing the need to defecate at normal times can lead to **constipation.** Constipation can also be caused by emotions such as anxiety, fear, or fright. Headaches and other symptoms that frequently accompany constipation result from the distension of the rectum, as opposed to toxins from the feces.

Treatment usually consists of eating proper foods, especially cereals, fruits and vegetables; drinking plenty of fluids; getting enough exercise; setting regular bowel habits; and avoiding tension as much as possible.

Carcinoma

Carcinoma, or cancer, may occur in any part of the digestive tract. The term "cancer" is a general word applied to a disease characterized by an abnormal and uncontrolled growth of cells. The resulting mass, or tumor, can invade and destroy surrounding normal tissues. Cancer cells from the tumor can spread, or **metastasize,** through the blood or lymph to start new cancerous growths in other parts of the body.

Stomach Cancer

The initial cancer cells that develop in the stomach quickly grow into masses of tissue known as tumors. Such tumors may be benign or malignant. A malignant growth, or tumor, is a cancer.

Benign tumors do not metastasize. They usually can be removed completely and are not likely to recur. A malignant stomach tumor, however, invades neighboring healthy stomach cells and organs.

Malignant stomach cancer cells can spread to other body parts, forming new growths or metastases. Even if the original tumor is surgically removed, the cancer may recur when malignant cancer cells have spread.

The initial symptoms of stomach cancer are much like those of other digestive disorders: heartburn, loss of appetite, persistent indigestion, slight nausea, a feeling of bloated discomfort after eating, and occasional mild stomach pain. Later symptoms include traces of blood in the feces, pain, weight loss, and vomiting.

Treatment involves surgical removal of the stomach tumor as soon as possible. Depending upon the size and the extent of growth of the tumor, part or all of the stomach may have to be removed.

If a stomach cancer has metastasized, surgical removal of the affected parts of neighboring organs, like the pancreas or spleen, is frequently required. But even with the most successful tumor excision, malignant cells can spread throughout the body via the blood. In such cases, **chemotherapy** (treatment with anti-cancer drugs) is prescribed. These drugs are administered into the bloodstream, circulating through the body to kill cancerous cells in any location of the body.

Radiation therapy plays a limited role in the treatment of stomach cancer. Very strong radiation doses are needed to kill the cancer cells, and they might also seriously damage neighboring healthy cells.

Further Study and Discussion

- Discuss problems which result from relieving symptoms such as heartburn and diarrhea with over-the-counter drugs instead of seeking medical advice.

Assignment

A. Match each disorder listed in column I with its description in column II.

Column I	Column II
_____ 1. cirrhosis	a. frequent liquid bowel movements
_____ 2. gastroenteritis	b. chronic liver disease
_____ 3. peptic ulcers	c. protrusion of the stomach into the esophagus
_____ 4. hiatal hernia	
_____ 5. heartburn	d. viral infection of the liver
_____ 6. diarrhea	e. inflammation of the abdominal cavity
_____ 7. cholecystitis	f. obstruction of the hepatic duct
_____ 8. infectious hepatitis	g. inflammation of the stomach and intestinal lining
_____ 9. pyloric stenosis	
_____ 10. peritonitis	h. inflammation of the gallbladder lining
	i. narrowing of sphincter in the stomach
	j. cardiospasm
	k. lesions which may result from acid secretion
	l. common symptoms characterized by a burning sensation

B. Briefly answer the following questions:

1. What are the two possible causes of enteritis?

2. Describe what colitis and appendicitis are.

3. What are the various ways serum hepatitis can be transmitted?

4. Name the various causes of jaundice.

DIGESTION OF FOOD

A. Label the structures in Figure SE6–A which make up the digestive system.

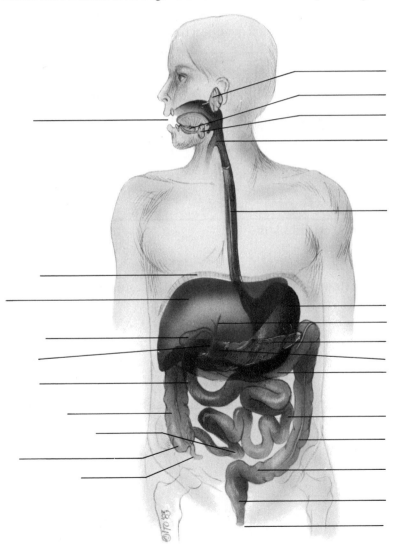

Figure SE6-A

B. Complete the following statements.

1. Substances which act upon foods to change them to simpler soluble forms are called _____ .

2. Teeth used for biting or cutting food are _____ ; those used for grinding are _____ ; and those used for tearing are _____ .

3. Digested food enters the bloodstream by passing through the _____ in the _____ intestine.

4. The main function of the large intestine is _____ and _____ .

5. The three juices which act upon food in the small intestine are _____ , _____ , and _____ .

C. Select the item which best completes the statement.

1. One part of the small intestine is the
   a. rectum   c. pancreas
   b. duodenum   d. appendix

2. The appendix is attached to the
   a. duodenum   c. cecum
   b. rectum   d. pylorus

3. Bile is secreted by the
   a. pancreas   c. stomach
   b. gallbladder   d. liver

4. A substance which requires further digestion to break it down is
   a. fatty acid   c. protein
   b. amino acid   d. glycerol

5. The salivary glands are situated
   a. in the small intestine   c. in the mouth
   b. in the pancreas   d. in the stomach

D. How does the blood differ in its composition before it enters the capillaries of the small intestine and after it leaves?

E. Explain the function of the liver and gallbladder in digestion.

F. Briefly answer the following questions.

1. List the five types of enzymes secreted by the small intestine and their related digestive action.

2. What is appendicitis and serum hepatitis?

3. What causes jaundice?

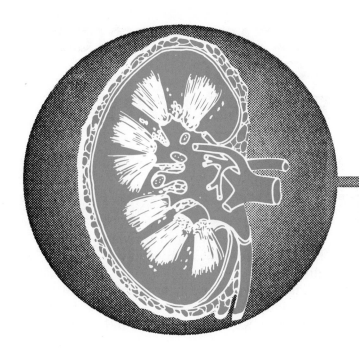

CHAPTER 7

ELIMINATION OF WASTE MATERIALS

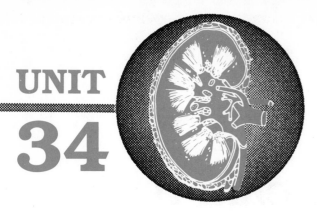

UNIT 34

INTRODUCTION TO THE EXCRETORY SYSTEM

KEY WORDS

excretion   metabolic wastes

OBJECTIVES

- Explain the function of the excretory organs
- List the parts of the body involved in elimination
- Relate the type of waste to the channel of excretion
- Define the Key Words related to this unit of study

Food is utilized through the process of digestion, absorption, and metabolism. These steps separate substances which can be digested from those which cannot. The blood and lymph transport products of digestion to the tissues where they are needed. After the cells of the tissues have used the food and oxygen needed for growth and repair, waste products formed by the process are taken away and excreted from the body. If they were left to accumulate in the body, the waste would act as poisons. The excretory organs eliminate the **metabolic wastes** and undigested food residue.

The channels through which elimination takes place include the kidneys, the skin, the intestines, and the lungs. The lungs, generally considered part of the respiratory system, serve an excretory function in that they give off carbon dioxide and water vapor during exhalation. The urinary system functions largely as an excretory agent of nitrogenous wastes, salts, and water, while the skin includes excretion of the dissolved wastes present in perspiration, mostly dissolved salts. The indigestible residue, water and bacteria are excreted by the intestines. The **excretion** of waste products is described and summarized in table 34–1.

Table 34–1 Elimination of Waste Products

ORGAN	PRODUCT OF EXCRETION	PROCESS OF ELIMINATION
Lungs	carbon dioxide and water vapor	exhalation
Kidneys	nitrogenous wastes and salts dissolved in water to form urine	urination
Skin	dissolved salts	perspiration
Intestines	solid wastes and water	defecation

Further Study and Discussion

- Discuss what may happen to a person if the body does not regularly excrete waste materials.

- Discuss which part of the excretory system performs the most important function.

Assignment

1. What is the function of the excretory organs?

2. What organs are involved in excretion?

3. How are waste products transported to the organs of excretion?

4. Name the excreted waste products of the body.

5. Explain the excretory function of the lungs.

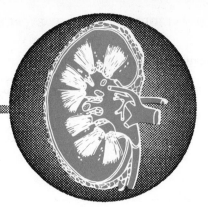

UNIT 35

URINARY SYSTEM

KEY WORDS

adipose capsule
afferent arteriole
antidiuretic
  hormone
Bowman's
  capsule
distal convoluted
  tubule
efferent arteriole
fibrous capsule
glomerulus
hilum (hilus, pl.)
kidney

loop of Henle
nephric filtrate
nephron
osmoreceptor
peritubular
  capillaries
proximal
  convoluted
  tubule
renal column
renal corpuscle
renal cortex

renal fascia
renal medulla
renal papilla
renal pelvis
renal pyramids
reservoir
retroperitoneal
ureter
urethra
urinary bladder
urinary meatus
vasopressin

OBJECTIVES

■ List the organs which make up the urinary system
■ Describe the way the kidneys excrete wastes from the body
■ Explain how the kidneys regulate the water balance
■ Define the Key Words related to this unit of study

The urinary system performs the main part of the excretory function in the body, see color plate 16A. The most important excretory organs are the **kidneys**. Their primary excretory function is removal of the nitrogenous waste products, the result of protein catabolism. If the kidneys fail to function properly, toxic wastes start to accumulate in the body. Toxic wastes accumulating in the cells cause them to "suffocate" and literally poison themselves.

The urinary system consists of two kidneys (that form the urine), two ureters, a bladder, and a urethra. Each kidney has a long, tubular **ureter** that carries urine to the **urinary bladder**. This is a temporary storage sac for urine, from which urine is excreted through the **urethra**.

KIDNEYS

The kidneys are bean-shaped organs resting high against the dorsal wall of the abdominal cavity; they lie on either side of the vertebral column, between the peritoneum and the back muscles. Because the kidneys are located behind the peritoneum (rather than inside with the digestive organs), they are said to be **retroperitoneal**. They are positioned between the twelfth thoracic and the third lumbar vertebrae. The right kidney is situated slightly lower than the left, due to the large area occupied by the liver.

Each kidney and its blood vessels is enclosed within a mass of fat tissue called the **adipose capsule**. In turn, each kidney and adipose capsule is covered by a tough, fibrous tissue called the **renal fascia**, or **fibrous capsule**.

282

Since the kidneys are located behind the peritoneal cavity, they can be surgically approached from the back. They are cushioned and protected by the adipose capsule.

There is an indentation along the concave medial border of the kidney called the **hilum**. The hilum is a passageway for the lymph vessels, nerves, renal artery and vein, and the ureter. At the hilum the fibrous capsule continues downward, forming the outer layer of the ureter. Cutting the kidney in half lengthwise reveals its internal structure. The upper end of each ureter flares into a funnel-shaped structure known as the **renal pelvis**.

Medulla and Cortex

The kidney is divided into two layers: an outer, granular layer called the **cortex**, and an inner, striated layer, the **medulla**. The medulla is red and consists of radially striated cones called the **renal pyramids**. The base of each renal pyramid faces the cortex, while its apex (**renal papilla**) empties into cuplike cavities called **calyces**. These, in turn, empty into the renal pelvis.

The cortex, reddish brown, is composed of millions of microscopic functional units of the kidney called **nephrons**. Cortical tissue is interspersed between renal pyramids, separating and supporting them. These interpyramidal cortical supports are the **renal columns**. The renal columns and the renal pyramids alternate with one another, see color plate 16B.

NEPHRON

The nephron is the basic structural and functional unit of the kidney. Most of the nephron is located within the cortex, with only a small, tubular portion in the medulla. Over a million nephrons comprise each kidney.

A nephron begins with the **afferent arteriole**, which carries blood from the renal artery. The afferent arteriole enters a double-walled hollow capsule, the **Bowman's capsule**.[1] Within the capsule the afferent arteriole finely divides, forming a knotty ball called the *glomerulus* which contains some fifty separate capillaries. The combination of the Bowman's capsule and the glomerulus is known as the **renal corpuscle**. The Bowman's capsule sends off a highly convoluted (twisted) tubular branch referred to as the **proximal convoluted tubule**.

Both the renal corpuscle and the proximal convoluted tubule are located in the cortex. The proximal convoluted tubule descends into the medulla to form the **loop of Henle**. In figure 35–1, observe that the loop of Henle has a straight descending limb, a loop, and a straight ascending limb. When the ascending limb of Henle's loop returns to the cortex, it turns into the **distal convoluted tubule**. Eventually this convoluted tubule opens into a larger, straight vessel known as the **collecting tubule**. Several distal convoluted tubules join to form this single straight collection tubule. The collecting tubule empties into the renal pelvis, then into the ureter.

As figure 35–1 shows, the walls of the renal tubules are surrounded by capillaries. After the **afferent** arteriole branches out to form the glomerulus, it leaves the Bowman's capsule as the **efferent** arteriole. The efferent arteriole branches to form the capillaries surrounding the renal tubules. All of these capillaries eventually join together to form a small branch of the renal vein which carries blood from the kidney.

1. Sir William Bowman (1816–1892), English anatomist and ophthalmologist

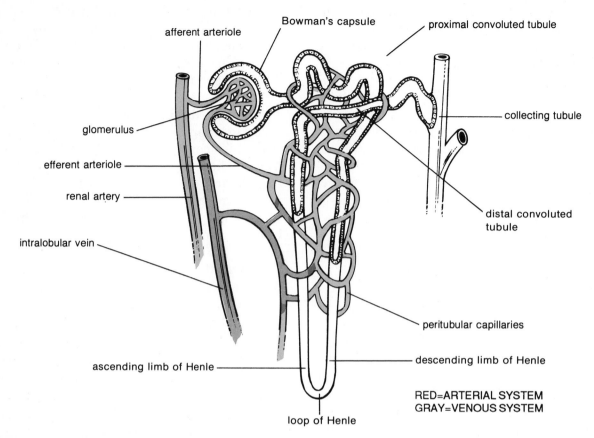

afferent arteriole

Bowman's capsule

proximal convoluted tubule

glomerulus

collecting tubule

efferent arteriole

renal artery

distal convoluted tubule

intralobular vein

peritubular capillaries

ascending limb of Henle

descending limb of Henle

RED=ARTERIAL SYSTEM
GRAY=VENOUS SYSTEM

loop of Henle

Figure 35-1   A nephron—the functional and structural unit of the kidney (From W. Schraer and R. Noelle, *A Learning Program for Biology*. Fairfield, New Jersey: Cebco Publishing Co.)

URINE FORMATION IN THE NEPHRON

The kidney nephrons form urine by three processes: (a) filtration by the glomerulus, (b) reabsorption within the renal tubules, and (c) secretion by the tubular cells.

Filtration

The first step in urine formation is filtration. In this process, blood from the renal artery enters the smaller afferent arteriole, which in turn enters the even smaller capillaries of the glomerulus. As the blood from the renal artery travels this course, the blood vessels grow narrower and narrower. This results in an increase in blood pressure. In most of the capillaries throughout the body, blood pressure is about 25 millimeters of mercury; in the glomerulus, it is between 60 and 90 millimeters.

This high pressure forces a plasma-like fluid to filter from the blood in the glomerulus into the Bowman's capsule. This fluid is called the **nephric filtrate**. It consists of water, glucose, amino acids, some salts, and urea. The nephric filtrate does not contain plasma proteins because they are too large to pass through the pores of the capillary membrane. The Bowman's capsule filters out 125 milliliters of fluid from the blood in a single minute. Thus in one hour, 7500 mL of filtrate leave the blood; this amounts to some 180,000 milliliters (180 liters) in a 24-hour period.

Obviously we cannot dispose of that much water each day. In fact, we only lose about a liter and a half per day because, as the nephric filtrate continues along the tubules, 99% of this water is reabsorbed back into the bloodstream.

Reabsorption

This process includes the reabsorption of useful substances from the nephric filtrate within the renal tubules into the capillaries around the tubules (**peritubular capillaries**). These substances are water, glucose, amino acids, vitamins, bicarbonate ions (HCO_3^-), and the chloride salts of calcium, magnesium, sodium and potassium. Reabsorption starts in the proximal convoluted tubules; it continues through the Henle's loop, the distal convoluted tubules, and the collecting tubules.

The proximal tubules reabsorb approximately 80% of the water filtered out of the blood in the glomerulus (180 liters). Water thus absorbed through the proximal tubules constitutes **obligatory** water absorption. This process occurs by osmosis. Simultaneously, glucose, amino acids, vitamins, and some sodium ions are actively transported back into the blood.

In the distal convoluted tubules about 10 to 15 percent of water is reabsorbed into the bloodstream, depending upon the needs of the body. This type of water absorption is called facultative (optional) reabsorption. It is controlled by the **antidiuretic hormone (ADH),** the hormone secreted from the posterior lobe of the pituitary gland, which is found at the base of the brain. ADH helps to maintain balance of body fluids by controlling the reabsorption of water in the nephron.

Secretion

The process of secretion is the opposite of reabsorption. Some substances are actively secreted into the tubules. Secretion transports substances from the blood in the peritubular capillaries into the urine in the distal and collecting tubules. Substances secreted into the urine include ammonia, hydrogen ions (H^+), potassium ions (K^+), and some drugs. Hydrogen and potassium ions, as well as drugs, are secreted from the blood into the urine by active transport. Ammonia is secreted by diffusion.

URETERS

Urine passes from the kidneys out of the collecting tubules into the renal pelvis, then down the ureter into the urinary bladder. There are two ureters (one from each kidney) carrying urine from the kidneys to the urinary bladder. They are long, narrow tubes, less than 1/4 inch wide and 10 to 12 inches long. Mucous membrane lines both renal pelves and the ureters. Beneath the mucous membrane lining of the ureters are smooth muscle fibers. When these muscles contract, peristalsis is initiated, pushing urine down the ureter into the urinary bladder.

URINARY BLADDER

The **bladder**, a hollow muscular organ, made of elastic fibers and involuntary muscle, acts like a reservoir. It stores the urine until about one pint is accumulated. The bladder then becomes uncomfortable and must be emptied. Emptying the bladder, or voiding, takes place by muscular contractions of the bladder which are involuntary, although they can be controlled to some extent through the nervous system. Contraction of the bladder muscles forces the urine through a narrow canal, the **urethra**, whichs extends to the outside opening, the **urinary meatus**.

The kidneys have the potential to work harder than they actually do. Under ordinary circumstances, only a portion of the glomeruli are used. Should one kidney not function, or have to be removed, more glomeruli and tubules open up in the second kidney to assume the work of the nonfunctioning or missing kidney.

CONTROL OF URINARY SECRETION

The control of the secretions of urine is under both chemical and nervous control.

Chemical Control

The reabsorption of water in the distal convoluted kidney tubules and the collecting ducts is influenced by the antidiuretic hormone (ADH) or **vasopressin**. ADH helps to increase the size of the cell membrane pores in the epithelial cells of the distal tubule and collecting ducts by increasing their permeability to water. The secretion and regulation of the ADH is under the control of the hypothalamus of the brain. In the hypothalamus, there are highly sensitive receptor cells called **osmoreceptors**. These osmoreceptors are sensitive to the osmotic pressure of blood plasma. For example, an increase in the osmotic blood pressure due to salt retention causes an increase in ADH secretion. This will inhibit normal urine formation, and water may also be held in the tissues. Figure 35–2 shows the effect of salt retention on human tissues.

There are other hormones involved in the reabsorption process. Aldosterone secreted by the adrenal cortex promotes the excretion of potassium and hydrogen ions and the reabsorption of sodium ions; chloride ions are also absorbed. In the absence of aldosterone, sodium and water are excreted in large amounts, and potassium is retained. Thus any dysfunction to the adrenal cortex produces pronounced changes in the salt and water content of body fluids.

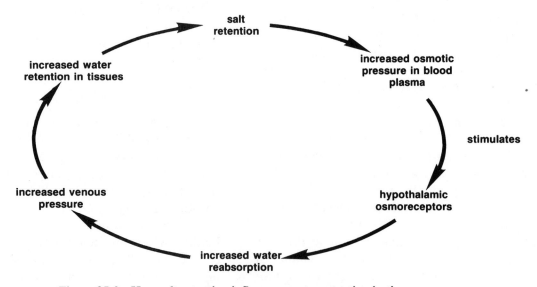

Figure 35-2 How salt retention influences water retention in tissues

Nervous Control _____

The nervous control of urine secretion is accomplished directly through the action of nerve impulses on the blood vessels leading to the kidney and on those within the kidney leading to the glomeruli. Indirect nerve control is achieved through the stimulation on certain endocrine glands, whose hormonal secretions will control urinary secretion.

Further Study and Discussion

• If laboratory facilities are available, obtain and examine several specimens of fresh, normal urine.

a. What is the color of the specimen?

b. Is it clear or cloudy?

c. Is the urine acid, alkaline or neutral?

To test, dip blue litmus paper into the urine. If acid is present, it will turn red. Dip red litmus paper in. If urine is alkaline, it will turn paper blue. If neither paper changes color, the urine is neutral.

d. What is the specific gravity of a specimen? To test, use a urinometer.

e. Is albumin present?

To test for albumin, place 10 milliliters of urine in a test tube. Add 3 drops of dilute acetic acid (2%). Hold the tube at the bottom and apply heat to the upper level of urine. If a cloud appears in the heated portion, albumin is present.

f. Is sugar (glucose) present?

To test for sugar, place 10 drops of urine in a Pyrex test tube. Add 5 milliliters of Benedict's solution. Mix thoroughly by shaking gently. Place in a water bath and boil for 3 minutes. As soon as the bubbling stops, interpret the test results as follows:

COLOR	INDICATION
No change in color	0 absent
Green	± trace of sugar
Greenish-yellow	+ one plus
Yellow	+ + two plus
Brown or brick red	+ + + three plus

- Using **Acetest** reagent tablets, examine the urine for acetone. Have the results and your interpretation checked by the instructor.

  Place the reagent tablet on a clean white sheet of paper. Place a drop of urine on the tablet. In 30 seconds, compare the resulting color with the color chart enclosed with the tablets. Record the result on the chart.

- Using **Clinitest** tablets and/or Clinistix reagent strips, test for sugar. Have the results and your interpretation checked by the instructor.

  Clinitest tablets: Place 5 drops of urine and 10 drops of water in a test tube. Add the Clinitest tablet. Observe the reaction. Then shake the test tube and compare the color of the solution with the color scale enclosed with the tablets. Record the result.

  Clinistix reagent strips: Dip the test end of the Clinistix in the urine and remove it. (Avoid contact with fingers or other objects because misleading results may occur.) If the moistened end turns blue, the result is *positive*. When sugar is present, the blue color will appear in less than one minute. Record the result.

- Using **Bumintest** reagent solution and/or Allritest tablets, test the urine for albumin. Have the results and your interpretation checked by the instructor.

  Bumintest: Dissolve 4 Bumintest reagent tablets in 30 milliliters of water in a test tube. (This makes a 5% solution). In another test tube, mix equal parts of urine and Bumintest solution and shake the tube gently. The amount of albumin is estimated by the degree of cloudiness (turbidity). Record the result.

  Allritest tablets: Place Allritest tablet on clean paper. Put one drop of urine on the tablet. When the urine has been absorbed, add 2 drops of water and allow the water to be absorbed before reading. Compare the color of the top of the tablet with the color photograph enclosed with each package of tablets. Record the result.

Assignment

A. Match each term in column I with its description in column II.

Column I	Column II
_____ 1. nephron	a. tubes which connect the kidney with the bladder
_____ 2. glomerulus	b. mass of capillaries
_____ 3. bladder	c. structure which absorbs wastes from the capillary mass
_____ 4. urethra	
_____ 5. ureter	

_____	6.	ADH
_____	7.	tubules
_____	8.	Bowman's capsule
_____	9.	kidney
_____	10.	renal vein

d. one of millions of tiny filtering units

e. returns blood to the inferior vena cava

f. hormone which regulates water reabsorption

g. contraction of bladder muscles

h. canal which opens to the outside of the body

i. primarily acts as a reservoir

j. allow urine to drain into the renal pelvis

k. bean-shaped organ

B. Briefly answer the following questions.

1. How do the kidneys function in excretion?

2. Of what value is it to the physician to have an exact measure of the patient's intake and output?

3. What is another important function of the kidneys besides the elimination of waste?

4. What is the function of the antidiuretic hormone?

5. How does aldosterone control urinary secretion?

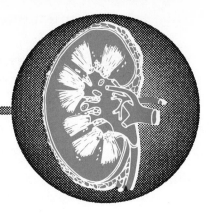

REPRESENTATIVE DISORDERS OF THE EXCRETORY SYSTEM

KEY WORDS

catheter
cystitis
• cystitis cystica
• cystitis em-
  physematosa
dermatophytosis
dysuria
hemodialysis

incontinence
micturition
nephritis
nephroptosis
neurogenic
  bladder
oliguria
pyelitis

pyelocystitis
pyelonephritis
uremia
urethritis
urethrocystitis
urinary calculi
  (kidney stones)

OBJECTIVES

■ List some disorders of the urinary tract
■ Describe the more common excretory system disorders
■ Define the Key Words related to this unit of study

The normal functioning of the excretory system has been described. Some disorders of the intestines were covered in unit 33. There are also malfunctions and disorders of the urinary tract and the skin with which the health care provider should be familiar.

DISORDERS OF THE URINARY TRACT

Acute kidney failure may be sudden in onset. Causes may be nephritis, shock, injury, bleeding, sudden heart failure, or poisoning. A common symptom is the absence of urine formation, which is termed **anuria**. Suppression of urine formation is dangerous; unless anuria is relieved, **uremia** will develop. Uremia is a toxic condition where the blood retains urinary waste products (like urea) because the kidneys fail to excrete them. Symptoms resulting from uremia are headaches, nausea, vomiting and in extreme cases, coma and death. When urine formation is diminished below the

normal amount, a condition known as **oliguria** results.

An artificial kidney machine may be used to remove wastes normally excreted by a healthy kidney. This process is called **hemodialysis**.

Cystitis is the inflammation of the mucous membrane lining of the urinary bladder. It can be caused by bacterial infection or kidney inflammation which has spread to the bladder. Inflammation of the urinary bladder is likely to be more obvious than a kidney infection, since it usually leads to frequent and painful urination. Proper treatment involves administration of large doses of antibiotics like erythrocin to kill the bacteria causing the inflammation.

Cystitis cystica is a chronic inflammation of the urinary bladder. It is characterized by the presence of small, translucent mucus-containing cysts.

Dysuria is difficult or painful urination.

Cystitis emphysematosa is a type of cystitis where spaces in the urinary bladder wall are filled with gas. This condition is caused by bacterial fermentation of sugar in the urine, as sometimes occurs in diabetes.

Incontinence is also known as **involuntary micturition** (urination). Here an individual loses voluntary control over urination. Incontinence occurs in babies prior to proper toilet training since they lack control over the external sphincter muscle of the urethra. Thus, urination occurs whenever the bladder fills. Similarly, a person who has suffered a stroke, or one whose spinal cord has been severed, has no bladder control. Such patients may require an indwelling **catheter**. This is a tube inserted into the neck of the bladder through the urethra. It diverts and directs urine into a convenient bag or other receptacle outside the body.

Pyelitis is inflammation of the pelvis of the kidney, usually due to an infection.

Pyelocystitis is the inflammation of the renal pelvis and urinary bladder, due to an infection. Treatment involves the use of antibiotics to destroy the bacteria.

Pyelonephritis is the inflammation of the kidney tissue itself along with its renal pelvis. This condition generally results from an infection that has spread from the ureters. One of the symptoms is pyuria, the presence of pus in the urine. The usual course of treatment includes the administration of antibiotics.

Nephritis is an inflammation of the kidney, causing damage to the kidney tissue. The result of this condition is that the kidneys are unable to carry on the task of excretion in an efficient manner. (It is also called Bright's disease.)

The kidney moves to a small degree in response to breathing movements and changes in body position. However, when the kidney movements are greater than normal, the disorder is called **nephroptosis** or movable kidney.

In extreme cases, it is called the wandering or floating kidney. Nephroptosis occurs more often in women than in men, and more often on the right side than on the left side.

A **neurogenic bladder** is caused by a damaged nerve that controls the urinary bladder. This results in dysuria, the inability to empty the bladder completely, and incontinence.

Acute nephritis usually occurs in children and young people. It may be a complication of a communicable disease, especially scarlet fever. The streptococcus organism may be the cause. **Chronic nephritis** is a kidney condition which develops gradually in older people. Usually high blood pressure is also present. Hardening of the renal blood vessels may be the cause, or the glomeruli and tubules may have been destroyed over an extended period of time.

Urethritis is inflammation of the urethra.

Urethrocystitis is the inflammation of the urethra and the urinary bladder, usually due to an infection. It is alleviated with antibiotics such as the tetracyclines, kanamycin, and sulfisoxazole.

Urinary calculi is another name for kidney stones. Some of the materials contained in urine are only slightly soluble in water. Therefore when stagnation of urine occurs, the microscopic crystals of calcium phosphate may clump together to form kidney stones. These kidney stones slowly grow in diameter. They eventually fill the renal pelvis and obstruct urine flow in the ureter. Their presence may be extremely uncomfortable; "passing a stone" during urination can cause excruciating pain. If it is not possible to re-dissolve or pass kidney stones, they must be surgically removed. There are various causes for the formation of these stones, including extended immobility, dehydration, renal infection, or hyperparathyroidism.

Tuberculosis of the kidney is a destructive kidney disease caused by the tubercle bacillus, *Mycobacterium tuberculosis*. Treatment involves the use of streptomycin.

Further Study and Discussion

- Explain the value of urinalysis in diagnosing cystitis or pyelitis.

- Visit a hemodialysis center. Ask for permission to read a patient's history. Write a short report to present to the class.

- Invite a staff member from a kidney transplant center to give a presentation to the class.

Assignment

1. What may cause cystitis or pyelitis?

2. What is a frequent result of nephritis?

3. How are kidney stones formed?

4. What is the value of hemodialysis to the patient whose kidneys are unable to remove waste products from the blood?

5. What is nephroptosis?

6. What is a neurogenic bladder? What causes it?

ELIMINATION OF WASTE MATERIALS

A. Match each description in column I with the correct term in column II.

Column I	Column II
_____ 1. waste product eliminated through lungs	a. anuria
_____ 2. blood filter	b. calculi
_____ 3. stones in the kidney	c. carbon dioxide
_____ 4. water and nitrogenous wastes	d. cystitis
_____ 5. inflammation of the mucous membrane lining the bladder	e. kidneys
	f. nephritis
_____ 6. kidney malfunction preventing elimination of metabolic wastes	g. perspiration
	h. uremia
_____ 7. helps regulate body temperature	i. ureter
_____ 8. urinary duct	j. urine
	k. urinometer

B. Label the parts indicated on figure SE7–A.

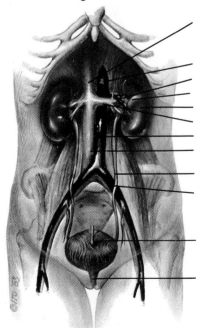

Figure SE7-A

C. Briefly answer the following questions.
   1. How does ADH control urinary secretion?

   2. Describe the following urinary disorders:
      a. dysuria

      b. neurogenic bladder

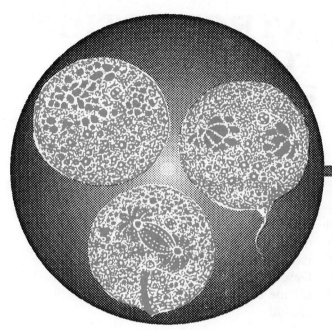

CHAPTER **8**

HUMAN REPRODUCTION

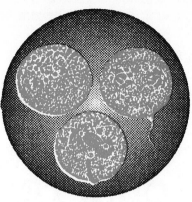

INTRODUCTION TO THE REPRODUCTIVE SYSTEM

KEY WORDS

autosome
cleavage
coitus
corona radiata
deoxyribonucleic
   acid
fertilization
   (internal)

gamete
gametogenesis
gonads
hyaluronic acid
hyaluronidase
meiosis
oogenesis
ova

ovaries
somatic cell
sperm
spermatogenesis
testes
zona pellucida
zygote

OBJECTIVES

- Contrast reproduction of simple cells and more complex forms of life
- Explain the process of fertilization
- Describe how physical traits are determined
- Define the Key Words related to this unit of study

All living organisms, whether unicellular or multicellular, small or large, must reproduce in order to continue their species. Humans and most multicellular animals reproduce new members of their species by sexual reproduction.

Specialized sex cells (**gametes**) must be produced by the **gonads** of both male and female sex organs before sexual reproduction can take place. The female gonads, called the **ovaries,** produce egg cells (**ova**). The male gonads, the **testes,** produce **sperm.** The formation of gametes within the gonads is known as **gametogenesis,** or **meiosis.** In the female, the specific meiotic process is called **oogenesis;** in the male, **spermatogenesis.**

In humans, the **somatic** (body) cells, including skin, fat, muscle, nerve, bone cells, etc. contain 46 chromosomes in the nucleus. Forty-four of these are **autosomes** (nonsex chromosomes). The remaining two are sex chromosomes. Each chromosome has a partner of the same size and shape so that they can be paired, figure 37–1. In the female, the somatic cells contain 22 pairs of autosomes, and a single pair of sex chromosomes (both are X chromosomes). In the male, the combination is also 22 autosomal pairs and a single pair of sex chromosomes. However, the male sex chromosomal pair consists of an X and a Y chromosome.

Oogenesis and spermatogenesis reduces the chromosome number of 46 to 23 in the gametes. All multicellular organisms start from a fusion of two gametes: the sperm (spermatozoan) from the male, and the ovum from the female. Figure 37–2 shows the structure of a spermatozoan and an ovum. During sexual intercourse, or **coitus,** sperm from the testes is deposited into the female vagina. Spermatozoa entering the female reproductive tract live for only a day or two at the most, though they

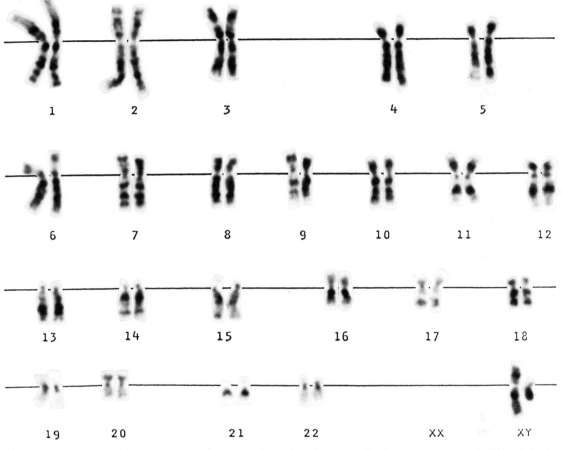

Figure 37-1   Karotype of human from a male somatic cell. A karotype is the arrangement of chromosome pairs according to shape and size.

may remain in the tract up to two weeks before degenerating. Approximately 100 million spermatozoa are contained in 1 milliliter (1cc) of ejaculated seminal fluid. They are fairly uniform in shape and size. If the count is less than 20 million per milliliter, the male is considered to be sterile. These millions of sperm cells swim towards the ovum that has been released from the ovary. The large quantity of sperm is necessary because a great number are destroyed before they even approach the ovum. Many die from the acidity of the secretions in the male urethra or the vagina. Some cannot withstand the high temperature of the female

abdomen, while others lack the propulsion ability to progress from the vagina to the upper uterine (fallopian) tube.

In order for a sperm to penetrate and fertilize an ovum, the **corona radiata** must first be penetrated. This is the layer of epithelial cells surrounding the **zona pellucida,** figure 37–2. Eventually, only one sperm cell penetrates and fertilizes an ovum. To accomplish this successfully, the sperm head produces an enzyme called **hyaluronidase.** Hyaluronidase acts upon **hyaluronic acid,** a chemical substance that holds together the epithelial cells of the corona radiata. As a result of the action of the hyalu-

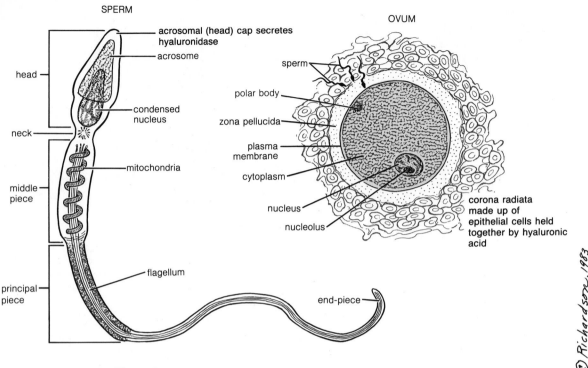

Figure 37-2 Diagrammatic representation of a human sperm and ovum

ronidase, the epithelial cells fall away from the ovum. This exposes an area of the plasma membrane for sperm penetration. Figure 37–3 illustrates the fertilization of an ovum by a sperm.

True fertilization occurs when the sperm nucleus combines with the egg nucleus to form a fertilized egg cell, or **zygote.** The type of fertilization that occurs in humans is referred to as **internal fertilization;** fertilization takes place within the female's body.

Fertilization restores the full complement of 46 chromosomes possessed by every human cell, each parent contributing one chromosome to each of the 23 pairs.

A substance called **deoxyribonucleic acid (DNA)** is found in the chromosomes. It contains the genetic code that is replicated and passed on to each cell as the zygote divides and redivides to form the embryo. The early pro-

cess whereby the zygote repeatedly divides to form an early embryo is known as **cleavage.** After early cleavage, actual embryonic development occurs until the fetus is completely formed.

All of the inherited traits possessed by the offspring are established at the time of fertilization. This is a point to remember when working with parents. A young mother-to-be may hope that her baby will be a girl with curly hair, or a prospective father may insist that he wants a son. The health care provider can assure them that the sex, and physical characteristics such as eye color and curly hair, are determined at the time of fertilization. These traits cannot be altered by wishful thinking. The sex chromosomes of the male parent determine the sex of the child but other characteristics are a combination of both parents.

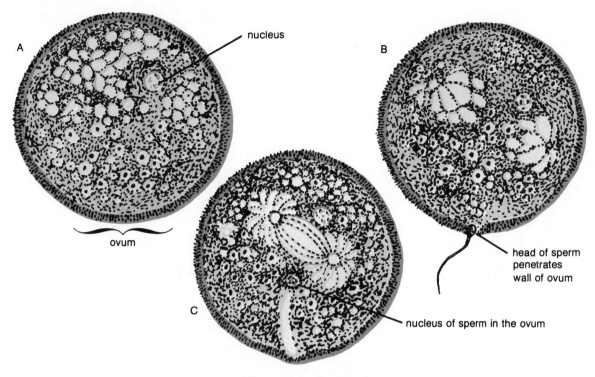

Figure 37-3   Fertilization

Further Study and Discussion

- Discuss recessive and dominant heredity traits. Give examples of each.
- Find out if mental illness, tuberculosis, or cancer is inherited. Research and submit a paper on one of these topics.

Assignment

1. When is the sex of the offspring determined?

2. What are chromosomes?

3. How many chromosomes are present in each body cell of the newborn child?

4. Where do these chromosomes come from?

5. What part does DNA play in hereditary characteristics?

UNIT 38

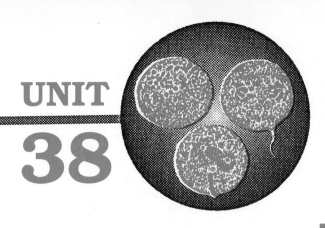

THE ORGANS OF REPRODUCTION

KEY WORDS

bulbourethral
  glands
  (Cowper's
  glands)
cells of Leydig
cervix
corpus luteum
cytogenic
cryptorchidism
ductus deferens
  (vas deferens)
ectopic pregnancy
ejaculatory ducts
endocrinic
endometrium
epididymis
estrogen
external os of
  cervix

fallopian tube
  (oviduct)
fimbrae
fundus
graafian follicle
infundibulum
internal orifice
  (os of the
  uterus)
interstitial tissue
lobule
maturation
menarche
menopause
myometrium
nongravid
ova
ovalution
penis

progesterone
prostate gland
prostatic urethra
puberty
rete testis
scrotum
seminal vesicles
seminiferous
  tubules
serosa of the
  uterus
sertoli cells
sperm
spermatic cord
testes
tunica albuginea
urethra
vagina

OBJECTIVES

- Identify the organs of the female reproductive system
- Identify the organs of the male reproductive system
- Describe the functions of the reproductive organs
- Define the Key Words relating to this unit of study

The function of the reproductive system is to provide for continuity of the species. In the human, the female reproductive system is composed of two ovaries, two fallopian tubes, the uterus, and the vagina. The male reproductive system is made up of two testes, seminal ducts, glands and the penis. The principal male organs are located outside the body in contrast to the female organs which are largely located within the body.

FEMALE REPRODUCTIVE SYSTEM

As shown in color plate 17, the female reproductive system consists of two ovaries, two fallopian tubes, the uterus, and the vagina. Ac-

cessory organs are the breasts. Placement of the female reproductive organs in the pelvic cavity are shown in figure 38–1.

The Ovaries

The ovaries are the primary sex organs of the female. They are located on either side of the pelvis, lateral to the uterus, in the lower part of the abdominal cavity. Each ovary is about the shape and size of a large almond, measuring about 3 centimeters long and from 1.5 to 3 centimeters wide. An **ovarian ligament,** a short fibrous cord within the **broad ligament,** attaches each ovary to the upper lateral part of the uterus.

Ovaries perform two functions. They produce the female gametes, or **ova,** and the fe-

303

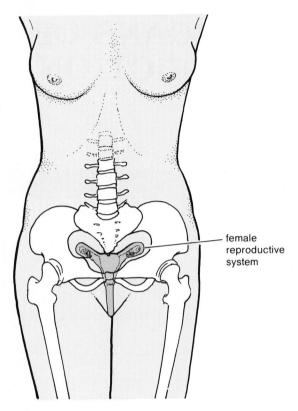

Figure 38-1 **Placement of the female reproductive system in the lower pelvic cavity**

Table 38–1 The Functions of Estrogen and Progesterone

HORMONE	FUNCTION
Estrogen	1. Repairs and thickens the uterine lining by stimulating the production of new epithelial cells 2. Develops and maintains the female secondary sex characteristics (breast development, feminine body contour, etc.)
Progesterone	1. Thickens the uterine lining so it can receive the developing embryo (provided estrogen has acted previously upon the uterine lining) 2. Decreases uterine contractions during pregnancy

male sex hormones, **estrogen** and **progesterone.** Thus the ovaries are said to be both **cytogenic** (cell-producing) and **endocrinic** (hormone-producing). Table 38–1 outlines the functions of the female sex hormones.

Each ovary contains thousands of microscopic hollow sacs called **graafian follicles** in varying stages of development. An ovum slowly develops inside each follicle. The process of development from an immature ova to a functional and mature ova inside the graafian follicle is called **maturation.** (In addition, the graafian follicle produces the hormone, estrogen.)

Usually a single follicle matures every twenty-eight days throughout the reproductive years of a woman. The reproductive years begin at the time of **puberty** and the **menarche** (initial menstrual discharge of blood). This usually occurs between ages 9 and 17 (the average is 12.5 years). The reproductive years end at the time of **menopause,** the cessation of menstruation. This usually occurs when the woman is about 45 to 50 years of age.

Occasionally two or more follicles may mature, thereby releasing more than one ovum. As the follicle enlarges, it migrates to the outside surface of the ovary and breaks open, releasing the ovum from the ovary. This process is called **ovulation;** it occurs about two weeks before the menstrual period begins. However, the time of ovulation may vary depending on emotional and physical health, state of mind, and age. During a woman's reproductive years, she produces about 400 ova. The two ovaries alternate in the maturation and ovulation of an ova. When an ovum is released from the ovary, it is about 0.09 millimeter in diameter and contains a very large nucleus.

The ovum also consists of cytoplasm and some yolk. This yolk is the initial food source for the growth of the early embryo. After ovulation, the ovum travels down one of the **fallo-**

female reproductive system

pian tubes, or **oviducts.** Fertilization of the ovum takes place only in the upper third of the oviduct. Therefore, the time of fertilization is limited to a day or two following ovulation. The ovum begins to deteriorate as it slowly travels down towards the lower part of the oviduct. If fertilization has not taken place, the ovum passes out of the body during menstruation.

The development of the follicle and release of the ovum occur under the influence of two hormones produced in the anterior lobe of the pituitary gland; they are the follicle-stimulating hormone (FSH) and the luteinizing hormone (LH). The follicle-stimulating hormone, FSH, also promotes the secretion of estrogen by the ovary. Estrogen promotes the rapid growth of the uterine lining (the **endometrium**) in preparation for possible implantation of a fertilized ovum.

Following ovulation the ruptured follicle enlarges, takes on a yellow fatty substance, and becomes the **corpus luteum** (yellow body). The corpus luteum secretes another ovarian hormone, progesterone, which functions to maintain the growth of the uterine lining. If the egg is not fertilized, the corpus luteum degenerates, progesterone production stops, and the thickened glandular endometrium sloughs off. The tiny blood vessels that supply the endometrium are ruptured, producing the characteristic blood flow of menstruation. Following menstruation the endometrium heals and then starts thickening again, marking the beginning of the new menstrual cycle.

Fallopian Tubes

The fallopian tubes, about 10 centimeters (4 inches) long, are not attached to the ovaries, figure 38–2 and color plate 17. The outer end of each oviduct curves over the top edge of each ovary and opens into the abdominal cavity. This position of the oviduct, nearest the ovary, is the **infundibulum.** Since the infundibulum is not attached directly to the ovary, it is possible for an ovum to accidentally slip into the abdominal cavity and be fertilized there. Such a condition is known as **ectopic pregnancy** (developing outside the uterine cavity). In addition, an infection occurring in the infundibulum and ovary can spread to the abdominal cavity.

The area of the infundibulum over the ovary is surrounded by a number of fringelike folds called **fimbrae.** Each oviduct is lined with mucous membrane, smooth muscle, and ciliated epithelium. The combined action of the peristaltic contractions of the smooth muscles and the beating of the cilia helps to propel the ova down the oviduct into the uterus.

Uterus

The **uterus** is a hollow, thick-walled, pear-shaped, and highly muscular organ. The **nongravid** (non-pregnant) uterus measures about 7.5 centimeters in length, 5 cm wide and 2.75 cm thick. This is about three inches long, two inches wide and about one inch thick. Its uterine cavity is extremely small and narrow. During pregnancy, however, the uterine cavity greatly expands in order to accommodate the growing embryo and a large amount of fluid.

The uterus is divided into three parts: (1) the **fundus,** the bulging, rounded upper part above the entrance of the two oviducts into the uterus; (2) the **body,** or middle portion; and (3) the **cervix,** or cylindrical, lower narrow portion that extends into the vagina. There is a short, cervical canal that extends from the lower uterine cavity (**internal orifice,** or **os of the uterus**) to the **external os** at the end of the cervix. The uterine wall is comprised of three layers:

- the outer **serous** layer

- an extremely thick, smooth, muscular middle layer, the **myometrium**

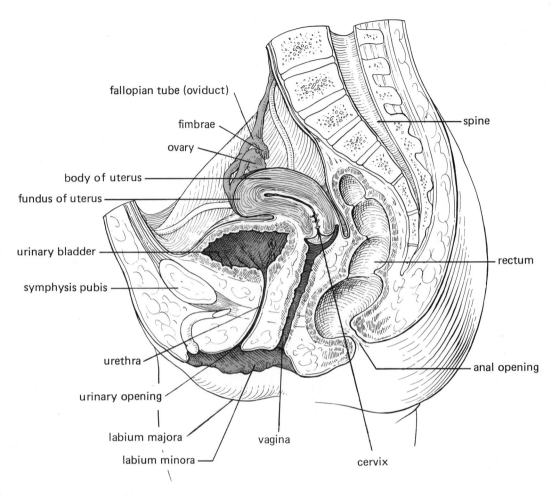

Figure 38-2 Longitudinal section of the female reproductive system (From *Human Anatomy and Physiology* by Joan G. Creager. © 1983 by Wadsworth, Inc. Reprinted by permission of Wadsworth Publishing Company, Belmont, California 94002.)

• an inner mucous layer, the **endometrium**

The endometrium, which lines the oviducts and the vagina, is also lined with ciliated epithelial cells, numerous, uterine glands, and many capillaries.

During development of the embryo-fetus, the uterus gradually rises until the top part is high in the abdominal cavity, pushing on the diaphragm. This may cause the expectant mother some difficulty in breathing during the late stages of pregnancy.

Vagina

The **vagina** is the short canal which extends from the cervix of the uterus to the vulva. It is muscular tissue which receives the sperm during sexual intercourse and stretches to assist in delivery during childbirth. See figure 38–3.

Breasts

The breasts are accessory organs to the female reproductive system, figure 38–4. They are composed of numerous lobes arranged in a

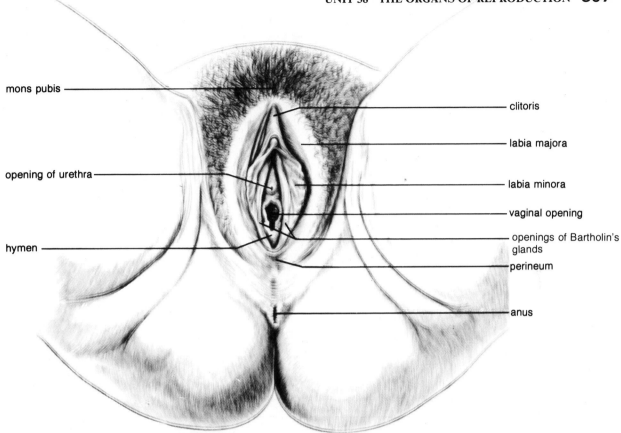

mons pubis

opening of urethra

hymen

clitoris

labia majora

labia minora

vaginal opening

openings of Bartholin's glands

perineum

anus

Figure 38-3   External female genitalia (From *Human Anatomy and Physiology* by Joan G. Creager. © 1983 by Wadsworth, Inc. Reprinted by permission of Wadsworth Publishing Company, Belmont, California 94002)

circular formation. Clusters of secreting cells surround tiny ducts. A single duct extends from each lobe to an opening in the nipple. The **areola,** the darker area which surrounds the nipple, changes to a brownish color during pregnancy. **Prolactin** from the anterior lobe of the pituitary gland stimulates the mammary glands to secrete milk following childbirth.

MALE REPRODUCTIVE SYSTEM

The male reproductive organs, figure 38–5, consist of the following structures:

1. The two **testes** produce the male gametes, spermatozoa, and the male sex hormone testosterone. They are suspended from the body wall by a **spermatic cord** and encased in a pouch called the **scrotum.**

2. A **system of ducts** helps to carry the sperm cells out of the testes to the outside of the male's body. These ducts are the **epididymus,** two seminal ducts (sing., **ductus deferens** or **vas deferens**), two **ejaculatory ducts,** and the **urethra.**

3. Accessory glands include the two **seminal vesicles,** two **bulbourethral glands** (Cowper's glands), and a **prostate gland.** These glands will add a viscous fluid to the sperm cells to form seminal fluid.

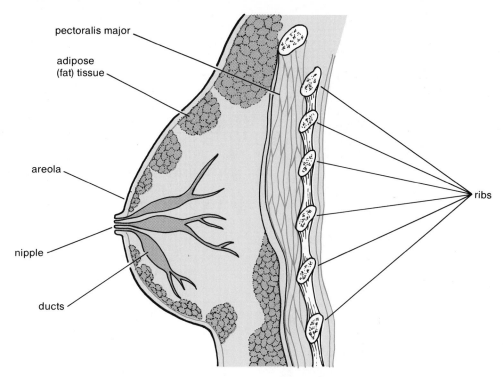

Figure 38-4   Sagittal section of the female breast

4. The **penis** is a copulatory structure that will transfer sperm cells to the female reproductive system.

Testes and Epididymus

The two testes are the primary male reproductive organs, figure 38–6. They are found in a pouch lying outside the male body called the scrotum. Each testis is about the size and shape of a small egg, approximately 4 centimeters long, 2.5 centimeters wide, and 2 centimeters thick. The testes are attached to an overlying structure called the epididymis. A fibrous tissue called the **tunica albuginea** covers the testes and sends incomplete partitions into the body of each testes. Each one of these partitions is called a **lobule,** and each testes contains 250 lobules.

Each testicular lobule contains one to four minute and highly convoluted (twisted)

seminiferous tubules. The seminiferous tubules are lined with specialized epithelial cells called **sertoli cells.** These sertoli cells help in sperm formation. All of the seminiferous tubules intertwine and join together to form a small mesh-like network of tubules called the **rete testis.** The rete testis unite to form the epididymis. The seminiferous tubules are supported by a type of tissue called **interstitial tissue.**

There are cells lining the interstitial tissue which will produce the male hormone testosterone. Testosterone is secreted in relatively steady amounts during the adult life of the male. These interstitial cells are also called **cells of Leydig.***

The epididymides connect the testes with the ductus deferens and help in the final development of the sperm cells.

---

*Franz von Leydig, German histologist (1821-1908).

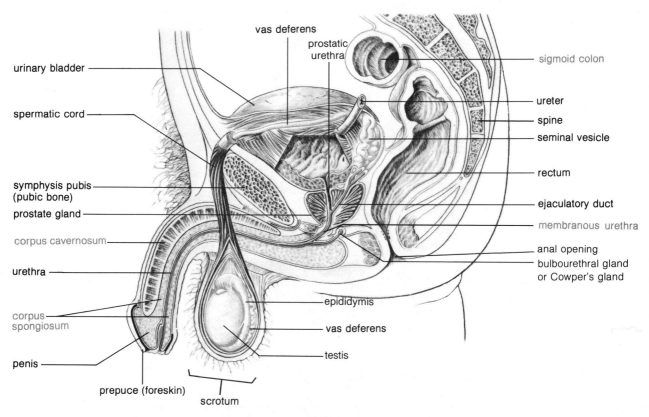

Figure 38-5   Longitudinal section of the male reproductive system (From *Human Anatomy and Physiology* by Joan G. Creager. © 1983 by Wadsworth, Inc. Reprinted by permission of Wadsworth Publishing Company, Belmont, California 94002.)

Descent of the Testes

In the embryo, the testes are formed and developed in the abdominal wall slightly below the kidneys. During the last three months of fetal development, the testes will migrate downward through the ventral abdominal wall into the scrotum. In its descent, each testis carries with it the ductus deferens, blood and lymphatic vessels, and autonomic nerve fibers. These structures and their fibrous tissue covering form the **spermatic cord.**

Occasionally, as in premature babies, the testes will not descend, though as a rule, they soon do. However, if the testes do not descend, this condition is known as **cryptorchidism.** (If one testis doesn't descend, it is called unilateral cryptorchidism. For two testes, it is called

bilateral cryptorchidism). If the testes stay inside the abdomen after puberty, spermatogenesis will be affected. The increased body temperature will destroy any sperm cells. A simple surgical procedure done before puberty can help this condition, however.

Scrotum

The scrotum is an external sac that contains the testes.

Ductus Deferens, Seminal Vesicles, and Ejaculatory Ducts

The right and left ductus deferens (vas deferens) are continuations of the epididymides. The ductus deferens has a dual function. It serves as a storage site for sperm cells and as

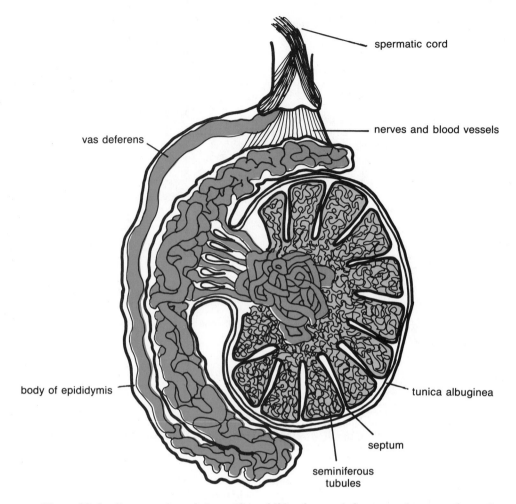

Figure 38-6 Cross-section of the testis, epididymis, vas deferens, and spermatic cord

the excretory duct of the testis. Each ductus runs from the epididymis up through the inguinal canal. It then runs downward and backward to the side of the urinary bladder. It then curves around the ureter and goes down to meet with the seminal vesicle duct on the posterior side of the bladder.

The **seminal vesicles** are actually two highly convoluted membranous tubes. A duct leads away from a seminal vesicle that joins to the ductus deferens to form the ejaculatory duct on either side. The seminal vesicles produce secretions containing amino acids, fructose, mucus, prostaglandins, and a small quantity of ascorbic acid. These substances found in the seminal fluid help to nourish and protect the sperm on its journey up the female reproductive system. At the precise moment of ejaculation, the seminal fluid is added to the sperm cells as they leave the ejaculatory ducts.

The ejaculatory ducts are short and very narrow. They begin where the ductus deferens and the seminal vesicle duct join. They then descend into the prostate gland to join with the urethra, into which they discharge their contents.

Penis

The external organs are the scrotum and the penis. Internally, the scrotum is divided into two sacs each containing a testis, epididymis, and lower part of the vas deferens. The penis contains erectile tissue that becomes enlarged and rigid during intercourse. Loose-fitting skin, called the **foreskin** or **prepuce,** covers the penis. The foreskin can be removed in a simple operation known as **circumcision.**

Prostate Gland

The prostate gland is located just under the urinary bladder, and it surrounds the opening of the bladder leading into the urethra. It surrounds the beginning portion of the urethra that is called the **prostatic urethra.** The prostate gland is about the shape, size, and consistency of a chestnut. It is covered by a dense fibrous capsule and contains glandular tissue surrounded by fibromuscular tissue that contracts during ejaculation. The prostate gland secretes a thin, milky alkaline fluid (pH 7.5) that enhances sperm motility. It also gives semen its characteristic strong musky odor. The fluid contains citric acid, magnesium, zinc, acid phosphatase, and a variety of other enzymes. Fluid in the ductus deferens is very acidic, and the female vaginal secretions are also quite acidic. Therefore, the alkaline prostatic fluid probably neutralizes the acidic semen and vaginal secretions. This consequently enhances the fertility and motility of the sperm cells.

Age Changes in the Prostate Gland. The prostate gland increases in size during adolescence along with the other reproductive organs due to the effect of the male hormones. It reaches full size during the twenties. As a man ages, occasionally the prostate gland increases in size. If this occurs, generally two out of every three men reaching age 70 suffer from some degree of blockage to urination. This blockage is caused by the narrowing of the diameter of the prostatic urethra.

Bulbourethral Glands. The **bulbourethral glands,** also known as **Cowper's glands,** are located on either side of the urethra below the prostate gland. They add an alkaline secretion to the semen that helps the sperm to live longer within the acid medium of the female reproductive tract.

Further Study and Discussion

- Discuss the relationship between ovulation, menstruation, and fertilization.

- Visit a prenatal clinic in your community. What do the examinations of a pregnant woman include on her first visit? On return visits?

- Discuss how oral and intrauterine contraceptives prevent pregnancy.

- Two blood tests which have been used to detect early pregnancy are the A-Z test and HCG test. How do they differ? What do the letters stand for?

- Investigate the value of using microsurgery techniques in ectopic or tubal pregnancies.

Assignment

A. Select the letter of the item which most correctly completes the statement.

1. One of the male hormones is
    a. progesterone
    b. luteinizing hormone
    c. follicle-stimulating hormone
    d. testosterone

2. Ovulation usually occurs
    a. the day before the menstrual period begins
    b. one week before the menstrual period begins
    c. three weeks before the menstrual period begins
    d. two weeks before the menstrual period begins

3. The ovaries contain
    a. thirty graafian follicles
    b. thousands of graafian follicles
    c. hundreds of graafian follicles
    d. six graafian follicles

4. The development of the follicle and release of the ovum are under the influence of
    a. the follicle-stimulating hormone and the luteinizing hormone
    b. estrogen and corpus luteum
    c. progesterone and the follicle-stimulating hormone
    d. estrogen and the luteinizing hormone

5. Which one of the following statements is *not* correct?
    a. The fallopian tubes are about four inches long.
    b. The fallopian tubes serve as ducts for the ovum on its way to the uterus.
    c. The fallopian tubes are also called oviducts.
    d. The fallopian tubes are attached to the ovaries.

B. Match each term in column I with its correct description in column II.

	Column I	Column II
_____	1. scrotum	a. secondary sex characteristics
_____	2. testosterone	b. external sac which holds the testes
_____	3. facial and pubic hair	c. excreted from the pituitary gland
_____	4. epididymis and penis	d. formed in the seminiferous tubules
_____	5. gonadotrophic hormone	e. male gamete
		f. secondary reproductive organs
		g. male hormone produced in the testes

C.   Briefly answer the following questions:

1.   What are the primary male reproductive organs?

2.   What is the function of the interstitial cells? What is another name for them?

3.   Why must the testes descend into the scrotum?

4.   Name the substances found in seminal fluid.

5.   What are the respective functions of the prostate gland and the bulbourethral glands?

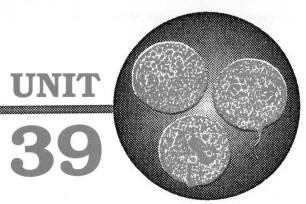

MENSTRUAL CYCLE AND MENOPAUSE

KEY WORDS

follicle stage
follicle-
  stimulating
  hormone
  (FSH)

irradiation
menstrual cycle
menstruation

negative
  feedback
ovulation stage
psychic

OBJECTIVES

■ Identify the stages of the menstrual cycle
■ Describe the major events occurring in the menstrual cycle
■ Explain menopause
■ List the anatomical, physiological, and psychic changes that occur to the menopausal female
■ Define the Key Words relating to this unit of study

THE MENSTRUAL CYCLE

In the mature human female, a mature egg develops and is ovulated from one of the two ovaries about once every 28 days. Before the mature egg is released from the ovary, a series of events occurs to thicken the uterine lining (endometrium). This is necessary to receive and hold a fertilized egg for embryonic development. If the egg is not fertilized, the endometrium starts to break down. Eventually the old unfertilized egg and the degenerated endometrium are discharged out of the female reproductive tract. The cycle then starts all over again with the development of another ovum and the buildup of the endometrium.

This cycle is called the **menstrual cycle.** The menstrual cycle starts at puberty. It can start as early as 9 years of age to as late as 18 or 19 years of age. Generally, the age range is between 12 and 15 (the average is 12.5 years).

The changes that occur during the menstrual cycle involve hormones from the pituitary gland and the ovaries.

The menstrual cycle is divided into four stages: the **follicle stage,** the **ovulation stage,** the **corpus luteum stage,** and the **menstruation stage.** (See figure 39–1 for a diagram of the menstrual cycle.)

Stages of the Menstrual Cycle

Follicle Stage. Follicle-stimulating hormone (FSH) is secreted from the anterior lobe of the pituitary gland. FSH is then circulated to an ovary via the bloodstream. When FSH reaches an ovary, it will stimulate several follicles. However, only one matures. As the one follicle grows in size, an egg cell also begins to grow inside the follicle, figure 39–2. As the follicle grows in size, it fills with a fluid containing estrogen. The estrogen stimulates the endome-

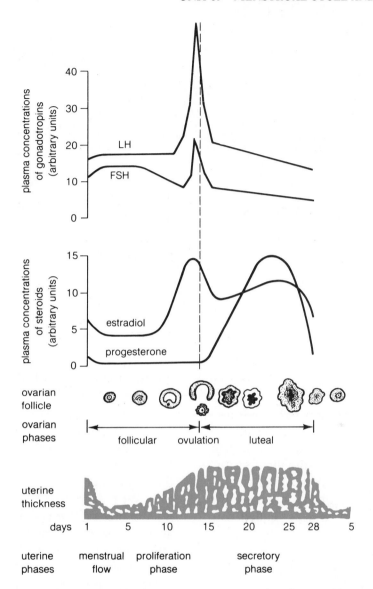

Figure 39-1   The menstrual cycle. This is a cycle of changes that occurs in the tissues of the female reproductive system. It results in the ovulation of mature ova, the preparation of the endometrium for a possible embryo implantation and pregnancy, and the return to the original state if no implantation occurs. The cycle is controlled by four interacting hormones and repeats itself about every 28 days. (From *Human Anatomy and Physiology* by Joan G. Creager. © 1983 by Wadsworth Inc. Reprinted by permission of Wadsworth Publishing Company, Belmont, California 94002.)

trium to thicken with mucus and a rich supply of blood vessels. These changes to the endometrium prepare the uterus for the implantation of an embryo. The follicle stage lasts about 10 days.

Ovulation Stage. When the concentration of estrogen in the female bloodstream reaches a high level, it causes the pituitary gland to stop FSH secretion. (This phenomenon is called **negative feedback.**) As this occurs, the lutein-

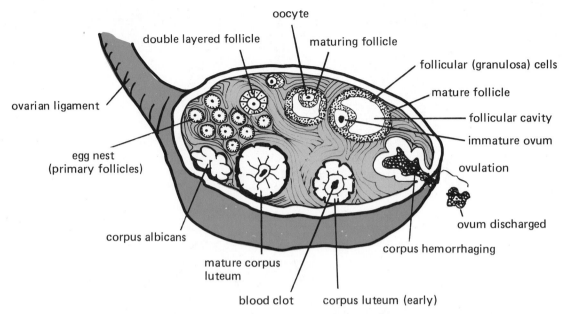

Figure 39-2   Cross section of an ovary showing the development of an ovum in a graafian follicle

izing hormone (LH) is secreted by the pituitary gland. At this point, there are three different hormones circulating in the female blood-stream — estrogen, FSH, and LH. Each hormone is present in different concentrations. Around the 14th day of the menstrual cycle, this hormonal combination somehow stimulates the mature follicle to break. When the follicle ruptures, a mature egg cell is released into the fallopian tube. This event is called **ovulation.**

Corpus Luteum Stage. After ovulation, LH stimulates the cells of the ruptured follicle to divide quickly. When this occurs, a mass of reddish-yellow cells called the corpus luteum is produced. The corpus luteum, in turn, secretes a hormone called progesterone. Progesterone helps to maintain the continued growth and thickening of the endometrium, so if an embryo happens to be implanted into the uterine lining, the pregnancy can be maintained. That is why progesterone is often called the "pregnancy hormone." Progesterone also prevents

the formation of new ovarian follicles by inhibiting the release of FSH. The corpus luteum stage lasts about 14 days.

Menstruation Stage. If fertilization does not occur and thus an embryo is not implanted in the uterus, the progesterone reaches a level in the bloodstream that inhibits further LH secretion. With decreased LH secretion, the corpus luteum breaks down causing a decrease in progesterone secretion as well. As the progesterone level decreases, the lining of the endometrium becomes progressively thinner and eventually breaks down. The extra layers of the endometrium, the unfertilized egg, and a small quantity of blood that comes from the ruptured capillaries as the endometrium peels away from the uterus are discharged from the female's body through the vagina. This causes the characteristic menstrual blood flow, and the menstruation stage starts around the 28th day of the cycle. The menstruation stage lasts about four days. While menstruation is occurring, the estrogen level in the bloodstream is decreasing. The anterior lobe of the pituitary gland is now stimulated to secrete FSH, consequently a new follicle starts to grow and the menstrual cycle starts again.

The relationship between the pituitary gland hormones and the ovarian hormones is one of feedback. That means, pituitary hormones control the functioning of the ovaries; in turn, the ovaries secrete hormones that control pituitary functioning. This is another example of the automatic regulation of many of the body's processes.

MENOPAUSE

Menopause is the time in a female's life when the monthly menstrual cycle comes to an end. This can occur any time between 35 to 55 years of age, but it frequently occurs between 45 and 50. Menopause signals the end of follicle growth and ovulation, consequently, it means the end of childbearing. However, a normal libido usually remains.

The menopausal female will experience the following anatomical changes:
1. Atrophy of the internal reproductive structures:
   a. uterus
   b. fallopian tubes
   c. ovaries
2. Atrophy of the external genitalia
3. Vagina becomes conical shaped
4. Atrophy of the vaginal mucous membranes
5. Reduction of the secretory activity of the glands associated with the reproductive organs

These changes do not occur overnight, they happen gradually over a period of years. There are also pronounced physiological changes that occur. These are "hot flashes," dizziness, headaches, rheumatic pains in joints, sweating, and susceptibility to fatigue. Depending upon the menopausal female, sometimes these physiological changes are also accompanied by **psychic** changes. These include abnormal fears, depression, excessive irritability, and a tendency to worry. Many of these physiological and psychic symptoms can be alleviated by the careful administration of female hormones. This can be helpful because a menopausal female experiences a very severe imbalance to her hormones.

Menopause can be induced prematurely (artificial menopause) by either deactivation or removal of ovarian tissue. This is done either by **irradiation** or surgery.

Further Study and Discussion

- Discuss the relationship between ovulation, menstruation, and fertilization.

Assignment

1. How many stages is the menstrual cycle divided into? What are the names of these stages?

2. Briefly describe the major events occurring in each of these stages.

3. What is meant by "negative feedback"?

4. What is menopause?

5. List four anatomical and physiological changes a menopausal female will experience?

6. What is artificial menopause and what causes it?

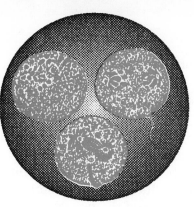

UNIT 40

GENETICS AND GENETICALLY LINKED DISEASES

KEY WORDS

amniocentesis
chromosomal
    mutation
Down's
    Syndrome
Duchenne's
    muscular
    dystrophy
gene
genetic mutation
genetics

Huntington's
    Disease
Klinefelter's
    Syndrome
lethal gene
mutagenic agent
mutation
phenylketonuria
    (PKU)
recombinant
    DNA

sickle-cell
    anemia
somatic cell
    mutation
Tay-Sachs
    Disease
trait
Trisomy 21
Turner's
    Syndrome

OBJECTIVES

- Define mutation
- Differentiate between the two basic types of mutations
- List at least six mutagenic agents
- Name three human genetic disorders and describe the cause and symptoms of each
- Define the Key Words relating to this unit of study

GENETICS

In sexual reproduction, a new individual is created from the union of the sperm cell and the egg cell. This process is called **fertilization,** and it creates a zygote, which is the cell resulting from the union of the egg and sperm. Contained in the nucleus of each gamete (the mature egg or sperm cell) are structures called **chromosomes.** The chromosomes contain DNA (deoxyribonucleic acid), the hereditary material referred to in unit 2, Chemistry of Living Things. The DNA is packaged in small functional units found along the length of a chromosome, called **genes.** A gene is an area of DNA which carries information for the cellular synthesis of a specific protein. These genes

are transmitted to the zygote, and will then control the development and characteristics of the embryo as it grows and matures. Eventually, due to the combined influence of all of the genes on all of the chromosomes, a new individual is formed. The new individual possesses all the necessary characteristics or **traits** needed for survival. Additionally, because the genes come from two parents, the offspring resemble both parents in some ways. However, it is also different from each parent. It has, for instance, all the characteristics of its species. Concurrently, it possesses its own unique traits that set it apart from all other members of its species.

Genetics is the branch of biology that studies how the genes are transmitted from parents to offspring. Occasionally, a gene or chromosome is changed, or **mutated,** in a gamete, and this mutated gene or chromosome is

Portions of this unit were contributed by Loretta Chiarenza, M.A., M.S., Associate Professor of Biology and Associate Dean, State University of New York at Farmingdale, Farmingdale NY 11735.

319

inherited by the offspring. The inheritance of such a mutated gene or chromosome will cause the appearance of a new and different trait, called a **mutation.** Sometimes the mutation is beneficial or harmless to an organism. Unfortunately, most inherited mutations are not beneficial. Still, it must be emphasized, that mutations in the genetic material are responsible for biological evolution on this planet.

TYPES OF MUTATIONS

There are two types of mutations. One type is called a **gene mutation.** When this mutation occurs, a new or altered gene is produced to replace a normal pre-existing gene. The other type is a **chromosomal mutation.** This mutation involves a change in the number of chromosomes found in the nucleus or a change in the structure of a whole chromosome.

Somatic Cell Mutation

Gene mutations occur occasionally at random in all cells of the human body. For instance, skin cells often undergo mutation as an individual ages. Mutations that occur in individual body (somatic) cells will not be transmitted to the offspring. This specific type of mutation is called a **somatic cell mutation.** A somatic cell mutation is not likely to affect other cells or the function of the organism as a whole. As an example, a single cell may lose the ability to make a certain protein and die without having an impact on the total organism.

Gametic Cell Mutation

Mutations that occur in the nucleus of the **gametes** (sperm and egg cell) will be passed on to the next generation. If either a gene or chromosomal mutation is present in a gamete at the moment of fertilization, all the cells of the embryo and the developed organism will have the mutation in at least half of their DNA.

LETHAL GENES

On the whole, inherited mutations are generally negative happenings to the individual. At times, they might even result in the formation of lethal genes. A **lethal gene** is a gene that results in death.

The time at which lethal genes exert their deadly influence varies. Some genes interfere with mitosis of the zygote and life ends before the zygote divides. Some lethal genes interfere with implantation of the fertilized egg in the uterus. Death would occur so early that a woman would never know that conception had even occurred. A lethal gene that prevents normal formation of the heart or normal blood production causes death at about three weeks after fertilization because this is the time when circulating blood becomes vital for continued existence. Others may kill at various times during development, depending on the time their products become vital for survival. Other lethal genes causing neonatal deaths involve abnormalities of the lungs and shifts in the circulatory system which must channel blood from the heart to the lungs instead of to the umbilical cord.

Some lethal genes do not exert their effects until later in life. Tay-Sachs Disease causes death several years after birth. Duchenne's muscular dystrophy causes death in the teens and early adulthood. Huntington's Disease usually brings about death at about forty to fifty years of age.

It is estimated that each person carries two or three different recessive lethal genes. Two similar recessive genes must be present in an individual in order for the gene to be expressed. Since there are so many kinds of lethal genes, one's chance of marrying someone with even one matching lethal is small. Statistically, should this happen, the lethal would be expressed in only one-fourth of the offspring.

When close relatives marry, the chance of the offspring inheriting two similar lethal genes increases. Persons with a common ancestry are more likely to share many genes than non-relatives. As a result, spontaneous abortions, still-births, neonatal deaths, and congenital deformities are higher among progeny of people sharing similar gene pools.

HUMAN GENETIC DISORDERS

Some diseases caused by gene mutations in humans are phenylketonuria (PKU), sickle-cell anemia, Tay-Sachs Disease, Duchenne's muscular dystrophy, and Huntington's Disease.

Phenylketonuria

PKU is a human metabolic disorder caused by an enzyme deficiency. The individual with the trait cannot break down the amino acid phenylalanine and, consequently, there is a buildup of this substance in the body. Excess phenylalanine disrupts the normal development of the brain. If a child born with the defect eats proteins containing phenylalanine

during childhood, mental retardation results. A newborn infant is tested for this defect, and, if the test is positive, a phenylalanine-restricted diet is prescribed. In most cases, this diet can be liberalized as the child grows older and brain development and maturation are completed.

Sickle-cell Anemia

Sickle-cell anemia is a blood disorder common in individuals of African descent. It is caused by a gene mutation resulting in an abnormal hemoglobin molecule in a red blood cell. Refer to figure 40–1. Especially in times of low oxygen availability, the shape of a red blood cell changes from that of a biconcave disc to a crescent shape. This is referred to as sickling. The sickle shape causes the cells to clump together, thus clogging small blood vessels and capillaries. Since a sickle cell has an abnormal hemoglobin (the pigment that combines with oxgen), it also carries less oxygen to the tissues, resulting in fatigue and listlessness. Breakage of these cells is also very common since their membranes are excessively fragile. See figure 40–2 for tissue damage and physiological effects caused by sickle-cell anemia.

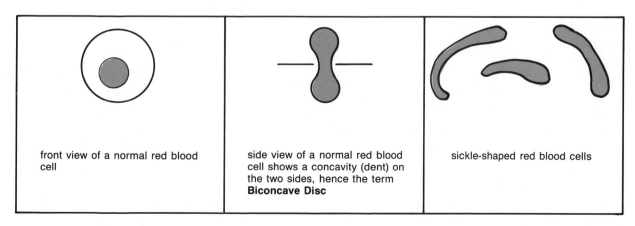

front view of a normal red blood cell

side view of a normal red blood cell shows a concavity (dent) on the two sides, hence the term **Biconcave Disc**

sickle-shaped red blood cells

Figure 40-1   Difference in shape between a normal red blood cell (biconcave disc) and a sickle-shaped red blood cell (crescent-shaped)

sickle-cell anemia

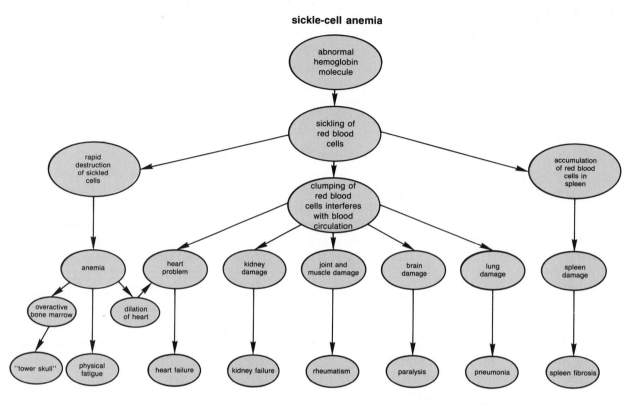

Figure 40-2   A series of damages and effects caused by sickle-cell anemia

Tay-Sachs Disease

Tay-Sachs is a genetic disorder caused by a mutation resulting in a deficiency of a lysosomal enzyme. The missing enzyme functions in breaking down lipid molecules in the brain. Without the enzyme, lipids accumulate in the brain cells and destroy them. This results in severe mental and motor deterioration leading to death several years after birth. This disorder is found most frequently among Jewish people of central European ancestry.

Huntington's Disease

Huntington's Disease is characterized by the degeneration of the central nervous system, which ultimately results in abnormal movements and mental deterioration. In this disorder, the product of an abnormal gene in- terferes with normal metabolism in nerve tissue.

Duchenne's Muscular Dystrophy

In muscular dystrophy, the muscles suffer a loss of protein and the contractile fibers are eventually replaced by fat and connective tissue, rendering skeletal muscle useless. As the weakening process of the disease continues, the teen or young adult is confined to a wheelchair. In many cases, the victim dies before the age of twenty from respiratory or heart failure.

Chromosomal Aberrations

Some mutations are caused by chromosomal aberrations. Some involve entire chromosomes and others involve parts of chromosomes. During **meiosis** (the cell division occurring during the formation of the gametes) a pair of chromosomes may adhere to each other and not pull apart at metaphase. As a result of this nondisjunction, duplicate chromosomes go to one daughter cell and none of this type of chromosome to the other. Nondisjunction of certain chromosomes referred to as sex chromosomes causes various abnormalities of sexual development such as Turner's Syndrome in females and Klinefelter's Syndrome in males.

One of the most common chromosomal abnormalities involves an extra chromosome designated as chromosome 21. In fact, this disorder is referred to as trisomy 21 or Down's Syndrome (Mongoloidism). The risk of bearing a child with Down's Syndrome significantly increases with the age of the mother. Many physicians therefore recommend amniocentesis for all women who become pregnant after thirty-five. Cells from the amniotic fluid will show trisomy 21 (as well as other chromosomal defects) if it is present. If a serious defect is detected prospective parents have the option of therapeutic abortion.

Mutagenic Agents

Although most gene or chromosomal mutations occur spontaneously, the rate or speed of mutations can be increased. This happens when a cell, a group of cells, or an entire organism is exposed to certain chemicals or radiations. Agents that speed up the occurrence of mutations are called **mutagenic agents.** Mutagenic agents can be radiations like cosmic rays, ultraviolet rays from the sun, X rays, and radiation from radioactive elements. Some muta-

genic chemicals are benzene, formaldehyde, phenol, and nitrous acid.

In recent times, the accelerated use of various chemical and physical agents with mutagenic properties has caused concern among some geneticists who fear possible significant alterations to genes and chromosomes that will be passed on to future generations. The increased use of ionizing radiation in medical diagnosis and the problem of the disposal of nuclear waste from reactors are examples. Certain chemical pollutants in the environment, such as herbicides and insecticides, are also suspect as causing genetic defects.

Since people are being exposed to more and more new substances, and since changes in genes are irreversible, caution should be the rule with regard to any unnecessary exposure to those suspected of being mutagens.

GENETIC ENGINEERING

Recent advances in the methods of gene transfer from the cell of one species to another offer exciting possibilities for the treatment of genetic deficiencies. Human insulin, human growth hormone, and human **interferons** (proteins that interfere with virus replication) are now being produced using the sophisticated technology of **recombinant DNA.** We can isolate a desired gene (to correct for a defective one) and grow millions of copies of it in the cells of bacteria and yeast which in turn produce the gene product on a commercial scale.

Some scientists even envision a time when we will have the ability to introduce copies of normal genes into humans whose genes are defective, thus alleviating a large segment of human suffering.

Further Study and Discussion

- Using library resources, investigate more fully the human genetic or chromosomal disorders such as Down's Syndrome, Klinefelter's Syndrome, Turner's Syndrome, and hemophilia.

Assignment

1. Explain the difference between a somatic cell and gametic cell mutation.

2. List at least 6 things that can cause mutations.

3. Describe the abnormalities characteristic of PKU, sickle-cell anemia, and Tay Sachs Disease, Duchenne's muscular dystrophy, and Huntington's Disease.

4. Give an example of genetic engineering.

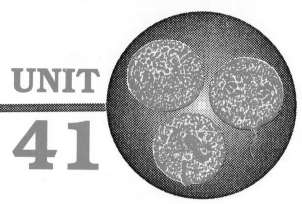

UNIT 41

REPRESENTATIVE DISORDERS OF THE REPRODUCTIVE SYSTEM

KEY WORDS

anorchidism	hysterectomy	prostatectomy
benign	leukorrhea	prostatitis
biopsy	mastectomy	retroversion of
carcinoma	metastasis	the uterus
dysmenorrhea	monorchidism	salpingitis
dyspareunia	orchitis	vaginismus
endocervicitis	palpate	vaginitis
epididymitis	pap smear	vesiculitis
fibroma	prolapsed uterus	

OBJECTIVES

- List some common disorders of the reproductive system
- Identify symptoms of some common disorders
- Define the Key Words related to this unit of study

Persons who are involved in health care should be familiar with the names and symptoms of the more common disorders of the reproductive system. Some representative disorders and their symptoms are briefly described in this unit.

FEMALE REPRODUCTIVE SYSTEM

A **carcinoma** is a malignant growth. Cancer cells multiply widely and invade normal cells and tissues. Carcinomas can develop in the breasts or uterus. As in other forms of cancer, early detection and treatment is vital to the patient's life. Breast carcinomas may sometimes be detected by self-examination. Periodically a woman should **palpate** (manipulate) her breasts in a circular motion. The purpose of this examination is to detect any developing lumps that may be lying below the surface. If a lump is discovered, a biopsy is usually performed to ascertain whether it is benign or malignant.

A **biopsy** is the removal of a small piece of tissue from the lump (or growth) for testing. If the lump is **benign,** surgery is the usual course of treatment. (A benign tumor is a noncancerous growth that does not invade and destroy normal tissue.) Should the lump prove to be malignant, however, the treatment may be more extensive. Frequently it necessitates complete removal of the carcinoma along with the entire breast. This surgical procedure is known as a **mastectomy.** The purpose of a mastectomy is to prevent the **metastasis,** or spread of the cancer, to nearby breast tissue.

Mastectomies are often followed by chemotherapy and/or radiation. Chemotherapy includes the use of anti-cancer drugs injected into the bloodstream. This procedure destroys any cancer cells that might have migrated into the lymph or bloodstream from the original carcinoma.

Cervical cancer is detected by the **Papanicolaou (PAP) smear.** Again, the usual course of treatment involves surgery. Surgical removal of the uterus is called a **hysterectomy.** Here, too, the operation may be followed by chemotherapy.

The chemotherapeutic drugs are the antimetabolites, cytotoxic or alkylating agents, antibiotics, and hormones.

An antimetabolite imitates the action of a hormone or nutrient needed by malignant cells for correct cell metabolism. Thus, the malignant cell erroneously ingests the antimetabolite and eventually dies.

Some examples of antimetabolites used to treat breast cancer are methotrexate, 5-fluorouracil, and vinblastine sulfate (Velban). Cytotoxic drugs are toxic (poisonous) to the cancer cells.

Dysmenorrhea is a term used for painful or difficult menstruation. Some different types of dysmenorrhea include:

- **Ovarian dysmenorrhea** — a form of dysmenorrhea due to disease of the ovaries

- **Spasmodic dysmenorrhea** — caused by severe and sudden uterine contractions

- **Uterine dysmenorrhea** — dysmenorrhea resulting from a uterine disease

Dysmenorrhea is generally characterized by abdominal pain, backache, headache, and occasionally nausea and vomiting.

Endocervicitis is an inflammation of the mucous membrane lining the cervix. Its key symptom is a white, muco-purulent discharge from the vagina, known as **leukorrhea.** Treatment consists of administration of antibiotics to combat the bacteria-causing cervicitis.

Fibroid tumor, or **fibroma,** is a benign tumor comprised mainly of fibrous connective tissue found in the uterus. Symptoms include backache and abnormal uterine bleeding. The general course of treatment is a **fibroidectomy,** or surgical removal of the uterine fibroma.

Prolapsed uterus is a disorder that results when the normal supportive structures weaken and allows the uterus to fall from its usual position.

Retroversion is a disorder of the uterus. The nongravid (nonpregnant) uterus normally tilts forward about 90 degrees in proportion to the vagina. Sometimes, however, the uterus may be abnormally tilted backward, a condition called **retroversion of the uterus.** Common symptoms, if any, may include backache, constipation, or dysmenorrhea.

Salpingitis is inflammation of the fallopian tubes. It is accompanied by lower abdominal tenderness and pain. There are several different types of salpingitis:

- **Gonococcic salpingitis** is an infection of the fallopian tubes, caused by the *gonococcus bacterium.*

- **Purulent salpingitis** produces a purulent (pus) discharge rather than mucus or serum.

- **Tuberculosis salpingitis** is brought about by infiltration of the uterine membrane lining and wall by tuberculous nodules.

Treatment of these and related inflammatory conditions generally necessitates the use of antibiotic chemicals.

Sterility is the inability to reproduce: it may occur in either sex.

Vaginismus is a condition that occurs when the vaginal muscles spasm or the muscles surrounding its entrance spasm. This prevents coitus or causes difficult or painful coitus (dyspareunia).

Vaginitis is an inflammation of the vagina caused by some type of infectious microorganism.

MALE REPRODUCTIVE SYSTEM

Anorchidism is a congenital absence of testes.

Epididymitis is a painful swelling in the groin and scrotum due to infection of the epididymis.

Monorchidism is the presence of only one testis.

Orchitis is inflammation of the testis. It may be a complication of mumps, influenza, or other infection. A symptom is the swelling of the scrotum, accompanied by elevated temperature and pain.

Both epididymitis and orchitis are treated by the administration of antibiotics.

Prostatitis is an inflammation of the prostate gland. By its pressure on the bladder, the prostate gland causes frequent, painful urination. If pressure on the urethra is severe, urinary retention may result. A **prostatectomy** is the surgical removal of all or part of the prostate gland.

Vesiculitis is an inflammation of a seminal vesicle.

Further Study and Discussion

- A woman of forty-seven years of age asks your advice concerning depression which she has experienced for several months. She has also had difficulty sleeping due to excessive perspiration during the night? How would you advise her?

- What is the Papanicolaou test? What is its value?

Assignment

A. Match each term in column I with its description in column II.

	Column I	Column II
_____	1. carcinoma	a. surgical removal of uterus
_____	2. endocervicitis	b. inflammation of fallopian tubes
_____	3. epididymitis	c. painful swelling in groin and scrotum
_____	4. hysterectomy	d. backward displacement of uterus
_____	5. mastectomy	e. may cause urine to be retained
_____	6. orchitis	f. surgical removal of breast
_____	7. prostatitis	g. inability to reproduce
_____	8. retroversion	h. inflammation in the lining or cervix
_____	9. salpingitis	i. cancer in breasts or uterus
_____	10. sterility	j. complication of disease or inflammation
		k. painful menstruation

B. Briefly answer the following questions:
   1. What is a prolapsed uterus?

   2. What causes vaginismus?

   3. How is anorchidism different from monochidism?

HUMAN REPRODUCTION

A.   Match each term in column I with its correct description in column II.

Column I	Column II
_____ 1. DNA	a. specialized sex cell of either sex
_____ 2. fertilization	b. male sex cell
_____ 3. gamete	c. conception
_____ 4. gonadotrophic hormone	d. determine hereditary characteristics
	e. reduction division
_____ 5. graafian follicle	f. microscopic sac
_____ 6. meiosis	g. female sex cell
_____ 7. ovum	h. stimulates testes to action
_____ 8. progesterone	i. a fertilized cell
_____ 9. sperm	j. prevents menstruation during pregnancy
_____ 10. zygote	k. study of genetics

B.   Complete the following statements.

1.   The tubes which receive the ova and allow them to pass into the uterus are the _____ .

2.   The cavity below the abdominal cavity is the _____ .

3.   The substance called _____ carries the inherited characteristics in the chromosomes.

4.   The unborn baby formed after the zygote divides is called a(an) _____ .

5.   The union of the ovum and sperm cell is called _____ .

C.   Briefly answer the following questions.

1.   Define mitosis.

2. Why is it important for the testes to descend into the scrotal pouch as a young boy enters puberty?

3. What is the function of the prostate gland?

4. How many stages is the menstrual cycle divided into? What are the names of these stages?

5. What is menopause?

6. Describe briefly the following disorders occurring to the human reproductive system:
   a. prolapsed uterus

   b. vaginitis

   c. anorchidism

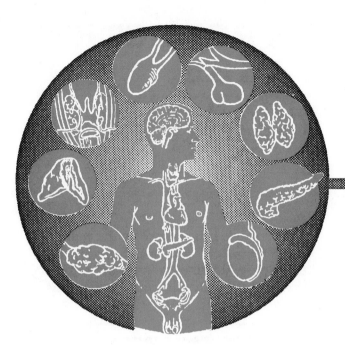

CHAPTER 9

REGULATORS OF BODY FUNCTIONS

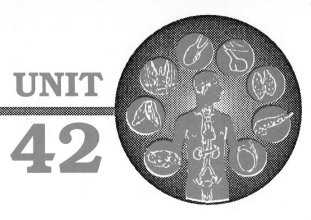

UNIT 42

INTRODUCTION TO THE ENDOCRINE SYSTEM

OBJECTIVES

■ List the glands which make up the endocrine system
■ Locate the endocrine glands in the body
■ Describe how each endocrine gland affects body activities

A gland is any organ that produces a secretion. **Endocrine glands,** figure 42–1, are organized groups of tissues which use materials from the blood or lymph to make new compounds called **hormones.** Endocrine glands are also called ductless glands and glands of internal secretion; the hormones are secreted directly into the bloodstream as the blood circulates through the gland. The secretions are then transported to all areas of the body where they have a special influence on cells, tissues, and organs.

One of the endocrine glands, the pancreas, has two major functions. The pancreas acts as a digestive gland in the production of **pancreatic fluid,** which passes through ducts to the digestive tract. Special groups of cells, known as islets of Langerhans, secrete the hormone **insulin** which is discharged directly into the bloodstream.

There are six important endocrine glands, or groups of glands, in the body:

- pituitary gland, at the base of the brain
- thyroid gland, in the neck
- parathyroid glands, near the thyroid gland
- pancreas, behind the stomach
- two adrenal glands, one over each kidney
- gonads, or sex glands: ovaries in the female lower abdomen, testes in the male scrotum.

Figure 42–1 shows the locations of the endocrine glands in the body. Each has specific functions to perform. Any disturbance in the functioning of these glands may cause changes in the appearance or functioning of the body. Sometimes both conditions arise.

332

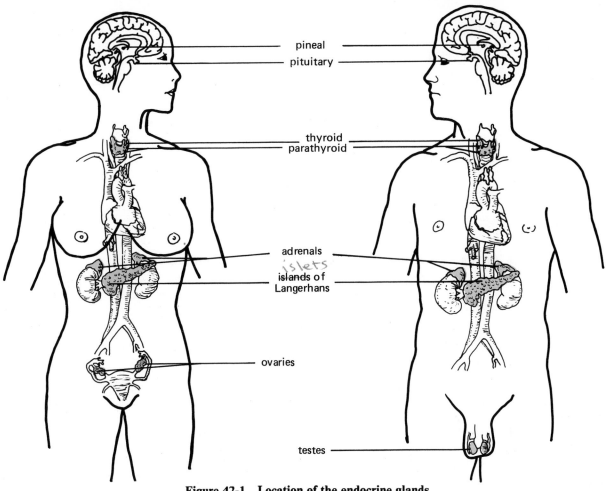

pineal
pituitary
thyroid
parathyroid
adrenals
islets
islands of
Langerhans
ovaries
testes

Figure 42-1   Location of the endocrine glands

Further Study and Discussion

• Discuss location, appearance, and inter-related activities of the endocrine glands.

• Determine from outside reading what secretions of the endocrine glands can be manufactured by artificial means (synthesis).

• A boy of four has shown no growth increase since the age of two years. He seems to have a low mentality. He usually holds his mouth open, and his tongue is large. His hair is dry and coarse. Which gland possibly may be responsible for this condition?

• Discuss other hormonal secretions and glandular structures: gastrin, secretin, placental, pineal, and thymus.

Assignment

1. Define "gland."

2. How do endocrine glands differ from other types of glands?

3. Give the general name of a secretion from an endocrine gland.

4. Name two secretions released from the pancreas.

5. Name the six important endocrine glands of the body.

6. What gland contains the islets of Langerhans?

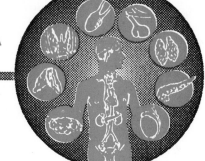

UNIT
43

THE PITUITARY GLAND

OBJECTIVES

- Locate the pituitary gland
- Describe the functions of the pituitary gland
- List the principal secretions of the pituitary gland
- Define the Key Words in this unit of study

The **pituitary** gland is also called the **hypophysis.** It is a tiny structure having a diameter of about 10mm and a weight of approximately .5 grams. It is located at the base of the brain within the **sella turcica,** a small bony depression in the sphenoid bone of the skull, figure 43–1. The pituitary gland is connected to the hypothalamus by a stalk called the **infundibulum.** The gland is divided into an **anterior lobe** and a **posterior lobe,** figure 43–2. It is called the master gland because it secretes several hormones into the bloodstream that affect other glands. These endocrine glands together with the pituitary gland secretions help maintain proper body functioning.

The **posterior lobe** or **neurohypophysis** does not produce any hormones of its own. However, it helps to store two hormones produced by the hypothalamus. These two hormones are **ADH (antidiuretic hormone)** and **oxytocin.** Figure 43–3 shows the hormones secreted by the pituitary gland.

The **anterior lobe** of the pituitary gland is also called the **adenohypophysis.** The tissue

structure of the adenohypophysis is much like other endocrine glands. It is composed of secretory cells and a large amount of capillaries to carry away its hormones. There are two types of secretory cells found in the adenohypophysis. They are the **acidophils** and **basophils.** The acidophils will secrete growth hormone and prolactin. The basophils secrete thyroid-stimulating hormone (TSH), adrenocorticotrophic hormone (ACTH), follicle-stim-

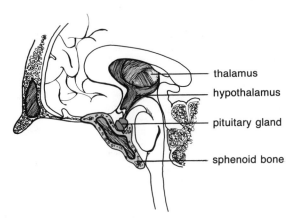

Figure 43-1   The pituitary gland in relation to the brain

335

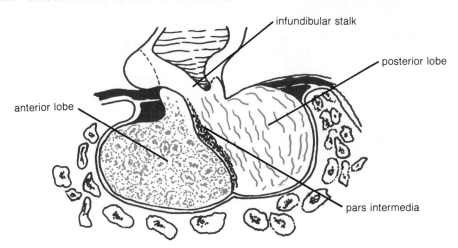

Figure 43-2   The pituitary gland

ulating hormone (FSH), luteinizing hormone (LH), and interstitial cell-stimulating hormone (ICSH). The release of these hormones is controlled by the hypothalamus, which releases chemicals called neurohumors. These neurohumors are carried via the bloodstream to the adenohypophysis. There they will stimulate the anterior lobe to function. These neurohumors do not act indiscriminately. There are several neurohumors produced, each one stimulating the secretion of only one hormone. In addition, there is one neurohumor that inhib-

Table 43–1 Pituitary Hormones and Their Known Functions

PITUITARY HORMONE		KNOWN FUNCTION
Anterior Lobe		
TSH	— Thyroid-Stimulating Hormone (Thyrotropin)	Stimulates the growth and the secretion of the thyroid gland
ACTH	— Adrenocorticotrophic Hormone	Stimulates the growth and the secretion of the adrenal cortex
FSH	— Follicle-Stimulating Hormone	Stimulates growth of new graafian (ovarian) follicle and secretion of estrogen by follicle cells in the female and the production of sperm in the male
LH	— Luteinizing Hormone (female)	Stimulates ovulation and formation of the corpus luteum
ICSH	— Interstitial Cell-Stimulating Hormone (male)	Stimulates testosterone secretion
LTH	— Lactogenic Hormone (Prolactin or luteotropin)	Stimulates secretion of milk and influences maternal behavior
GH	— Growth Hormone (Somatotropin, STH)	Accelerates body growth
Posterior Lobe		
VASOPRESSIN (Antidiuretic Hormone, ADH)		Maintains water balance by reducing urinary output. It acts on kidney tubules to reabsorb water into the blood more quickly
OXYTOCIN		Promotes milk ejection and causes contraction of the smooth muscles of the uterus

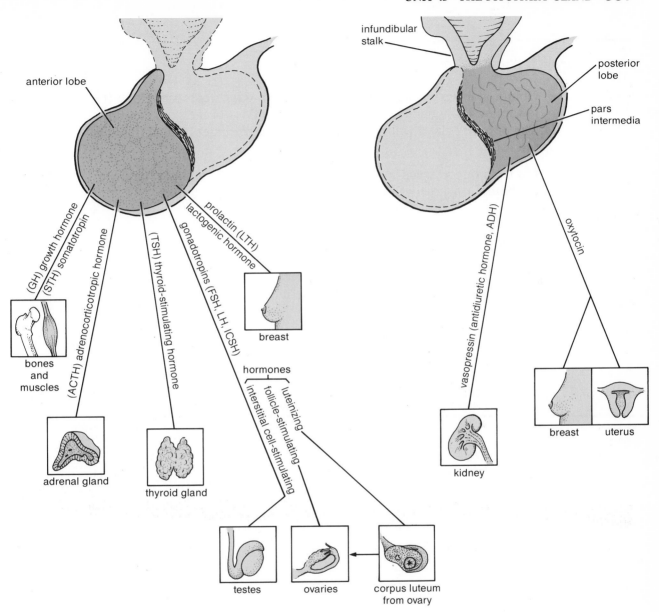

Figure 43-3   Pituitary hormones secreted by the anterior and posterior lobes of the pituitary gland

its the secretion of growth hormone, still another inhibits prolactin secretion.

To briefly summarize, the pituitary gland is responsible for the growth of the long bones; thus, it controls the height of the individual. Circus giants are often the result of overgrowth of the long bones caused by oversecretion by the pituitary gland. The organs of reproduc-

tion are influenced by it as pituitary secretions are essential to pregnancy and lactation. The pituitary is responsible for maintaining the water balance of the body and affects the use of starches and sugars by the body. It secretes ACTH, one of the hormones used in the treatment of arthritis. Table 43–1 lists the pituitary hormones and their known functions.

Further Study and Discussion

- Obtain a sheep's head from the butcher or slaughterhouse. Have the lower jaw and tongue removed. Remove the floor of the skull carefully. The pituitary gland will be found in a bony encasement called the sella turcica.

- If a fresh or preserved specimen is not available, use a plastic model of the brain or a large wall chart to locate the pituitary gland.

Assignment

A. Briefly answer the following questions.

1. Why is the pituitary gland called the master gland?

2. Describe the principal functions of the pituitary, or hypophysis, gland.

3. Why may a hormone be thought of as a chemical messenger?

4. What is the name of the small depression in the sphenoid bone within which the pituitary gland is located?

5. Name the two lobes of the pituitary gland.

6. How does the pituitary gland control height in an individual?

7. Give the functions of the two hormones secreted from the posterior lobe of the pituitary gland.

8. What is the approximate size of the pituitary gland?

9. What effects does estrogen have on the female breasts, fallopian tubes, and pelvis?

10. How is the uterus affected by progesterone?

B. Match each of the hormones listed in column I with its function in column II. More than one function may be selected.

Column I	Column II
_____ 1. thyroid-stimulating hormone	a. stimulates secretion of estrogen in the female and sperm production in the male
_____ 2. luteinizing hormone	
_____ 3. follicle-stimulating hormone	b. stimulates testosterone secretion
	c. stimulates growth and secretion of the adrenal cortex
_____ 4. lactogenic hormone	
_____ 5. interstitial cell-stimulating hormone	d. maintains water balance through kidney reabsorption
_____ 6. adrenocorticotrophic hormone	e. stimulates secretion of milk in the mother
_____ 7. growth hormone	f. accelerates body growth
_____ 8. somatotropin	g. stimulates both the growth and secretion of the thyroid gland
_____ 9. thyrotropin	
_____ 10. prolactin	h. causes contraction of smooth muscle in the uterus.

THE THYROID AND PARATHYROID GLANDS

KEY WORDS

calciferol
  (vitamin D)
calcitonin
hypercalcemia
isthmus of
  thyroid
  gland
osteoblast

osteoclast
parathormone
parathyroid gland
thymus
thyroglobulin
thyroid gland,
  intermediate
  lobe

TSH (thyroid-
  stimulating
  hormone)
thyroxine
triiodothyronine

OBJECTIVES

- Locate the thyroid, parathyroid, and thymus glands
- Describe the important functions of the thyroid gland
- Describe the functions of the parathyroid and thymus glands
- Define the Key Words related to this unit

The thyroid and parathyroid glands are located in the neck, close to the cricoid cartilage ("Adam's apple"). The thyroid regulates body metabolism. The parathyroid maintains the calcium-phosphorus balance.

The thymus gland is located anterior to and above the heart. It is involved with the development of an immune response in the newborn. The gland grows until puberty at which time the original lymphoid tissue is replaced with adipose and connective tissue.

THYROID GLAND

The **thyroid gland** is a butterfly-shaped mass of tissue located in the anterior part of the neck, figure 44–1. It lies on either side of the larynx, over the trachea. Its general shape is that of the letter "H," figure 44–2. It is about two inches long, with two lobes joined by strands of thyroid tissue called the **isthmus.**

Coming from the isthmus is a finger-like lobe of tissue known as the **intermediate lobe.** This intermediate lobe projects upward toward the floor of the mouth, as far up as the hyoid bone. The thyroid gland has a rich blood supply. In fact, it has been estimated that about 4 to 5 liters (some 8 1/2 to 10 1/2 pints) of blood pass through the gland every hour.

The thyroid gland secretes three hormones: **thyroxine, triiodothyronine,** and **calcitonin.** The first two are iodine-bearing derivatives of the amino acid, tyrosine. Triiodothyronine is 5 to 10 times more active than thyroxine, but its activity is less prolonged. However, the two have the same effect. Both hormones are produced in the follicle cells of the thyroid gland. These cells are stimulated to secretory activity by a hormone from the anterior lobe of the pituitary gland. This hormone, **TSH (thyroid-stimulating hormone),**

341

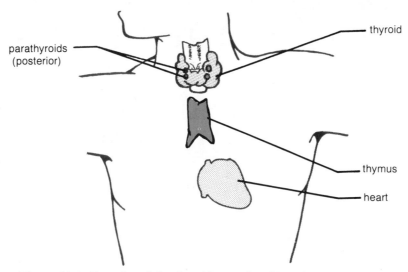

Figure 44-1   Location of the thyroid, parathyroid, and thymus glands

controls the production and secretion of the thyroid hormone from the thyroid gland. The thyroid hormones contain iodine.* Most of the iodine needed for their synthesis comes from the diet. Iodides are circulated to the thyroid gland, where they are "trapped." Here the iodides combine with the amino acid tyrosine to form the thyroglobulin molecule. Prior to being secreted into the bloodstream, thyroglobulin is chemically converted into triiodothyronine (T_3), and finally into thyroxine (T_4). T_3 is the major active form of the hormone at the cellular level.

Under normal circumstances, the presence of these two hormones (T_3 and T_4) in the bloodstream serves to regulate the system. On the other hand, an excess would suppress TSH secretion. Consequently, the thyroid gland secretes less of these two hormones. When the concentration of thyroid hormones is lowered in the bloodstream, the pituitary gland secretes more TSH. This, in turn, stimulates thyroid gland activity. (The consequences of hypose-

cretion and hypersecretion of the thyroid hormones is discussed in unit 47, *Representative Disorders of the Endocrine System*).

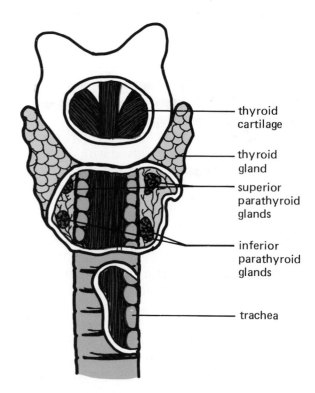

Figure 44-2   Thyroid and parathyroid glands

---

*In its pure elemental form, iodine is a violent cellular poison. It exists, however, within the human body in minute amounts as iodides. Half of the body's total iodine supply (about 50 milligrams) is found in the thyroid as *thyroglobulin* (a combination of tyrosine and iodine).

Thyroxine controls the rate of metabolism, heat production, and oxidation of all cells, with the possible exception of the brain and spleen cells. We have already noted the thyroid's role in regulating physical growth, mental development, sexual maturity, and the distribution and exchange of water and salts within the body. It can speed up or slow down the activities of the body as needed. In the liver, the two thyroid hormones affect the conversion of glycogen from sources other than sugar. It also helps to change glycogen into glucose, raising the glucose level of the blood. Figure 44–3 shows how the level of thyroxin in the bloodstream is controlled.

To summarize, the functions of thyroxin are as follows:

1. Thyroxin is a diuretic; it promotes water loss through urine.
2. Thyroxin stimulates protein synthesis and thus helps in tissue growth.
3. Thyroxin stimulates the breakdown of liver glycogen.
4. Thyroxin stimulates the cellular breakdown of glucose.

Calcitonin

Calcitonin is another hormone produced and secreted by the thyroid gland. It controls the calcium ion concentration in the body by maintaining a proper calcium level in the bloodstream.

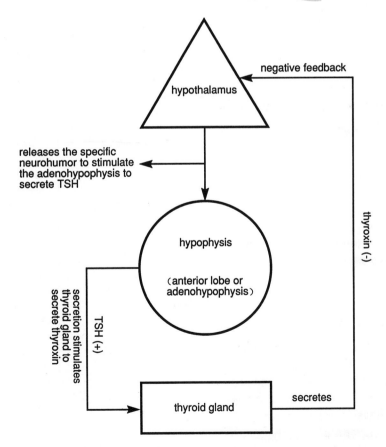

Figure 44-3   How the concentration of thyroxin is controlled in the bloodstream.

Calcium is an essential body mineral. Approximately 99% of the calcium in the body is stored in the bones. The rest is located in the blood and tissue fluids. Calcium is necessary for blood clotting, holding cells together, and neuromuscular functions. The constant level of calcium in the blood and tissues is maintained by the action of calcitonin and parathormone (produced by the parathyroid gland).

When blood calcium levels are higher than normal, calcitonin secretion is increased. Calcitonin lowers the calcium concentration in the blood and body fluids by decreasing the rate of bone resorption or osteoclastic activity and by increasing the calcium absorption by bones or osteoblastic activity. Proper secretion of calcitonin into the blood stream prevents a harmful rise in the blood calcium level, or hypercalcemia.

THYMUS GLAND

The **thymus gland** is both an endocrine gland and a lymphatic organ. It is located under the sternum, anterior and superior to the heart. Fairly large during childhood, it begins to disappear at puberty. Recent research has discovered that the thymus gland secretes a large number of hormones. These hormones help to stimulate the lymphoid cells that are responsible for the production of antibodies against certain diseases. Table 44–1 lists the thymus gland hormones and their functions.

PARATHYROID GLANDS

The **parathyroid** glands, usually four in number, are tiny glands the size of grains of rice. These are attached to the posterior surface of the thyroid gland, and secrete the hormone, **parathormone.** Parathormone, like calcitonin, also controls the concentration of

Table 44–1 Thymus Gland Hormones and Their Related Functions

HORMONE	FUNCTION
1. Homeostatic Thymic Hormone (HTH)	Helps the bone marrow cells to maintain its immunological abilities.
2. Thymic Factor (TF)	• Stimulates the thymus gland to differentiate and develop T-cells • Increases the antigen activity of the thymus gland.
3. Thymic Humoral Factor (THF)	• It is a protein; it will *stimulate mitosis.* • THF secretion diminishes with age, by disease, by toxins, and by radiation.
4. Thymic Replacing Factor (TRF)	• Restores the immune activity of T-cell-deprived structures
5. Thymosin	• Enhances the development of T-cells • Helps specifically in the growth and differentiation of thymus lymphoid cells • Stimulates the secretion of the luteinizing hormone releasing factor (LHRF).
6. Thymopoietin	Once called thymin, it stops neuromuscular nerve message transmission
7. Thymosterin	Inhibits tumor growth and lymph cell formation.
8. Lymphocytosis Stimulating Hormones (LSHr and LSH$_R$)	• Stimulates lymphocyte production • Enhances antigen-antibody response

calcium in the bloodstream. When the blood calcium level is lower than normal, parathormone secretion is increased.

Parathormone stimulates an increase in the number and size of specialized bone cells referred to as **osteoclasts**. Osteoclasts quickly invade hard bone tissue, digesting large amounts of the bony material containing calcium. As this process continues, calcium leaves the bone and is released into the bloodstream, increasing the calcium blood level.

Bone calcium is bonded to phosphorus in a compound called calcium phosphate $(CaPO_4)$. So when calcium is released into the bloodstream, phosphorus is released along with it. Parathormone stimulates the kidneys to excrete any excess phosphorus from the blood; at the same time, it inhibits calcium excretion from the kidneys. Consequently, the concentration of blood calcium rises.

Thus parathormone and calcitonin have opposite, or antagonistic effects to one another (see figure 44–4 for a summary of their actions). Parathormone, however, acts much more slowly than calcitonin. It may be hours before the effects of parathormone become apparent. In this manner, the secretion of parathormone and calcitonin serve as complementary processes controlling the level of calcium in the bloodstream.

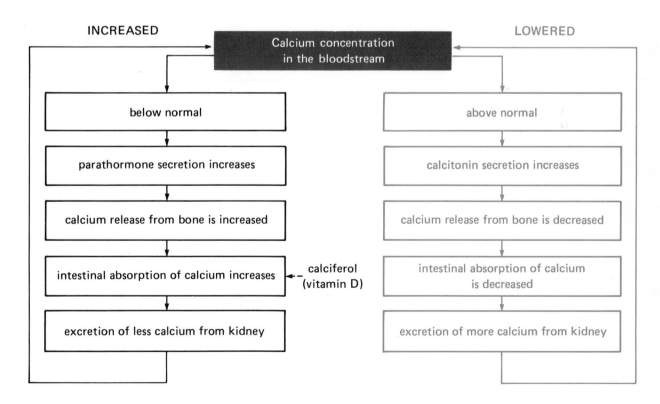

Figure 44-4   Effects of parathormone and calcitonin on the level of calcium in the blood

Further Study and Discussion

- Locate the thyroid, parathyroids, and thymus glands using classroom models or wall charts.

- Relate the function of the thyroid gland to the process of metabolism.

Assignment

1. Locate and describe the thyroid gland.

2. Locate and describe the parathyroid glands.

3. Describe the functions of the thyroid, parathyroid, and thymus glands.

4. Label figure 44–5.

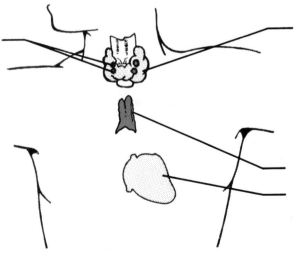

Figure 44-5

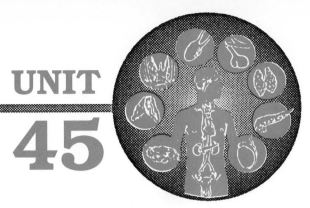

UNIT 45

THE ADRENAL GLANDS AND GONADS

KEY WORDS

androgens   glucocortocoids   progesterone
epinephrine   mineralcorticoids   testosterone

OBJECTIVES

- Locate the adrenal glands and gonads
- Describe functions of the adrenals and gonads
- Name the secretions of the adrenals and gonads
- Define the Key Words related to this unit of study

One of the two **adrenal** glands is located on top of each kidney, figure 45–1. Each gland has two parts, the **cortex** and the **medulla**. Adrenocorticotrophic hormone (ACTH) from the pituitary glands stimulates the activity of the cortex of the adrenal gland. The hormones secreted by the adrenal cortex are known as **corticoids.** The corticoids are very effective as anti-inflammatory drugs.

The cortex secretes three groups of corticoids, each of which is of great importance:

- **Mineralcorticoids (M-Cs)** affect the kidney tubules by speeding up the reabsorption of sodium into the blood circulation and increasing the excretion of potassium from the blood. They also speed up the reabsorption of water by the kidneys. Aldosterone (M-C) is used in the treatment of Addison's Disease to replace deficient secretion of mineralcorticoids.

- **Glucocorticoids (G-Cs)** increase the amount of glucose in the blood. This is

presumably done by (1) conversion of the protein brought to the liver into glycogen, followed by (2) breakdown of the glycogen into glucose. These glucocorticoids also help the body resist the aggravations caused by various everyday stresses. Both cortisone and hydrocortisone are G-Cs.

- **Androgens** are male sex hormones which, together with similar hormones from the gonads, bring about masculine characteristics. They also promote protein anabolism and body growth.

The medulla of the adrenal gland secretes **epinephrine** and **norepinephrine**, table 45–1. Epinephrine (generic name), or Adrenalin (trade), is a powerful cardiac stimulant. It functions by bringing about a release of more glucose from stored glycogen for muscle activity; and increasing the force and rate of the heartbeat. This chemical activity increases cardiac output and venous return, and raises the systolic blood pressure.

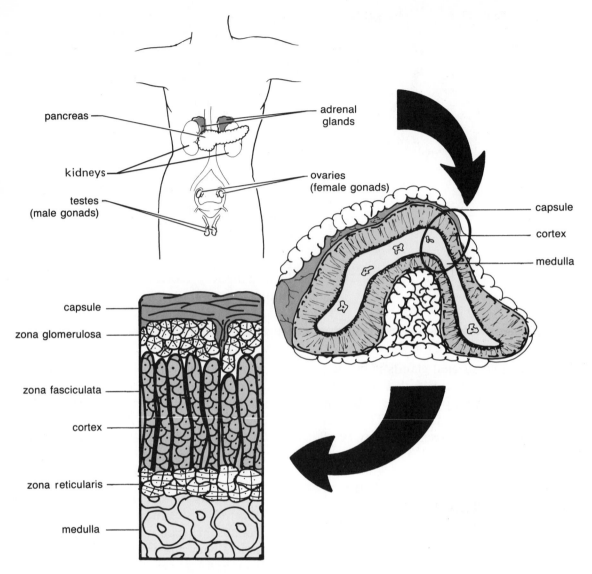

Figure 45-1 Location of adrenals and gonads

The gonads, or sex glands, include the ovaries in the female and the testes in the male. The ovaries are located in the pelvic cavity, one on either side of the uterus. The testes are located in the scrotum.

The secretions of the ovaries, **estrogen** and **progesterone**, are necessary for ovulation and the characteristic female appearance, table 45–2. The secretion of the testes, **testosterone**, is essential to the development of the male sex characteristics. The gonads are responsible for fertility and reproduction in both sexes. Review Unit 38 for further details about the reproductive organs.

Table 45-1 Comparison of the Effects Between Epinephrine and Norepinephrine

EPINEPHRINE	NOREPINEPHRINE
1. Bronchial relaxation	No effect
2. Dilation of iris	No effect
3. Excitation of central nervous system	No effect
4. Increased conversion of stored glycogen to glucose	Much less effect
5. Increased heart rate	Little effect
6. Increased cardiac output and venous return	Slight effect
7. Increased blood flow to muscles	Vasoconstriction in muscle
8. Increased myocardial strength	About the same
9. Increased basal metabolic rate (BMR)	Much less effect
10. Increased systolic blood pressure	Raises both systolic and diastolic blood pressure
11. Increased lipolytic effects; frees fatty acids from fat deposits	Slightly greater effects
12. Relaxation of uterine myometrial muscles	Pilomotor contraction

Table 45-2 Effects of Estrogen and Progesterone on the Female System

HORMONE	PLACE OF ACTION	EFFECT
Estrogen	Breasts	Stimulates breast development
	Fallopian tubes and endometrium	Causes glandular cells to grow
	Pelvis	Widens the pelvis and increases the size of the vagina
	Skeleton	Increases osteoblastic activity at puberty. There is a rapid growth rate.
	Skin	Causes skin to develop a soft, smooth texture and increases its blood vessel supply
Progesterone	Breasts	Enlarges breasts; promotes final development of breast alveoli and lobular tissue; stimulates growth and function of secretory cells
	Fallopian tubes	Stimulates secretions of the fallopian tube mucosa
	Uterus	Promotes secretory changes and storage of nutrients in the endometrium. This prepares the uterus for eventual embryo implantation.

Further Study and Discussion

- There are many instances on record of individuals performing superhuman feats during emergencies. Perhaps you have had such an experience yourself. What is the explanation for such strength at these times?

- Secure a lamb kidney with the adrenal gland attached. Make a long incision through the adrenal gland. Notice that it has an outer area and an inner area. Each part contributes its own secretion. Compare the lamb's adrenal gland with a picture or model of the human gland, noticing shape, size, and color.

- If frogs are available to you for laboratory work, inject about 9.2 milliliters of adrenalin chloride (1:100 000 solution) into the ventricle of the heart of an anesthetized frog. Count the heartbeat before the injection and after the injection. What did the adrenalin do to the heart? What was the quality of the heartbeat before and after injection?

- Describe the use of adrenalin for hemorrhage and asthma control.

Assignment

1. Describe the location of the adrenal glands.

2. Summarize the functions and secretions of the adrenals and the gonads, using the following chart.

GLAND	SECRETION	FUNCTION
Adrenals	Cortex	
	Medulla	
Gonads	Ovaries	
	Testes	

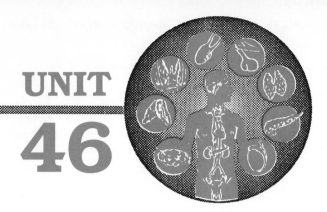

UNIT
46

THE PANCREAS

KEY WORDS

alpha cells
antagonistic
beta cells
diabetes mellitus

glucagon
insulin
islets of
   Langerhans

pancreas
pancreatic
   juice

OBJECTIVES

■ Describe the endocrine functions of the
   pancreas
■ Explain the body's need for insulin
■ Define the Key Words relating to this unit of
   study

The *pancreas* is an organ located behind the stomach. The glandular cells of the pancreas regulate the production of **pancreatic juice**, a digestive juice. The islet cells secrete the hormone *insulin*. Therefore the pancreas is a gland of both external and internal secretion.

The islet cells (mostly beta cells) are distributed throughout the pancreas. These cells were named the **islets of Langerhans** after the doctor who discovered them, figure 46–1. **Beta cells** produce insulin which: (1) promotes the utilization of glucose in the cells, necessary for maintenance of normal levels of blood glucose,

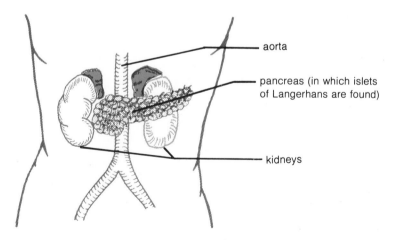

aorta

pancreas (in which islets
of Langerhans are found)

kidneys

Figure 46-1   Location of islets of Langerhans

(2) promotes fatty acid transport and fat deposition into cells, **(3)** promotes amino acid transport into cells, and **(4)** facilitates protein synthesis. Lack of insulin secretion by the island (islet) cells causes **diabetes mellitus**.

The **alpha cells** contained in the islets of Langerhans secrete the hormone **glucagon**. The action of glucagon is **antagonistic** or opposite to that of insulin. Glucagon's function is to increase the level of glucose in the bloodstream. This is done by stimulating the conversion of liver glycogen to glucose. The control of glucagon secretion is achieved by negative feedback. Low glucose levels in the bloodstream stimulate the alpha cells to secrete glucagon, which quickly increases the glucose level in the bloodstream.

Further Study and Discussion

- If laboratory facilities are available, obtain a sheep or beef pancreas. Prepare a thin section for use with the microscope.
  a. Focus the slide under low power to show the arrangement of the islets. Discuss what you see.
  b. Focus the slide under high power to observe the arrangement of the cells in the islets and the pancreas in general.

- Obtain several specimens of urine to test for the presence of sugar. Pour 5 milliliters (cc) of Benedict's solution into a test tube. Using a medicine dropper, and 10 drops of urine to the solution. Shake well to mix thoroughly. Boil the solution in a test tube in water bath for 3-5 minutes. Note the color.

COLOR	INDICATION
Blue	Sugar free
Green	+ present, trace
Greenish yellow	1 +
Yellow	2 +
Brown or red	3 + to 4 +

Your instructor may have new tablet testing devices for the presence of sugar. Try these simplified methods as well as the Benedict's solution method.

- Research and discuss whether insulin may be considered a cure for diabetes.

Assignment

1. What is meant by the statement that the pancreas is a gland of external as well as internal secretion?

2. Where is the pancreas located?

3. Where in the pancreas is insulin produced?

4. What are the functions of insulin?

5. What condition is caused by a lack of insulin in the bloodstream?

6. Why is the action of the hormone glucagon antagonistic to that of insulin?

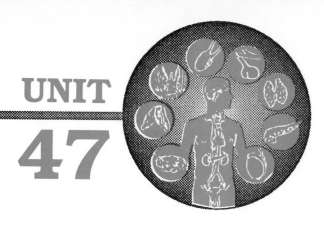

UNIT 47

REPRESENTATIVE DISORDERS OF THE ENDOCRINE SYSTEM

KEY WORDS

acidosis
acromegaly
Addison's
  disease
cretinism
Cushing's
  syndrome

diabetes
  mellitus
electrolyte
exophthalmos
gigantism
glycosuria
goiter

hyperthyroidism
ketone body
myxedema
pituitary
  dwarfism
tetany

OBJECTIVES

■ List causative factors of endocrine gland disorders
■ Recognize certain endocrine gland disorders which interfere with body functions
■ Relate treatment to some of the more common types of gland disorders
■ Define the Key Words related to this unit of study

Endocrine gland disturbances may be caused by several factors, such as disease of the gland itself, infections in other parts of the body, and dietary deficiencies. Most disturbances result form (1) hyperactivity of the glands, causing oversecretion of hormones, or (2) hypoactivity of the gland, resulting in undersecretion of hormones.

THYROID DISORDERS

Since the thyroid gland controls metabolic activity, any disorder will affect other structures besides the gland itself. Signs and symptoms of the disorders most frequently seen are discussed in this unit.

Hyperthyroidism

Hyperthyroidism is due to the overactivity of the thyroid gland. Thus too much thy-

roxin is secreted (hypersecretion), leading to enlargement of the gland. An increase in the basal metabolic rate (BMR) also occurs. In hyperthyroidism, an individual's BMR may be 50 to 75% higher than normal. People with hyperthyroidism consume large quantities of food, but nevertheless suffer a loss of body fat and weight. They may suffer from increased blood pressure and heartbeat, hand tremors, perspiration, and irritability. In addition, the liver releases excess glucose into the bloodstream, increasing the blood sugar level and causing a mild case of **glycosuria**. The most pronounced symptoms of hyperthyroidism include enlargement of the thyroid gland (**goiter**), bulging of the eyeballs (**exophthalmos**), dilation of the pupils, and wide-opened eyelids.

The immediate cause of exophthalmos is not completely known, figure 47–1. It is not directly caused by the hyperthyroidism, because

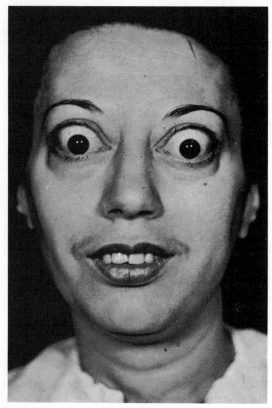

Figure 47-1 Hyperthyroidism (Reproduced with permission from S.L. Robbins and R.S. Cotran, *Pathological Basis of Disease*. Philadelphia: W. B. Saunders)

removal of the thyroid does not always cause the eyeballs to return to their normal state. Treatment of hyperthyroidism includes total or partial removal of the thyroid, and administration of drugs like propylthiouracil and methylthiouracil to reduce the thyroxin secretion.

Determination of the basal metabolism rate (BMR) is an aid in diagnosing thyroid function. The test is performed by measuring the amount of oxygen a person uses at rest; from this the basal body metabolism rate can be calculated. Another diagnostic test is the protein-bound iodine test (P.B.I.). This blood test determines the concentration of thyroxin in the bloodstream. Other thyroxin level tests are the T_3 and T_4. These tests are more accurate than the P.B.I. but are more difficult to perform.

The **radioactive iodine uptake** test measures the activity of the thyroid gland. Dilute radioactive iodine is given orally. The amount which accumulates in the thyroid gland is calculated by use of a Geiger counter. Simple goiter is an enlargement of the thyroid gland due to a deficiency of iodine in the diet.

Hypothyroidism

Hypothyroidism is a condition in which the thyroid gland does not secrete sufficient thyroxin (hyposecretion). This is manifested by a low metabolic rate and decelerated body processes. Depending upon the time hypothyroidism strikes its victims, two different sets of disorders may occur, cretinism or myxedema.

Cretinism. This disorder develops in early infancy or childhood. It is characterized by a lack of mental and physical growth, resulting in mental retardation and malformation (dwarfism or **cretinism**). The sexual development and physical growth of cretins do not proceed beyond that of 7- or 8-year-old children.

In treating cretinism, thyroid hormones or thyroid extract may restore a degree of normal development if administered in time. In most cases, however, normal development cannot be completely restored once the affliction has set in.

Myxedema. This condition is similar to cretinism, although it develops during later childhood or in adult life. **Juvenile myxedema** commonly results in a short, squat physique. The young person suffers from dry skin, an enlarged head, a short and heavy neck, and a dull and vacant facial expression.

Adult myxedema produces edema, lethargy, obesity, decreased heartbeat and lowered intelligence. The hair and skin grow coarse. Victims tend to feel cold due to a greatly diminished metabolic rate.

The treatment for thyroid deficiency usually consists of administering oral thyroid extract so as to restore a normal metabolism.

PARATHYROID DISORDERS

The parathyroid glands regulate the use of calcium and phosphorus. Both of these minerals are involved in many of the body systems.

Hyperfunctioning of the parathyroid glands may cause an increase in the amount of blood calcium, thereby increasing the tendency for the calcium to crystallize in the kidneys as **kidney stones**. Excess amounts of calcium and phosphorus are withdrawn from the bones; this may lead to eventual deformity. So much calcium can be removed from the bones that they become honeycombed with cavities. Afflicted bones become so fragile that even walking can cause fractures.

Hypofunctioning of the parathyroid glands leads to a condition known as **tetany**. In this case, severely diminished calcium levels affect the normal function of nerves. Convulsive twitchings develop, and the afflicted person dies of spasms in the respiratory muscles. Treatment consists of administering vitamin D, calcium, and parathormone to restore a normal calcium balance.

PITUITARY DISORDERS

Disturbances of the pituitary gland may produce a number of body changes. This gland is chiefly involved in the growth function. However, as the master gland, the pituitary indirectly influences other activities.

Gigantism

Hyperfunctioning of the pituitary gland (often due to a pituitary tumor) causes hyper-secretion of the pituitary growth hormone. When this occurs during preadolescence it causes **gigantism**, an overgrowth of the long bones leading to excessive tallness. The most famous giant was Robert Wadlow (1919-1940) of Alton, Illinois. Wadlow grew to 8'-10 3/4" in height and weighed 495 lbs. (He wore a size 37 shoe!)

If hypersecretion of the growth hormone occurs during adulthood, **acromegaly** results. This is an overdevelopment of the bones of the face, hands and feet, figure 47–2. In adults whose long bones have already matured, the growth hormone attacks the cartilaginous regions and the bony joints. Thus the chin protrudes, and the lips, nose, and extremities enlarge disproportionately. Lethargy and severe headaches frequently set in as well.

Treatment of acromegaly and gigantism is difficult due to the inaccessibility of the pituitary gland. If a pituitary tumor is responsible for the hypersecretion of growth hormones, surgery or bombardment with X rays may offer some relief.

Hypofunctioning of the pituitary gland during childhood leads to **pituitary dwarfism**.

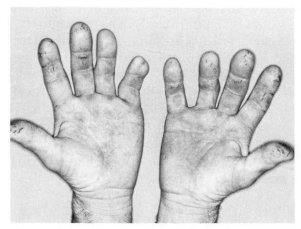

Figure 47-2   Effects of acromegaly on fingers and hands (Armed Forces Institute of Pathology, negative 72-14615)

Growth of the long bones is abnormally decreased by an inadequate production of growth hormone. Despite the small size, however, the body of a dwarf is normally proportioned and intelligence is normal. Unfortunately, the physique remains juvenile and sexually immature. Treatment involves early diagnosis and injections of human growth hormone. The treatment period is 5 years or more.

Other disorders caused by pituitary hypofunctioning include diabetes insipidus and menstrual problems.

ADRENAL DISORDERS

Overactivity of the adrenal gland may result in virilism and Cushing's syndrome. Virilism is the development of male secondary characteristics in a woman (facial hair, broad shoulders, small breasts).

Cushing's syndrome results from the hypersecretion of the glucocorticoid hormones from the adrenal cortex. This hypersecretion may be caused by an adrenal cortical tumor. (Oddly enough, more women than men tend to develop this endocrine disorder.) Symptoms include high blood pressure, muscular weakness, obesity, poor healing of skin lesions, and a tendency to bruise easily. The most noticeable characteristics are a rounded "moon" face and a "buffalo hump" that develops from the redistribution of body fat. Therapy consists of surgical removal of the adrenal cortical tumor.

Hypofunctioning of the adrenal cortex can also lead to **Addison's disease**. Persons with Addison's disease exhibit the following symptoms:

- Excessive pigmentation, prompting the characteristic "bronzing" of the skin
- Decreased levels of blood glucose, causing carbohydrate imbalance
- A severe drop in blood pressure, leading to kidney malfunction
- Pronounced muscular weakness and fatigue
- Gastrointestinal malfunction, resulting in diarrhea, weight loss and vomiting
- Retention of water in the body tissues
- A severe drop of sodium in the blood and tissue fluids, causing a serious imbalance of **electrolytes**

The medical treatment of Addison's disease is focused on the replacement of the deficient hormones.

GONAD DISORDERS

Disturbances in the ovaries may consist of cysts and tumors, abnormal menstruation, and menopausal changes. Turner's syndrome may occur in either the male or female; this is a chromosomal disorder.

PANCREATIC DISORDERS

Diabetes mellitus is a condition caused by decreased secretion of insulin from the islet cells of the pancreas. As a result, carbohydrate metabolism is disturbed; this has an adverse effect on protein and fat metabolism.

Insulin deficiency causes glucose to accumulate in the bloodstream, rather than be transported to the cells and converted into energy. Eventually the excess becomes too much for the kidneys to reabsorb, and the excess glucose is excreted in the urine. Excretion of excess glucose requires an accompanying excretion of large amounts of water. This occurs to insure that the sugar concentration does not rise too high. Diabetics are constantly thirsty because the lost water must be replaced.

Since insufficient glucose is available for cellular oxidation in such cases, the body starts to burn up protein and fats. The diabetic is constantly hungry and usually eats voraciously, but loses weight nonetheless.

When fats are utilized as a fuel source, they are rapidly but incompletely oxidized. One product of this abnormal rate of fat oxidation is **ketone bodies**. Ketone bodies are highly toxic; the type most commonly formed is acetoacetic acid. These keto acids accumulate in the blood, promoting the development of **acidosis**, giving the breath and urine an odor of "sweet" acetone. If acidosis is severe, **diabetic coma** and death may result. Prolonged diabetes leads to atherosclerosis, heart disease, and kidney damage. Therapy consists of daily insulin injections, or (in some cases) daily antidiabetic tablets and a controlled diet. Most diabetics live active, normal lives when properly treated.

Diabetes insipidus is caused by the malfunctioning of the posterior lobe of the pituitary gland. It is characterized by excessive loss of body fluids, by a larger output of urine (which, however, contains no sugar), and by **polydipsia** (excessive thirst). Diabetes insipidus is due to a lack of the antidiuretic hormone, which is secreted by the hypothalamus and stored in the posterior lobe of the pituitary gland.

Further Study and Discussion

- Discuss how a disturbance in the pituitary gland can affect the functioning of other endocrine glands.

- Discuss some of the symptoms of diabetes mellitus.

- Discuss the treatments available to a diabetic.

Assignment

1. What is the meaning of each of the following terms?

    a. hyperfunctioning

    b. hypofunctioning

2. What symptoms indicate hyperfunctioning of the thyroid gland?

3. What conditions may result from hypofunctioning of the pituitary gland?

4. Complete the following chart.

GLAND	HORMONE	NORMAL FUNCTION	DISORDERS
Pituitary			
Thyroid			
Parathyroid			
Thymus			
Adrenals			
Gonads			
Pancreas			

5. What are the characteristics of diabetes insipidus?

6. What causes diabetes insipidus?

SELF-EVALUATION

REGULATORS OF BODY FUNCTIONS

A. Match each term in column I with its correct description or function in column II.

	Column I	Column II
_____	1. ACTH	a. master gland of the endocrine system
_____	2. adrenals	b. any gland of internal secretion
_____	3. cortisone	c. a hormone secreted by adrenals
_____	4. gonad	d. regulates use of calcium
_____	5. endocrine	e. the secretion of any endocrine gland
_____	6. hormone	f. helps body meet emergencies
_____	7. insulin	g. sex gland
_____	8. parathyroid	h. regulates body metabolism
_____	9. pituitary	i. one of the hormones secreted by pituitary gland
_____	10. thyroid	j. a hormone which regulates carbohydrates and metabolism
		k. hypofunction of endocrine glands

B. Identify the labelled glands in figure SE9–A.

① _____

② _____

③ _____

④ _____

⑤ _____

⑥ _____

⑦ _____

⑧ _____

⑨ _____

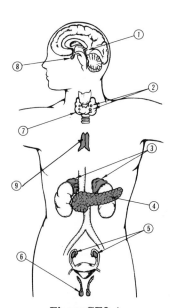

Figure SE9-A

C. Briefly answer the following questions.

  1. How many lobes is the pituitary gland divided into? What are the names of these lobes?

  2. What types of hormones are secreted from the different lobes of the pituitary gland?

  3. List the functions of thyroxin.

  4. What effects do estrogen and progesterone have on the following structures found in the female reproductive system?

     a. breasts

     b. fallopian tubes

  5. What cells in the pancreas secrete the hormone glucagon? What is its function?

6.   What causes diabetes insipidus and what are its symptoms?

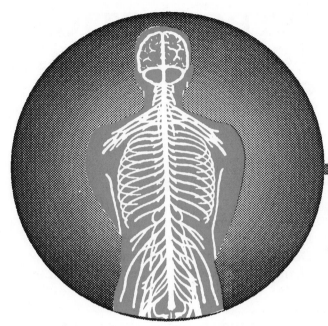

CHAPTER 10

COORDINATION OF BODY FUNCTIONS

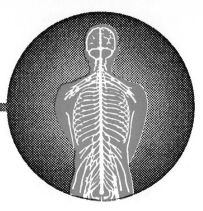

INTRODUCTION TO THE NERVOUS SYSTEM

KEY WORDS

associative
  (connecting)
  neuron
autonomic
  nervous
  system
axon

central nervous
  system
conductivity
dendrites
impulse
irritability

motor neuron
neuron
peripheral
  nervous
  system
sensory neuron

OBJECTIVES

- Describe the functions of the nervous system
- List the main parts of the nervous system
- Describe three types of neurons
- Define characteristics of the nerve cells
- Define the Key Words related to this unit of study

The study of body functions reveals that the body is made up of millions of small structures that perform a multitude of different activities; these are coordinated and integrated into one harmonious whole. The two main communications systems are the endocrine system and the nervous system. They send chemical messengers and nerve impulses to all of the structures. The endocrine system and hormonal regulation have been discussed in earlier units. Hormonal regulations is slow, while neural regulation is comparatively rapid.

The nervous system is the most highly organized system of the body, consisting of the brain, spinal cord, and nerves. The structural and functional unit, as in other systems, is the cell. The nerve cell, or **neuron**, is especially constructed to carry out its function of com-

munication. In addition to the nucleus, cytoplasm, and cell membrane, the neuron has extensions of cytoplasm from the cell body. These extensions, or processes, are called **dendrites** and **axons**. There may be several dendrites, but only one axon. These processes, or **fibers**, as they are often called, are paths along which nerve impulses travel, figure 48–1.

All neurons possess the characteristics of being able to react when stimulated and of being able to pass the nerve impulse generated on to other neurons. These characteristics are **irritability** (the ability to react when stimulated) and **conductivity** (the ability to transmit a disturbance to distant points). The dendrites receive the impulse and transmit it to the cell body, and then to the axon where it is passed on to another neuron or to a muscle or gland. There are three types of neurons:

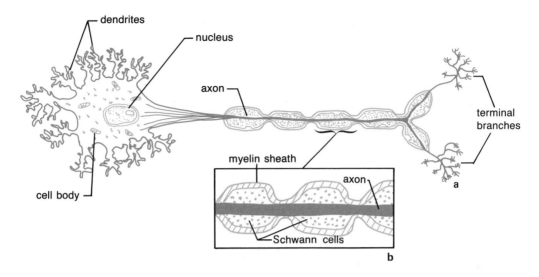

dendrites

nucleus

axon

terminal branches

myelin sheath

axon

cell body

Schwann cells

a

b

Figure 48-1   (a) A neuron; (b) A longitudinal section of a myelinated axon

- **Sensory neurons** which emerge from the skin or sense organs and carry messages, or **impulses**, toward the spinal cord and brain

- **Motor neurons** which carry messages from the brain and spinal cord to the muscles and glands

- **Connecting, associative,** or **internuncial neurons** which carry impulses from one neuron to another

Classification of neurons is illustrated in figure 48–2A. Different types of neurons are shown in figure 48–2B.

The nervous system can be divided into three divisions: the central, the peripheral, and the autonomic nervous system.

1.   The **central nervous system** consists of the brain and spinal cord

2.   The **peripheral nervous system** is made up of the nerves of the body consisting of twelve pairs of cranial nerves extending out from the brain and thirty-one pairs of spinal nerves extending out from the spinal cord

3.   The **autonomic nervous system** peripheral nerves and ganglia (a group of cell bodies outside the central nervous system that carry impulses to involuntary muscles and glands)

Where decision is called for and action must be considered, the central and peripheral nervous systems are involved. They carry information to the brain where it is interpreted, organized, and stored. An appropriate command is sent to organs or muscles. The autonomic nervous system supplies heart muscle, smooth muscle, and secretory glands with nervous impulses as needed. It is usually involuntary in action.

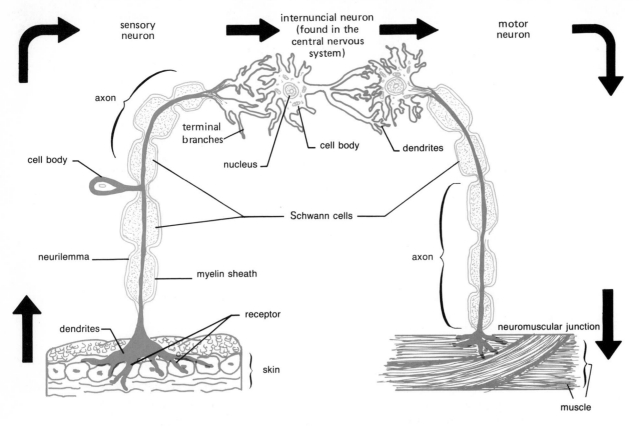

Figure 48-2A Classification of neurons according to function

Further Study and Discussion

- Using library reference materials prepare a brief report on the following types of behavior:

    - Conditioned reflex

    - Habit

    - Instinct

    - Reflex

    - Voluntary action

- Include in the report a description of the behavior and examples of that type of behavior.

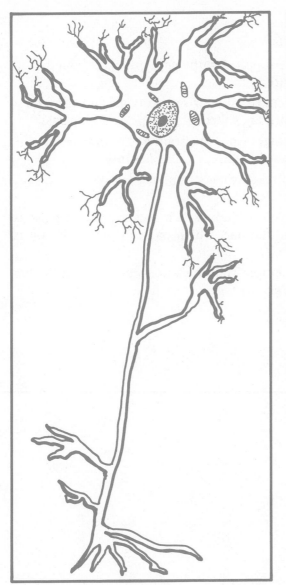

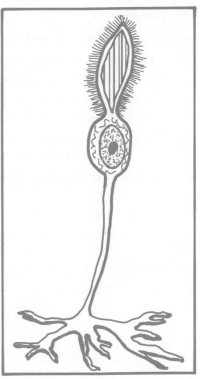

sensory neuron

motor neuron

Figure 48-2B   Representative types of neurons

Assignment

Complete the following statements.

1. Two types of muscle tissue supplied with nerve impulses from the autonomic nervous system are _____ and _____ .

2. Neurons which emerge from the skin or sense organs and carry messages toward the spinal cord are called _____ neurons.

3. Neurons which carry messages from the brain and spinal cord to the muscles and glands are called _____ neurons.

4. The ability of a neuron to react when stimulated is called _____ .

5. The extension of the nerve cell body which receives the impulse is called the _____ and the part which passes the impulse on is called the _____ .

6. Glands that receive stimulation from the autonomic nervous system are called _____ glands.

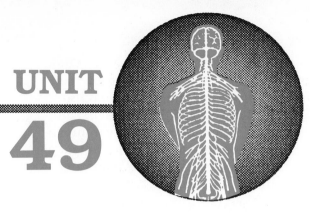

UNIT 49

THE CENTRAL NERVOUS SYSTEM: BRAIN AND SPINAL CORD

KEY WORDS

arachnoid
arachnoid villi
blood-brain
 barrier
brainstem
central fissure
 (fissure of
 Rolando)
cerebellum
cerebral aqueduct
 (aqueduct of
 Sylvius)
cerebral
 ventricles
cerebrospinal
 fluid
cerebrum
choroid plexus
convolutions
corpus callosum

cortex
diencephalon
 (interbrain)
dura mater
ependymal cells
exudate
fissure
foramen of
 Magendie
fourth ventricle
frontal lobe
gyrus (plural,
 gyri)
hypothalamus
interventricular
 foramen
lateral fissure
 (fissure of
 Sylvius)
lateral ventricle

longitudinal
 fissure
lumbar puncture
medulla
meninges
occipital lobe
parietal lobe
parieto-occipital
 fissure
pia mater
pons
sensory
 (somesthetic)
 area
sulcus (plural,
 sulci)
temporal lobe
thalamus
third ventricle
transverse fissure

OBJECTIVES

- Identify the parts of the brain
- Describe the structure of the brain and spinal cord
- Relate functions to the various parts of the brain
- Identify the Key Words related to this unit of study

The adult human brain is a highly developed, complex, and intricate mass of soft nervous tissue. It weighs about 1400 grams (3 lbs). The brain is protected by the bony cranial cavity; further protection is afforded by three membranous coverings called **meninges,** and the cerebrospinal fluid.

The three meninges are the dura mater, arachnoid, and the pia mater, see color plate 18. The **dura mater** is the outer brain covering, which lines the skull on one side. This is a tough, dense membrane of fibrous connective tissue, containing an abundance of blood vessels. The **arachnoid (mater)** is the middle layer. It resembles a fine cobweb with fluid-filled spaces. Covering the brain surface itself is the **pia mater,** comprised of blood vessels held together by fine areolar connective tissue. The space between the arachnoid and pia mater is filled with cerebrospinal fluid, produced within the ventricles of the brain. This fluid acts both as a shock absorber and a source of nutrients for the brain.

VENTRICLES OF THE BRAIN

The brain contains four lined cavities filled with cerebrospinal fluid. These cavities are called **cerebral ventricles.** Each ventricle is lined with ependymal cells. The ventricles lie deep within the brain. The two largest, located within the cerebral hemispheres, are known as the right and left **lateral ventricles.** Each lateral ventricle is subdivided into four parts, or horns. An **anterior horn** is located in the frontal lobe; a middle, or **body,** is found in the parietal lobe; an **inferior,** or **temporal,** horn is positioned in the temporal lobe; and an **occipital,** or **posterior,** horn is situated in the occipital lobe.

The **third ventricle** is placed behind and below the lateral ventricles. It is connected to the two lateral ventricles via the **interventicular foramen,** or foramina of Monro.[1] The **fourth ventricle** is situated below the third, in front of the cerebellum, and behind the pons and the **medulla oblongata.** The third and fourth ventricles are interconnected via a narrow canal called the **cerebral aqueduct,** or aqueduct of Sylvius.[2] In the roof of the fourth ventricle is an opening known as the **foramen of Magendie.**[3] The lateral wall of the fourth ventricle contains two openings called the foramina of Luschka.[4]

Each of the four ventricles contains a rich network of blood vessels of the pia mater referred to as the **choroid plexus.** The choroid plexus is in contact with the ependymal cells lining the ventricles, which helps in the formation of cerebrospinal fluid.

Cerebrospinal Fluid and Its Circulation

Cerebrospinal fluid is a substance that forms inside the four brain ventricles from the blood vessels of the choroid plexuses. This fluid serves as a liquid shock absorber protecting the delicate brain and spinal cord. It is formed by filtration from the intricate capillary network of the choroid plexuses. The fluid transports nutrients to, and removes metabolic waste products from, the brain cells.

Choroid plexus capillaries differ significantly in their selective permeability from capillaries in other areas of the body. A potential result is that drugs within the bloodstream may not effectively penetrate brain tissue, rendering infections (such as meningitis) difficult to cure. This phenomenon is commonly referred to as the **blood-brain barrier.**

After filling the two lateral ventricles of the cerebral hemispheres, the cerebrospinal fluid seeps into the third ventricle via the foramen of Monro. From here it flows through the aqueduct of Sylvius into the fourth ventricle. The fluid then passes through the foramen of Magendie and the two lateral foramina of Luschka, into the small, tubelike central canal of the cord and into the subarachnoid spaces. The subarachnoid spaces are thus filled with cerebrospinal fluid which bathes the brain and the spinal cord. Ultimately the cerebrospinal fluid returns to the bloodstream via the venous structures in the brain, called **arachnoid villi.**

The formation and circulation of cerebrospinal fluid is used by members of the health team to detect any defects or disease of the brain. For example, inflammation of the cranial meninges quickly spreads to the meninges of the spinal cord. This leads to an increased secretion of cerebrospinal fluid which collects in the confined bony cavity of the brain and spinal column. The accumulation of excess fluid causes headaches, reduced pulse rate, slow breathing, and partial or total unconsciousness.

Removal of cerebrospinal fluid for diagnostic purposes is accomplished with a **lumbar puncture.** The needle used to withdraw the cerebrospinal fluid is inserted between the third and fourth lumbar vertebrae. The fluid, or **exudate** withdrawn contains by-products of the inflammation and the organisms causing it.

---

1. Alexander Monro (Primus) (1697–1767), Scottish anatomist
2. Francois Sylvius (1614–1672), French anatomist
3. Francois Magendie (1783–1855), French physiologist
4. Hubert von Luschka (1820–1875), German anatomist

Therefore, a lumbar puncture is helpful in diagnosing such diseases as cerebral hemorrhage, increased pressure, intracranial tumors, meningitis, and syphilis. It also serves to alleviate the pressure caused by meningitis, and especially hydrocephalus. Occasionally it may be used for the introduction of antimeningitis sera or drugs.

Brain tissue is made up of gray and white matter. The outer surface of the brain is grayish, the center is white. The cortex is the highest center of the brain and is made up of so-called gray matter. The gray matter really consists of millions of nerve cell bodies and naked nerve fibers. The white matter contains millions of nerve cell fibers with myelin sheaths, which accounts for the difference in appearance.

The brain is divided into three parts: the cerebrum, cerebellum, and brainstem. The brainstem is further divided into three parts, the medulla, pons, and the midbrain, see color plate 18.

CEREBRUM

The **cerebrum** is the largest and highest part of the brain. It occupies the whole upper part of the skull and weighs about two pounds. Covering the upper and lower surfaces of the cerebrum is a layer of gray matter called the **cerebral cortex.**

The cerebrum is divided into two hemispheres, right and left, by a very deep groove known as the **longitudinal fissure.** The cerebral surface is completely covered with furrows and ridges. The deeper furrows, or grooves, are referred to as **fissures,** and the shallower ones, **sulci.**

The elevated ridges between the sulci are the **gyri,** also known as **convolutions,** figure 49–1. These convolutions serve to increase the surface area of the brain, resulting in a proportionately larger amount of gray matter. The arrangement of the gyri and sulci on the brain's surface varies from one brain to another. Certain fissures, however, are constant and represent important demarcations. They help to localize specific functional areas of the cerebrum, and to divide the hemipsheres into four lobes.

Each cerebral hemisphere is divided into a **frontal, parietal, occipital,** and **temporal** lobe. These lobes correspond to the cranial bones by which they are overlaid, figure 49–1.

The five major fissures dividing the cerebral hemispheres include:

- **Longitudinal fissure** — a deep groove divides the cerebrum into two hemispheres. The middle region of the two hemispheres is held together by a wide band of axonal fibers called the **corpus callosum.**

- **Transverse fissure** — divides the cerebrum from the cerebellum

- **Central fissure,** or **fissure of Rolando** — located beneath the coronal suture of the skull, dividing the frontal from the parietal lobes.

- **Lateral fissure** or **fissure of Sylvius** — situated on the side of the cerebral hemispheres, dividing the frontal and temporal lobes

- **Parieto-occipital fissure** — the least obvious of all the fissures, serves to separate the occipital lobe from the parietal and temporal lobes. There is, however, no definite demarcation between these two lobes.

Cerebral Functions

Each lobe of the cerebral hemispheres controls different types of functions.

1. **Frontal lobe** — The cerebral cortex of the frontal lobe controls the **motor**

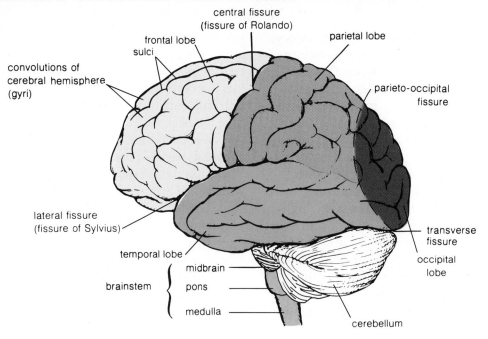

central fissure
(fissure of Rolando)

frontal lobe

sulci

parietal lobe

convolutions of
cerebral hemisphere
(gyri)

parieto-occipital
fissure

lateral fissure
(fissure of Sylvius)

transverse
fissure

occipital
lobe

temporal lobe

midbrain

brainstem { pons

medulla

cerebellum

A. LATERAL VIEW

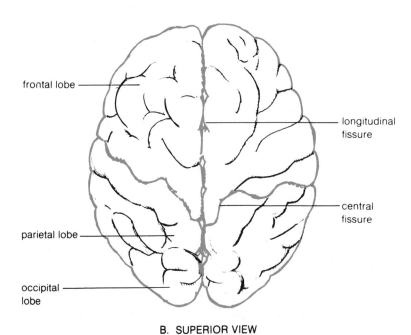

frontal lobe

longitudinal
fissure

central
fissure

parietal lobe

occipital
lobe

B. SUPERIOR VIEW

Figure 49-1   External view of the brain showing some of the fissures and convolutions (From *Human Anatomy and Physiology* by Joan G. Creager. © 1983 by Wadsworth, Inc. Reprinted by permission of Wadsworth Company, Belmont, California 94002.)

functions of humans. The **motor area** occupies a long band of cortex, just in front of the fissure of Rolando, in the posterior part of the frontal lobe. This motor area controls the voluntary muscles. Cells in the right hemisphere activate voluntary movements which occur in the left side of the body; the left hemisphere controls voluntary movements of the right side. The frontal lobe also includes two areas which control speech.

2. **Parietal lobe** — The parietal lobe comprises the **sensory (somesthetic)** area. It is found behind the fissure of Rolando, in front of the parietal lobe. This area receives and interprets nerve impulses from the sensory receptors for pain, touch, heat, and cold. It further helps in the determination of distances, sizes, and shapes.

3. **Occipital lobe** — The occipital lobe, located over the cerebellum, houses the **visual area,** controlling eyesight.

4. **Temporal lobe** — The upper part of the temporal lobe contains the **auditory area;** the anterior part of the lobe is occupied by the **olfactory (smell) area.**

The cerebral cortex also controls conscious thought, judgment, memory, reasoning, and will power. This high degree of development makes the human the most intelligent of all animals.

The **diencephalon** is located between the cerebrum and the midbrain. It is composed of two major structures, the thalamus and the hypothalamus. The **thalamus** is a spherical mass of gray matter. It is found deep inside each of the cerebral hemispheres, lateral to the third ventricle. The thalamus acts as a relay station for incoming and outgoing nerve impulses. It receives direct or indirect nerve impulses from the various sense organs of the body (with the exception of olfactory sensations). These nerve impulses are then relayed to the cerebral cortex. The thalamus also receives nerve impulses from the cerebral cortex, cerebellum, and other areas of the brain. Damage to the thalamus may result in increased sensibility to pain, or total loss of consciousness.

The **hypothalamus** lies below the thalamus. It forms part of the lateral walls and floor of the third ventricle. A bundle of nerve fibers connects the hypothalamus to the posterior pituitary gland, the thalamus, and the midbrain. Eight vital functions are performed by the hypothalamus:

- **Autonomic nervous control** — Regulates the parasympathetic and sympathetic systems of the autonomic nervous system.

- **Cardiovascular control** — Controls blood pressure by regulating the constriction and dilation of blood vessels and the beating of the heart.

- **Temperature control** — Helps in the maintenance of normal body temperature (37°C or 98.6°F).

- **Appetite control** — Assists in regulating the amount of food we ingest. The "feeding center," found in the lateral hypothalamus, is stimulated by hunger "pangs," which prompt us to eat. In turn, the "satiety center" in the medial hypothalamus becomes stimulated when we have eaten enough.

- **Water balance** — Within the hypothalamus, certain cells respond to the osmotic pressure (osmolality) of the blood. When osmolality is high, due to water deficiency, the antidiuretic hormone (ADH) is secreted. ADH is produced in the hypothalamus and secreted by the posterior pituitary gland. Secreted into the bloodstream, ADH causes the kidneys to conserve water; this, in turn, keeps the blood from becoming too concentrated. A "thirst area" is found near the satiety area, becoming stimulated when the blood's osmolality is high. This causes us to consume more liquids.

- **Gastrointestinal control** — Increases intestinal peristalsis and secretion from the intestinal glands.

- **Emotional state** — Plays a role in the display of emotions such as fear and pleasure.

- **Sleep control** — Helps keep us awake when necessary.

CEREBELLUM

The **cerebellum** is located behind the pons and below the cerebrum (see figure 49–2). It is composed of two hemispheres or wings—the right cerebellar hemisphere and the left cerebellar hemisphere. These two hemispheres are connected to a central portion called the **vermis.** The cerebellum consists of gray matter on the outside and white matter on the inside. The cerebellar surface is marked by many gyri and sulci. The white matter on the inside of the cerebellum is marked with a tree-like pattern. This pattern is called **arbor vitae** (tree of life).

The cerebellum communicates with the rest of the central nervous system by three pairs of tracts. These tracts are called the inferior, middle, and superior **cerebellar peduncles** (see figure 49–3). The inferior peduncle connects the cerebellum to the lower brainstem and the spinal cord. The middle peduncle connects the cerebellum to the pons, and the superior one links the cerebellum to the midbrain, thalamus, and cerebrum. These three peduncles are composed of "incoming" axons that carry nerve messages into the cerebellum and "outgoing" axons that transmit messages out of the cerebellum. The incoming axons carry messages to the cerebellum regarding movement within joints, muscle tone, position of the body, and the tightness of ligaments and tendons. Thus any and all information relating to skeletal muscle activity is carried to the cerebellum. This information reaches the cerebellum directly from sensory receptors or indirectly from other brain areas. The "outgoing" axons carry nerve messages to the different parts of the brain that control skeletal muscles.

Cerebellar Function

The cerebellum controls all body functions that have to do with skeletal muscles.

1. **Maintenance of balance.** If the body is imbalanced, sensory receptors in the inner ear send nerve messages to the cerebellum. There the cerebellum carries impulses to the motor controlling areas of the brain. These brain areas, in turn, stimulate muscle contraction that restores balance.

2. **Maintenance of muscle tone.** The cerebellum transmits nerve impulses to the red nucleus that, in turn, relays them to the spinal cord and then to the skeletal muscles.

3. **Coordination of secretory movements.** Any voluntary movement is initiated in the cerebral cortex. However, once the movement is started, its smooth execution is the role of the cerebellum. The cerebellum allows each muscle to contract at the right time, with the right strength, and for the right amount of time so that the overall movement is smooth and flowing. This is important when doing complex

Figure 49-2   Cross section of the brain, showing the arachnoid villi and subarachnoid space as well as other structures (From *Human Anatomy and Physiology* by Joan G. Creager. © 1983 by Wadsworth, Inc. Reprinted by permission of Wadsworth Publishing Company, Belmont, California 94002.)

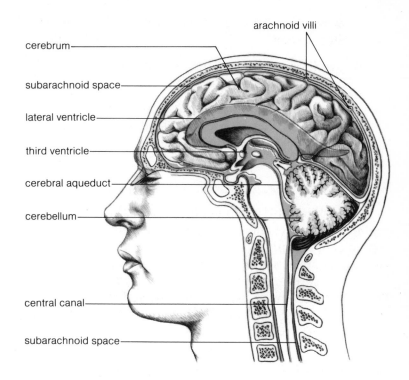

or skilled movements such as speaking, walking, writing; even simple movements need the coordinating abilities of the cerebellum. A simple action such as raising the hand to the face to avoid a blow requires the synchronized action of 50 or more muscles. These muscles then act on 30 separate bones of the arm and hand.

The removal of or injury to the cerebellum results in motor impairment.

BRAINSTEM

The **brainstem** is made up of three parts: the midbrain, pons, and the medulla. The **pons** is located in front of the cerebellum, between the midbrain and the medulla oblongata. It contains interlaced transverse and longitudinal myelinated, white nerve fibers mixed with gray matter. The pons serves as a two-way con-

ductive pathway for nerve impulses between the cerebrum, cerebellum, and other areas of the nervous system. In this way, nerve impulses are transmitted between the two cerebellar hemispheres, from the cerebellum to the midbrain and cerebrum, and from the cerebellum to the medulla and spinal cord. The pons is also the site for the emergence of four pairs of cranial nerves, and it contains a center that controls respiration.

The **medulla oblongata** is a bulb-shaped structure found between the pons and the spinal cord. It lies inside the cranium, above the foramen magnum, in the occipital bone. The medulla is white on the outside, just like the pons, because of myelinated nerve fibers. Its functions include:

- Serving as a passageway for nerve impulses between the spinal cord and the brain

- Slowing the heart rate via the **cardiac inhibitory center**

- Controlling the rate and depth of respiration via the **respiratory center**

- Causing the dilation and constriction of blood vessels, thereby affecting blood pressure via the **vasoconstrictor center**

SPINAL CORD

The spinal cord continues down from the medulla. It is white and soft and lies within the vertebrae of the spinal column. Like the brain, the spinal cord is submerged in cerebrospinal fluid and is surrounded by the three meninges. The gray matter in the spinal cord is located in the internal section; the white matter composes the outer part, figure 49–3. In the gray matter of the cord, connections can be made between incoming and outgoing nerve fibers which provide the basis for reflex action. The spinal cord functions as a reflex center and as a conduction pathway to and from the brain.

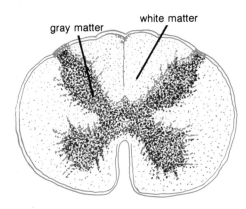

Figure 49-3   Cross section of the spinal cord

Further Study and Discussion

- If laboratory facilities are available, make arrangements to observe the dissection of the brain of a sheep or calf. Locate the cerebrum, cerebellum, medulla, convolutions, hemispheres.

- From memory, draw a diagram of the brain and identify the structures. Compare it with color plate 17 upon completion.

- Make up a chart listing the parts of the brain and spinal cord. Do outside research and add functions which may not have been covered in this unit.

Assignment

Match each term in column I with its description in column II.

Column I	Column II
_____ 1. meninges	a. the innermost covering of brain tissue
_____ 2. cortex	b. separates the other two meninges
_____ 3. arachnoid	c. matter which contains naked nerve fibers
_____ 4. cerebellum	d. fluid made in the ventricles of the brain
_____ 5. pia mater	e. largest of 3 parts of the brain
_____ 6. white matter	f. nerve fibers covered with myelin sheath
_____ 7. cerebrum	g. part of the brain which coordinates movements
_____ 8. gray matter	h. the highest center of the brain
_____ 9. dura mater	i. the outer meninge
_____ 10. cerebrospinal fluid	j. regulates heartbeat, respiration, and coughing
	k. three membranes that cover the brain

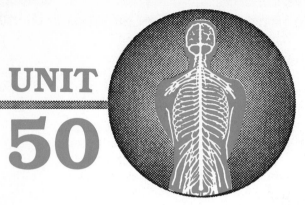

THE PERIPHERAL AND AUTONOMIC NERVOUS SYSTEMS

KEY WORDS

afferent nerve
autonomic
  nervous system
connecting
  neuron
efferent nerve

effector
mixed nerve
motor nerve
peripheral
  nervous system

receptor
reflex act
reflex arc
sensory nerve
stimulus

OBJECTIVES

■ Relate the functions of the sympathetic and parasympathetic nervous systems
■ Explain how a simple reflex act is carried out by the nervous system
■ Define the terms associated with a reflex action
■ Define the Key Words related to this unit of study

A nerve is composed of bundles of nerve fibers enclosed by connective tissue. If the nerve is composed of fibers that carry impulses from the sense organs to the brain or spinal cord, it is called a **sensory,** or **afferent,** nerve; if it is composed of fibers carrying impulses from the brain or spinal cord to muscles or glands, it is known as a **motor,** or **efferent,** nerve; and if it contains both sensory and motor fibers, it is referred to as a **mixed nerve.**

Certain of the twelve pairs of cranial nerves (such as the facial nerve) are mixed nerves; some (as the optic nerve) contain only sensory fibers; and others are entirely motor nerves. All thirty-one pairs of spinal nerves are mixed nerves. Each of them divides into branches. These go either directly to a particular body segment, or they form networks with adjacent spinal nerves known as **plexuses.**

PERIPHERAL NERVOUS SYSTEM

The **peripheral nervous system** includes all the nerves of the body, see figure 50–1. It connects the central nervous system to the various body structures. The **autonomic nervous system** is a specialized part of the peripheral system; it controls the involuntary, or automatic, activities of the vital internal organs.

AUTONOMIC NERVOUS SYSTEM

The autonomic nervous system includes nerves, ganglia, and plexuses which carry impulses to all smooth muscle, secretory glands, and heart muscle, figure 50–2. It thus regulates the activities of the **visceral organs** (heart and blood vessels, respiratory organs, alimentary

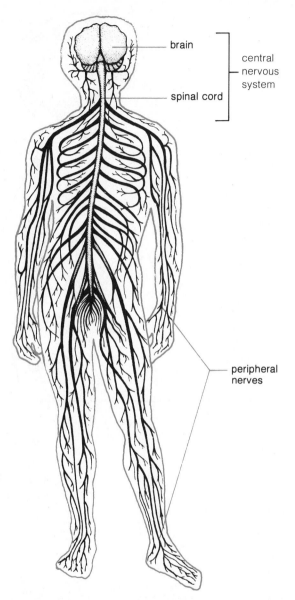

Figure 50-1 The peripheral nervous system connects the central nervous system to the various structures of the body. Messages are relayed from these structures back to the brain via the spinal cord. Spinal nerves leave the spinal cord through openings in the vertebrae, extending, dividing, and branching out into an intricate and complicated network reaching every structure of the body. Thirty-one pairs of spinal nerves pass between the vertebrae and branch out to all parts of the body. (Courtesy of CPR, Teaneck, New Jersey)

canal, kidneys and urinary bladder, and reproductive organs). The activities of these organs are usually automatic and not subject to conscious control.

The autonomic system is comprised of two divisions: the **sympathetic** and the **parasympathetic.** These two divisions are antagonistic in their action. For example, the sympathetic system may accelerate the heartbeat in response to fear, whereas the parasympathetic slows it down. Normally the two divisions are in balance; the activity of one or the other becomes dominant as dictated by the needs of the organism.

The sympathetic nervous system consists primarily of two cords, beginning at the base of the brain and proceeding down both sides of the spinal column. These are made up of nerve fibers and ganglia of nerve cell bodies. The cord between the ganglia is a cable of nerve fibers, closely associated with the spinal cord. Sympathetic nerves extend to all the vital internal organs, including the liver and pancreas, as well as innervating the heart, stomach, intestines, blood vessels, the iris of the eye, sweat glands, and the bladder.

The parasympathetic system is composed of two important active nerves: the vagus and the pelvic nerves. The vagus nerve, which extends from the medulla and proceeds down the neck, sends branches to the chest and neck. The pelvic nerve, emerging from the spinal cord around the hip region, sends branches to the organs in the lower part of the body.

Both the sympathetic and parasympathetic are strongly influenced by emotion. During periods of fear, anger, or stress, the sympathetic division acts to prepare the body for action. The effects of the parasympathetic are generally to counteract the effects of the sympathetic. For example, the sympathetic nervous system increases the rate of heart muscle contraction, and the parasympathetic de-

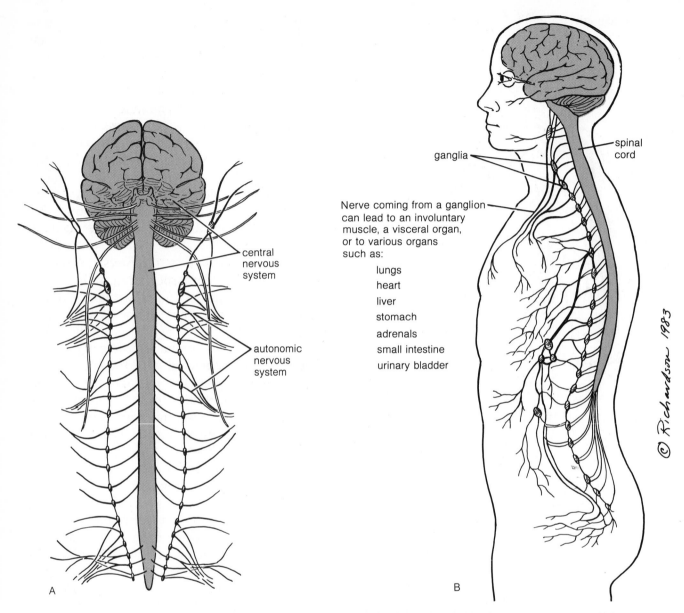

Figure 50-2 The autonomic nervous system (involuntary nervous system) governs those functions that are carried out automatically, without conscious thought, such as regulation of heart beat, digestion of food, etc.

creases the rate. The two systems operate as a pair, striking a nearly perfect balance when the body is functioning properly.

The Reflex Act

The simplest type of nervous response is the **reflex** act, which is unconscious and involuntary. The blinking of the eye when a particle of dust touches it, the removing of the finger from a hot object, the secretion of saliva at the sight or smell of food, the movements of the heart, stomach, and intestines, are all examples of reflex actions.

Every reflex act is preceded by a stimulus. Any change in the environment is called a **stimulus.** Examples of stimuli are sound waves, light waves, heat energy, and odors. Special structures called **receptors** pick up these stimuli. For example, the retina of the eye is the receptor for light; special cells in the inner ear are receptors for sound waves; and special structures in the skin are the receptors for heat and cold.

Reaction to a stimulus is called the **response.** The response may be in the form of movement; in which case, the muscles are the **effectors,** or responding organs. If the response is in the form of a secretion, the glands are the effectors. Reflex actions involving the skeletal muscles are controlled by the spinal cord. They involve only sensory, **connecting,** and motor neurons. This pathway is known as the **reflex arc,** figure 50–3.

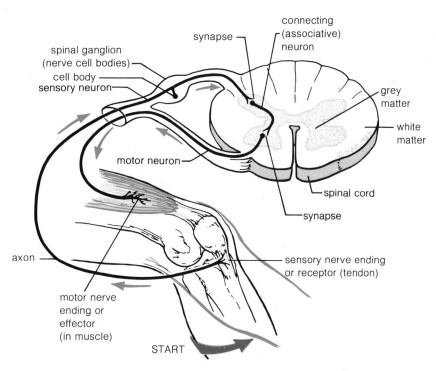

Figure 50-3   The reflex arc. In this example, tapping the knee (patellar tendon) results in extension of the leg, producing the knee jerk reflex.

Further Study and Discussion

- Discuss the action of the autonomic nervous system when a person is served an appetizing lunch.

- List ten reflex acts.

Assignment

A. Complete the following statements.

1. A nerve is composed of small blood vessels and of bundles of fibers called _____ .

2. A nerve composed of fibers carrying impulses from sense organs to the brain or spinal cord is called a _____ or _____ nerve.

3. A nerve composed of fibers which carry impulses from the brain or spinal cord to muscles or glands is called a _____ or _____ nerve.

4. A mixed nerve contains both _____ and _____ fibers.

5. The autonomic nervous system is a specialized part of the peripheral system and controls _____ .

6. The autonomic nervous system has two parts which counterbalance each other; these are the _____ and _____ systems.

B.   Identify the structures on figure 50–4. Enter your answers below it.

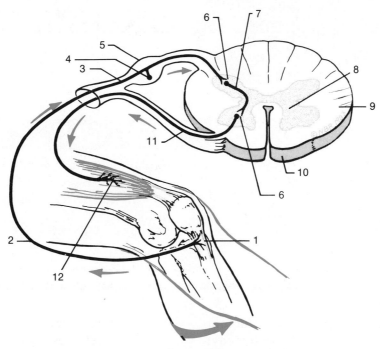

Figure 50-4

① _____   ⑦ _____

② _____   ⑧ _____

③ _____   ⑨ _____

④ _____   ⑩ _____

⑤ _____   ⑪ _____

⑥ _____   ⑫ _____

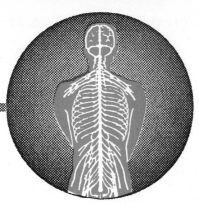

UNIT 51

SPECIAL SENSE ORGAN: THE EYE

KEY WORDS

anterior chamber
choroid coat
cones
cornea
dilator pupillae
extrinsic muscles
intrinsic muscles

iris
lens
orbital socket
posterior
  chamber
pupil
retina

rods
sclera
sphincter
suspensory
  ligament
vitreous humor

OBJECTIVES

- Explain how stimulation of a sense organ results in sensation
- Identify the parts of the eye, and relate them to their function
- Define the Key Words that relate to this unit of study

Sensory receptors are special structures which are stimulated by changes in the environment. Sensory receptors (touch, pain, temperature, and pressure) are found all over the body, located either in the skin or connective tissues. Special sensory receptors include the taste buds of the tongue, special cells in the nose, the retina of the eye, and the special cells in the inner ear which make up the organ of Corti. When a sense organ is stimulated, the impulse travels along nerve pathways to the brain, where it is registered in a certain area. Sensation actually takes place in the brain, but it is mentally referred back to the sense organ. This is called **projection** of the sensation.

THE EYE

The human eye is a tender sphere about 1″ in diameter (about 2.5 cm). It is protected by the **orbital socket** of the skull. The eyeball is moved by muscles. The eye is protected by the

bone surrounding it and by the eyebrows, eyelids, and eyelashes, figure 51–1.

The location of the eyes in front of the head allows for superimposition of images from each eye. This enables us to see stereoscopically, in three dimensions (length, width, and depth). The eye's optical system for detecting light is similar to that of a camera.

The wall of the eye is made up of three concentric layers, or coats, each with its specific function. These three layers are the sclera, the choroid, and the retina, see color plate 19.

Sclera

The outer layer is called the **sclera,** or white of the eye. It is a tough, unyielding fibrous capsule which maintains the shape of the eye and protects the delicate structures within. Muscles responsible for moving the eye within the orbital socket are attached to the outside of the sclera. These muscles are referred to as the **extrinsic muscles,** figure 51–2.

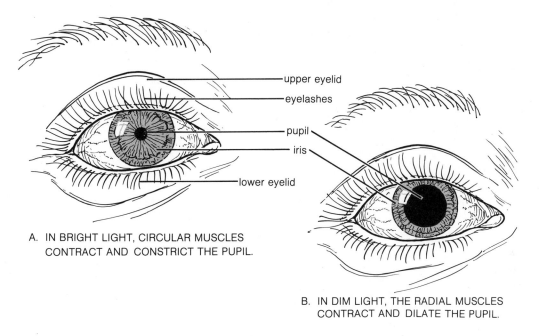

A. IN BRIGHT LIGHT, CIRCULAR MUSCLES
   CONTRACT AND CONSTRICT THE PUPIL.

B. IN DIM LIGHT, THE RADIAL MUSCLES
   CONTRACT AND DILATE THE PUPIL.

Figure 51-1   External view of the eye

They include the superior, inferior, lateral, medial rectus, and the superior and inferior oblique. See table 51–1 for a listing of the extrinsic eye muscles and their functions.

Cornea

In the very front center of the sclerotic coat lies a circular, clear area called the **cornea.** The cornea is sometimes referred to as the "window" of the eye. It is transparent to permit light rays to pass through it. This transparency is due to the lack of blood vessels. Thus corneal cells are fed by the movement of lymph through interstitial, or lymph spaces. The cornea is composed of five layers of flat cells arranged much like sheets of plate glass. Possessing pain and touch receptors, it is sensitive to any foreign particles that come in contact with its surface. An injury to the cornea causes scarring and impaired vision.

Choroid Coat and the Iris

The middle layer of the eye is the **choroid coat.** It contains blood vessels to nourish the eye, and a non-reflective pigment rendering it dark and opaque. The pigment provides the choroid coat with a deep, red-purple color; this darkens the eye chamber, preventing light reflection within the eye. In front, the choroid coat has a circular opening called the **pupil.** A colored, muscular layer surrounds the pupil; this is the **iris,** or colored part of the eye. The iris may be blue, green, gray, brown, or black. Eye color is related to the number and size of melanin pigment cells in the iris. If there is little melanin present, the eye is blue, because light is scattered to a greater extent. With increasing quantities of melanin, eye color ranges from green to black. The total absence of melanin results in a pink eye color, characteristic of albinism. Such irises are pink be-

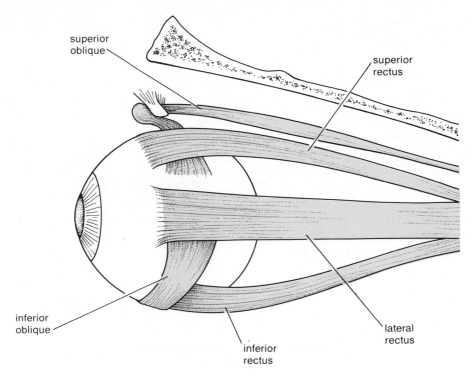

Figure 51-2 Extrinsic eye muscles

Table 51–1 Extrinsic and Intrinsic Eye Muscles

EYE MUSCLE	FUNCTION
A. Extrinsic	
1. Superior rectus	Rolls eyeball upward
2. Inferior rectus	Rolls eyeball downward
3. Lateral rectus	Rolls eyeball laterally
4. Medial rectus	Rolls eyeball medially
5. Superior oblique	Rolls eyeball on its axis, moves cornea downward and laterally
6. Inferior oblique	Rolls eyeball on its axis, moves cornea upward and laterally
B. Intrinsic	
1. Sphincter pupillae	Constricts pupil
2. Dilator pupillae	Dilates pupil

cause the blood inside the choroid blood vessels shows through the iris.

Within the iris are two sets of antagonistic, smooth muscles, the **sphincter** and the **dilator pupillae.** These muscles help the iris to control amounts of light entering the pupil. When the eye is focused on a close object or stimulated by bright light, the sphincter pupillae muscle contracts, rendering the pupil smaller. Conversely, when the eye is focused on a distant object or stimulated by dim light, the dilator pupillae muscle contracts. This causes the pupil to grow larger, permitting as much light as possible to enter the eye. In this way the eye may be compared to a camera; the iris corresponds to the shutter or diaphragm.

Lens and Related Structures

The **lens** is a crystalline structure located behind the iris and pupil. It is composed of concentric layers of fibers and crystal-clear proteins in solution. It is an elastic, disc-shaped structure with anterior and posterior convex surfaces, thus forming a biconvex lens. However, the posterior surface is more curved than that of the anterior. The curvature of each surface alters with age. During infancy, the lens is spherical; in adulthood, medium convexed; and almost flattened in old age. The capsule surrounding the lens also loses its elasticity over a period of time. The lens is held in place behind the pupil by **suspensory ligaments** from the **ciliary body** of the choroid body.

The lens is situated between the **anterior** and **posterior chambers.** The anterior chamber is filled with a watery fluid referred to as the **aqueous humor,** and it is constantly replenished by blood vessels behind the iris. **Vitreous humor,** a transparent jellylike substance, fills the posterior chamber. Both of these substances help to maintain the eyeball's spherical shape, refracting (bending) light rays as they pass through the eye.

Retina

The **retina** of the eye is the innermost, or third coat of the eye. It is located between the posterior chamber and the choroid coat. The retina does not extend around the front portion of the eye. It is upon this light-sensitive layer that light rays from an image are formed.

After the image is focused on the retina, it travels via the optic nerve to the visual part of the cerebral cortex. This is found towards the back of the head, just above the neck. If light rays do not focus correctly on the retina, the condition may be corrected with properly fitted contact lenses, or eyeglasses, which bend the light rays as required.

The retina contains pigment and specialized cells known as **rods** and **cones,** figure 51-3, which are sensitive to light. The part of the retina where the nerve fibers enter the optic nerve to go to the brain does not have these specialized cells; therefore, it is most sensitive to light. For this reason, it is often called the "blind spot."

The Optic Disc and the Fovea. Viewing the retina through an ophthalmoscope, one can observe a yellow disc known as the **macula lutea.** Within this disc is the fovea centralis, which contains the cones for color vision, see color plate 19. The area around the fovea centralis is the **extrafoveal** or **peripheral region.** This is where the rods for dim and peripheral vision can be found.

Slightly to the side of the fovea lies a pale disc called the **optic disc** or **blind spot.** Nerve fibers from the retina gather here to form the nerve. The optic disc contains no rods or cones; therefore, it is devoid of visual reception.

See figure 51-4 to help you locate your blind spot.

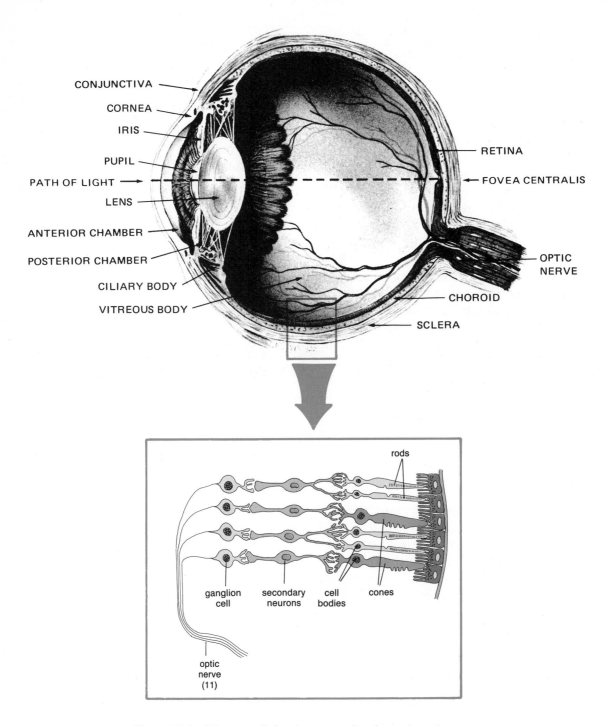

Figure 51-3   Diagram of visual neurons showing rods and cones

1. Close your left eye and focus your right eye on the <u>cross</u>.
2. Move the page slowly away from your eye and then slowly toward your eye.
3. At a distance of about 6–8 inches the black <u>circle</u> "disappears."

Figure 51-4   Testing for the blind spot

Further Study and Discussion

-   Using an eye model, identify the chief structures in the eye. Explain their functions.

-   Using color plate 19, trace the path of light rays from the time they strike the cornea until the sensation of sight is registered in the brain.

Assignment

1. Name the three structural coats found in the eye. Give the function of each one.

2. Explain how refraction of light is important to vision.

3. Identify the structures in figure 51–5 and write your answers in the spaces provided.

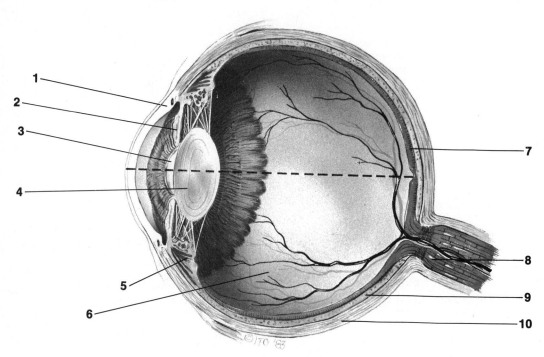

Figure 51-5

① _____		⑥ _____	
② _____		⑦ _____	
③ _____		⑧ _____	
④ _____		⑨ _____	
⑤ _____		⑩ _____	

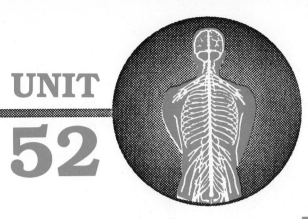

SPECIAL SENSE ORGAN: THE EAR

KEY WORDS

anvil (incus)	organ of Corti
cochlea	semicircular
cochlea duct	canals
eustachian tube	stirrup (stapes)
hammer	tympanic
(malleus)	membrane

OBJECTIVES

- List the parts of the ear and relate them to their function
- Define the Key Words that relate to this unit of study

THE EAR

The ear is a special sense organ which is especially adapted to pick up sound waves and send these impulses to the auditory center of the brain, located in the temporal area just above the ears. The receptor for hearing is the delicate **organ of Corti,** which is located within the cochlea of the inner ear.

The ear has three parts: the outer or external ear, the middle ear, and the inner ear, see figure 52–1. The outer ear consists of the visible portion and a canal which leads to the ear drum (**tympanic membrane**).

The middle ear is really the cavity in the temporal bone. It connects with the pharynx by means of a tube called the **eustachian tube.** This tube serves to equalize the air pressure in the middle ear with that of the outside atmosphere. A chain of three tiny bones is found in the middle ear: the **hammer** (malleud), the **anvil** (incus), and the **stirrup** (stapes); they transmit sound waves from the ear drum to the inner ear.

The inner ear consists of several membrane-lined channels which lie deep within the temporal bone. The special organ of hearing is a spiral-shaped passage known as the **cochlea,** which contains a membranous tube called the **cochlear duct.** The duct is filled with fluid that vibrates when the sound waves from the stirrup bone strike against it. Located in the cochlear duct are delicate cells which make up the organ of Corti. These hairlike cells pick up the vibrations caused by sound waves against the fluid, then they transmit them through the auditory nerve to the hearing center of the brain.

Three **semicircular canals** also lie within the inner ear, figure 52–2. They contain a liquid, and delicate hairlike cells which bend when the liquid is set in motion by head and body movements. These impulses are sent to the brain, helping to maintain body balance, or equilibrium. They have nothing to do with the sense of hearing.

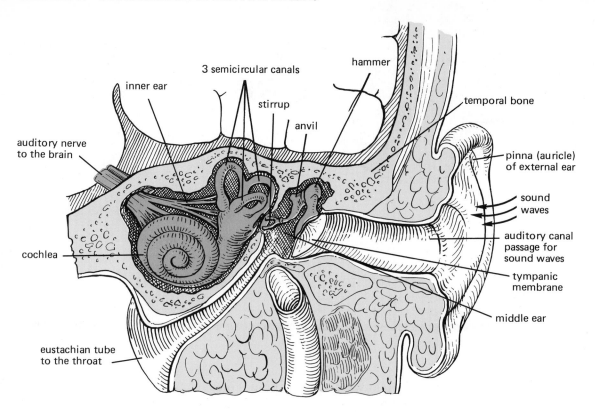

Figure 52-1   The ear and its structures

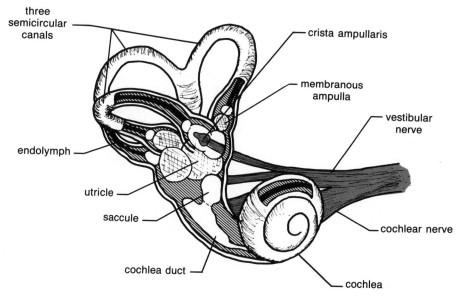

Figure 52-2   Enlargement of the inner ear showing the three semicircular canals

Further Study and Discussion

- Using an ear model, identify the chief structures in the ear. Explain their functions.

- In figure 52–1, trace the path of sound waves from the time they strike the ear drum until the sensation of hearing is registered in the brain.

Assignment

1. How many main parts is the ear divided into?

2. What are the names of these parts and list the important structures found in each part?

3. What is the organ of Corti?

4. What is the function of the semicircular canals?

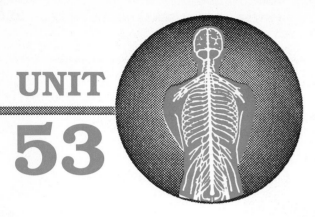

UNIT 53

REPRESENTATIVE DISORDERS OF THE NERVOUS SYSTEM

KEY WORDS

anticonvulsant   paresthesia   topically
arbovirus   spastic   unilateral
herpetic neuralgia   quadriplegia
miotic

OBJECTIVES

■ Recognize symptoms of some common ailments of the nervous system
■ Relate treatment to some common nervous system diseases
■ List common ear and eye disorders and related treatment
■ Identify the Key Words in this unit of study

The health care provider must become familiar with symptoms and treatments for disorders of the nervous system. Some of the more common ones are mentioned here.

Chorea is a nervous system disorder characterized by involuntary muscular twisting and writhing movements of the arms, face, and legs. The symptoms frequently appear following streptococcal infection. The disease may last from three to six months. Treatment consists of rest, nourishing food, and avoidance of excitement of any kind. The disorder is also known as **chorea minor, dancing chorea, St. Vitus' dance,** or **Sydenham's chorea.**

Shingles or **herpes zoster** is an acute viral nerve infection. It is characterized by a unilateral (one-sided) inflammation of cutaneous nerves. Although intercostal nerves are commonly affected, the course of nerve inflammation can spread virtually to any nerve. Symptoms include extremely painful vesicular eruptions of the skin and mucous membranes along the route of the inflamed nerve. The extreme pain resulting from shingles is known as **herpetic neuralgia.** Shingles is often found in elderly or debilitated persons. The afflicted area, typically the chest or abdomen, must be treated by protecting it from air and from clothing irritation.

Neuralgia is a sudden severe, sharp, stabbing pain along the pathway of a nerve. The pain is often brief, usually a symptom of a disease. The various forms of neuralgia are named according to the nerve that they affect. For instance, neuralgia of the trigeminal nerve (sensory nerve of the face and head) is called **trigeminal neuralgia.** The pain from trigeminal neuralgia and other forms of neuralgia can be relieved with analgesics and/or narcotics.

Neuritis is the inflammation of a nerve trunk. This condition can cause extreme pain, hypersensitivity, loss of sensation, muscular atrophy, paralysis, weakness and **paresthesia** (tingling, burning and crawling of the skin). The different types of neuritis are named according to their cause, location and pathology. They include four major types:

1. **alcoholic neuritis** — neuritis deriving from chronic alcoholism, presumably a result of thiamine deficiency because of insufficient and improper diet.

2. **ascending neuritis** — neuritis that extends from the periphery of a nerve to the spinal cord or brain.

3. **infectious neuritis** — an acute multiple neuritis caused by a viral disease.

4. **sciatic neuritis** or **sciatica** — this is a form of neuralgia or neuritis of the sciatic nerve of the body.

The pain from these various forms of neuritis can be relieved by administering pain killers or analgesics.

Poliomyelitis, or **infantile paralysis,** is a viral infectious disease of the nerve pathways in the spinal cord. The muscles which are controlled by these diseased nerve paths become paralyzed. Death may result. Treatment consists of hot packs, exercises given by a trained professional, and special exercises given under water. The patient may have to be placed in an "iron lung" if the muscles of respiration are involved. The Sister Kenny method of treatment is administered by trained specialists. Vaccines (Salk and Sabin) are now available to protect against polio, and all children should be immunized against this crippling disease.

Encephalitis is a viral disease characterized by inflammation of the brain. There are several causes of encephalitis in addition to viruses, including various other organisms and certain chemical substances. A number of viruses have been isolated and identified as the major causative factors. Encephalitis results primarily from the bite of a mosquito carrying the encephalitis virus; hence the term **arbovirus** (arthropod-borne virus). The different forms of encephalitis are all characterized by fever, lethargy, extreme weakness, and visual disturbances. No adequate preventive immunization methods have yet been developed, nor is there a specific treatment for the infections. A strain known as *California encephalitis* has been reported throughout the United States. This severe disease, which primarily affects children, is accompanied by coma and convulsions; fortunately the prognosis is excellent.

Cerebral palsy is a disturbance in voluntary muscular action due to brain damage. Definite causes are unknown. It may result from birth injuries, intracranial hemorrhage, or infections such as encephalitis. The most pronounced characteristic of cerebral palsy is **spastic quadriplegia.** Spastic quadriplegia involves spastic paralysis of all four limbs, though it is most pronounced in the legs.

Hydrocephalus is an increased volume of cerebrospinal fluid within the cavity of the brain. This causes enlargement of the skull and prominence of the forehead.

Convulsions, characterized by violent muscle contractions, may occur because of high fever, calcium imbalance or brain tumors; during convulsions brain tissue discharges abnormal nerve signals.

Acute bacterial meningitis is the inflammation of the membranes, or meninges, of the brain or spinal cord. The different types of meningitis are classified according to their causative organisms: tuberculosis meningitis, pneumococcal meningitis, or meningococcus meningitis. The latter, meningococcus meningitis, is caused by *Neisseria meningitidis.*

Epidemics of this disease occur infrequently, although isolated cases do come up. It is endemic to such close-living groups as residents of college dormitories and members of the armed services. These groups may suffer frequent outbreaks due to the introduction of new carriers, or susceptibles. In the military, these outbreaks range from 200 to 500 cases a year.

Symptoms of meningococcus meningitis include headache, fever, nasal secretions, sore throat, back and neck pain, loss of mental alertness, and rashes. Treatment by intravenous injection of immune serum (or injection directly into the spinal canal) has met with limited success. Immunity of unpredictable duration follows recovery from the inflammation. Chemotherapy with penicillin, rifampin, sulfanomides, sulfadiazine, and other antibiotics is fairly successful. However, even this method of treatment has its limitations due to the possible development of drug-resistant strains. Another problem is that drugs do not readily pass through the meninges to reach the invading bacteria.

Epilepsy is a disorder of the brain, characterized by a recurring and excessive electrical discharge from neurons. Approximately one person out of 200 in the United States suffers from some form of epilepsy. Epileptic seizures are believed to be a result of spontaneous, uncontrolled, reverberating cycles of electrical activity in the neurons of the brain. One portion of the brain stimulates another, setting off a cycle of activity that accelerates and runs its course until the neurons become fatigued. When such electrical reverberations occur, the subject may suffer hallucinations and a seizure. The confused neuronal electrical circuitry leads to a loss of consciousness; the neuronal fatigue induces sleep. **Grand mal,** or severe seizure, is less frequent than the **petit mal** (milder seizure). In petit mal, some of the victims see flashes of light. There may be odor and sound sensations, even a blackout of consciousness. Most epileptic persons can lead normal lives with regular medication.

Medications used to control seizures are referred to as **anticonvulsants.** Diphenylhydantoin (Dilantin) helps to control grand mal seizures. Trimethadione (Tridione) and paramethadione (paradione) control petit mal.

EAR DISORDERS

Otitis media is an infection of the middle ear. It usually causes earache. This disorder is often a complication of the common cold in children. Treatment with antibiotics will cure the infection.

Otosclerosis is a chronic, progressive disorder in which the bone in the region of the oval window first becomes spongy and then hardens. This causes the stirrup or stapes to become fixed or immovable. Otosclerosis is a common cause of deafness in young adults. This condition can be alleviated by an operation called **stapes mobilization.** In this operation, the stirrup is freed and hearing often is restored. Another procedure removes the stapes, and they are replaced by a tissue graft.

Tinnitis is a sensation of ringing or buzzing that is perceived in the ear in the absence of an actual sound stimulus. It may be caused by impacted wax, otitis media, otosclerosis, blockage of normal blood supply to the cochlea, or the effects of various drugs like the salicylates (painkillers) and quinine (once a cure for malaria).

Cauliflower ear is an enlarged and abnormally disfigured ear. This condition is commonly seen in boxers and wrestlers. It develops from hematomas that become calcified.

EYE DISORDERS

Conjunctivitis is an inflammation of the conjunctival membranes in front of the eye. Redness and discharge of mucus occur. Since it may be contagious, conjunctivitis should be promptly treated by a physician. Treatment includes eye washes, or irrigations, to flush the conjunctiva. Eye irrigations cleanse and relieve the inflammation and the pain. These solutions usually consist of weak solutions of normal isotonic saline and/or boric acid.

Glaucoma is an eye condition in which the aqueous humor does not circulate properly within the eye and pressure increases within the eyeball. If untreated, glaucoma leads to blindness because it damages the retina and optic nerve. With prompt treatment, total blindness may be avoided. Early detection is most important, and treatment usually prevents progress of the disease.

Treatment involves the use of **miotics** (drugs causing constriction of the pupil). Miotic drugs lower eyeball pressure. These include pilocarpine nitrate (Pilocarpine Hydrochloride), the effects of which last only several hours, and demercarium bromide (Humorsol), with effects that last from 5 to 10 days.

A **cataract** is a condition characterized by a lack of transparency of the lens. Light cannot pass through the clouded lens; therefore the person cannot see. The vision is corrected with eyeglasses or surgery; the opaque lens is removed and replaced by a synthetic lens.

A **sty** is a tiny abscess at the base of an eyelash. It is due to inflammation of one of the sebaceous glands of the eyelid. Various antibiotics can be used as a curative. Bacitracin is especially useful as an ophthalmic anti-infective, because it is non-irritating to the eye and produces no known side effects. Few microorganisms are able to develop a resistance to bacitracin. It is administered topically in an ophthalmic ointment.

Further Study and Discussion

- Discuss the procedure that should be followed in caring for a patient seized by an epileptic attack. What observations should be reported?

- Prepare for a panel discussion on rehabilitation of cerebral palsy patients. Include family and social problems.

- Explain how deafness can be helped or treated.

- Discuss the reason for the infrequency of poliomyelitis today.

Assignment

A.   Match each of the terms in column I with its description in column II.

Column I	Column II
_____ 1. acute bacterial meningitis	a. disease which may be characterized by convulsions
_____ 2. poliomyelitis	b. infection of the brain membranes
_____ 3. epilepsy	c. middle ear infection
_____ 4. glaucoma	d. viral disease for which there is now a vaccine
_____ 5. cataract	e. a clouded or opaque lens
	f. condition caused by increased pressure within the eyeball

B. Answer the following questions.
    1. What is the difference between neuralgia and neuritis?

    2. What is sciatica?

    3. What disease results when the membranes of the brain become inflamed?

    4. What are the hazards of untreated glaucoma?

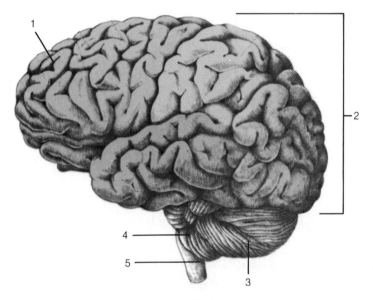

Figure SE10-A

① _____

② _____

③ _____

④ _____

⑤ _____

B. Trace the path of the impulse in figure SE10–B. Identify the numbered parts and describe the action.

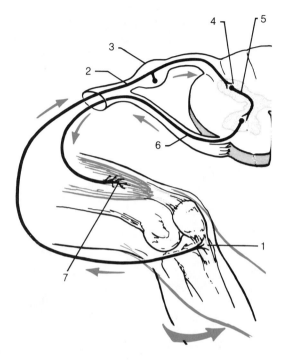

Figure SE10-B

① _____

② _____

③ _____

④ _____

⑤ _____

⑥ _____

⑦ _____

C. Place the correct answers in the blank spaces.

1. The unit of structure in nervous tissue is the _____.

2. There are two chief types of neurons, the _____ or _____ which carries messages to the brain and the _____ or _____ which convey messages away from the central nervous system to peripheral areas.

3. Axons of nerve cells have a protective covering around them called the _____.

4. The brain and spinal cord are covered by three _____. They are, from the center out, _____, _____, and _____.

5. The three main divisions of the brain include the _____, _____, and _____.

6. The spinal cord lies within the _____.

7. Connections between the brain and surrounding structures are established by _____ nerves.

8. Connections between the spinal cord and other structures are established by _____ nerves.

9. The _____ is the largest part of the human brain.

10. The four receptors for sensation which are found in the skin are those for touch, cold, heat, and _____.

D. Briefly answer the following questions.

1. Briefly describe the three functions of the cerebellum.

2. What is the organ of Corti?

3. What is the function of the semicircular canals?

4. What condition will stapes mobilization cure and how is this accomplished?

5. What is tinnitis?

6. List some of the symptoms of tinnitis.

7. What ear disorder is commonly seen in boxers and wrestlers?

GLOSSARY

A

abdomen (ab'-do-mun): portion of body lying between thorax and pelvis

abdominal hernia (ab-dom'-i-nul hur'-nee-uh): abnormal protrusion of an organ, or part of an organ, through abdominal wall

abduction (ab-duck'-shun): movement away from midline or axis of body

abscess (ab'-sess) pus-filled cavity

absolute zero (ab'-suh-lewt zee'-row): complete absence of heat or about − 273.2°C (− 459.8°F)

absorption (ub-sorp'-shun): passing of a substance into body fluids and tissues

accessory digestive organs (ack-sez'-uh-ree di-jes'-tiv or'-gunz): structures helping in mechanical digestion of food; glands producing secretion to assist chemical digestion in mouth, stomach, small intestine. Accessory organs include teeth, tongue, salivary glands, pancreas, liver, and gallbladder

acetabulum (as''-e-tab'-you-lum): a cup-shaped cavity in the innominate bone receiving the head of the femur

Achilles tendon (ack-i-'-leez ten'-dun): cord at rear of the heel

acid (as'-id): chemical compound that ionizes to form hydrogen ions (H^+) in aqueous solution

acidophil (a-sid'-o-fil): type of secretory cell found in the anterior lobe of the pituitary gland. Acidophil cells secrete the growth hormone and prolactin

acidosis (as''-i-do'-sis): disturbance in the acid-base balance from excess acid, or excessive loss of bicarbonate; depletion of alkaline reserve

active transport (ack'-tiv tranz'-port): process by which solute molecules are transported across a membrane against a concentration gradient, from an area of low concentration to one of high concentration

adduction (a-duck'-shun): movement of part of body or limb toward the midline of body; opposite of abduction

adenohypophysis (ad''-e-no-high-pof'-i-sis): another name for the anterior lobe of the pituitary gland. The adenohypophysis secretes several hormones: growth hormone, prolactin, thyroid-stimulating hormone (TSH), adenocorticotrophic hormone (ACTH), follicle-stimulating hormone (FSH), luteinizing hormone (LH), and interstitial cell-stimulating hormone (ICSH)

adenoids (ad'-e-noydz): pair of glands composed of lymphoid tissue, found in nasopharynx; also called *pharyngeal tonsils*

adenosine diphosphate (ADP) (a-den'-o-seen dye-fos'-fate): chemical compound consisting of one molecule of adenine, one of ribose, two of phosphoric acid. Intermediary compound in the production of energy for cellular and muscular activity

adenosine triphosphate (ATP) (a-den'-o-seen try-fos'-fate) chemical compound consisting of one molecule of adenine, one of ribose, three of phosphoric acid

adipose (ad'-i-pose): fatty or fat-like

afferent nerve (af'-ur-unt nurv): a nerve that carries nerve impulses from the periphery to the central nervous system; also known as a *sensory nerve*

agglutinin (a-gloo'-ti-nin): antibody found in normal or immune serum, causing antigen and cellular clumping

agglutinogen (a-gloo'-tin-o-jen): chemical substance (antigen) which stimulates the formation of a specific agglutinin

agranulocyte (ay-gran'-yoo-lo-site): nongranular, white blood cell; known as *agranular leukocyte*

albinism (al'-bi-nizm): partial or total absence of melanin pigment from eyes, hair, and skin

albuminuria (al-bew"-mi-new'-ree-uh): excess of albumin protein in urine

alimentary canal (al"-i-men'-tuh-ree kuh-nal'): entire digestive tube from mouth (ingestion) to anus (excretion)

alkalosis (al"-kuh-lo'-sis): excessive alkali; disturbance in acid-base balance from excess loss of acid

alveoli (al-vee'-o-li): air cells found in lung

ameboid (a-mee'-boyd): resembling amoeba in form or movement

amenorrhea (a-men"-o-ree'-uh): absence of menstruation

ampulla of Vater (am-pul'-uh of vah-ter): a junction or common passageway formed from the common bile duct of the liver and the pancreatic duct. It helps to empty bile into the duodenum. It is named after the German anatomist who discovered it

anal sphincter (ay'-nul sfink'-tur): muscles surrounding anal opening

anemia (uh-nee'-mee-uh): blood disorder characterized by reduction in number of red blood cells or hemoglobin

aneurysm (an'-you-rism): a widening, or sac, formed by dilation of a blood vessel

angina pectoris (an-ji'-nuh peck'-to-ris): attacks of tightness, choking or suffocation, often accompanied by severe chest pain radiating to left shoulder and arm; caused by inadequate blood and oxygen supply to heart

ankylosis (ank"-i-lo'-sis): abnormal immobility and consolidation of a joint

anorchidism (an-or'-kih-dizm): congenital absence of testes

anorexia (an"-o-rek'-see-uh): loss of appetite

anterior chamber (an-teer'-ee-ur chame'-bur): space between cornea and iris

antibody (an'-tih-bod"-ee): substance produced by the body, that inactivates a specific foreign substance which has entered the body

anticoagulant (an"-tih-ko-ag'-yoo-lunt): chemical substance that prevents or slows down blood clotting (like heparin)

anticonvulsant (an"-tih-kun-vul'-sunt): therapeutic agent that stops or prevents convulsions

antidiuretic hormone (an"-tih-dye-yoo-ret'-ik hor'-mone): hormone secreted by the posterior pituitary gland, which prevents or suppresses urine excretion

antigen (an'-tih-jin): substance stimulating formation of antibodies against itself

antiprothrombin (an"-tih-pro-throm'-bin): chemical substance that directly or indirectly reduces or retards action of prothrombin (such as heparin)

antithromboplastin (an"tih-throm'-bo-plas'-tin): chemical substance inhibiting clot-accelerating effect of thromboplastins

anus (ay'-nus): outlet from rectum

anvil (an'-vil): middle ear bone, or ossicle, in a chain of three ossicles of the middle ear

aorta (ay-or'-tuh): largest artery in body, rising from left ventricle of the heart; its branches distribute oxygenated blood to all parts of the body

aortic-semilunar valve (ay-or'-tik sem"-ee-loo'-nur-valv): made up of three half-moon-shaped cups, located between junction of aorta and left ventricle of heart

apex (ay'-peks): top of object; point or extremity of a cone

apex of lung (ay'-peks of the lung): upper extremity of lung, behind border of the first rib

aphasia (a-fay'-zhuh): loss of ability to speak, may be accompanied by loss of verbal comprehension

apnea (ap'-nee-uh): temporary stoppage of breathing movements

aponeurosis (ap"-o-new-ro'-sis): flattened sheet of white, fibrous connective tissue; serves as attachment for flat muscles, or as sheet enclosing/binding muscle groups

appendicitis (a-pen"-di-si-tis): inflammation of appendix

appendicular skeleton (ap"-en-dik'-yoo-lur skel'-uh-tun): part of skeleton consisting of pectoral and pelvic girdles, and limbs

arachnoid (uh-rak'-noyd): weblike middle membrane of meninges

arbor vitae (ahr'-bur vye'-tee): white matter on the inside of the cerebellum is marked with a tree-like pattern. This pattern is called arbor vitae

arbovirus (ahr"-bo-vye'-rus): any of over 200 arthropod-borne viruses transmitted to susceptible vertebrate hosts by blood-sucking arthropods

areola (a-ree-o'-luh): pigmented ring around nipple; any small space in tissue

arrhythmia (a-rith'-mee-uh): absence of a normal rhythm in heartbeat arteriole (ahr-teer′-ee-ole): small branch of artery

arteriosclerosis (ahr-teer″-ee-o-skleh-ro′-sis): hardening of arteries, resulting in thickening of walls and loss of elasticity

artery (ahr′-tur-ee): blood vessel which carries blood away from heart

arthritis (ahr-thry′-tis): inflammation of a joint

ascites (a-si′-teez): accumulation of fluid in the peritoneal cavity

assimilation (a-sim″-i-lay′-shun): process of changing food into form suitable for absorption by the circulatory system, and subsequent transformation into body tissue

astral rays (as′-trul rais): short cytoplasmic fibers that radiate out of the centriole

ataxia (ay-tak′-see-uh): muscle incoordination, particularly of muscle groups involved in walking or reaching for objects

atlas (at′-lus): first cervical vertebra; articulates with axis and occipital skull bone

atrial fibrillation (ay′-tree-ul fib″-ri-lay′-shun): cardiac arrhythmia, characterized by rapid, irregular atrial impulses and ineffective atrial contractions; heartbeat varies from 60 to 180 per minute and is highly irregular in rhythm and intensity

atrioventricular or A-V node (ay″-tree-o-ven-trik′-yoo-lur node): small mass of interwoven conducting tissue underneath right atrial endocardium

atrioventricular valves (ay″-tree-o-ven-trik′-yoo-lur valvz): tricuspid and mitral (bicuspid) valves of heart

atrium (ay′-tree-um): upper chamber of heart

atrophy (a′-truh-fee): wasting away of tissue

auricle (aw′-ri-kul): (1) pinna, or ear flap of external ear; (2) atrium of the heart

autoimmune (aw″-to-eh-mewn′): self-produced attack by the body's own cells

autonomic (aw″-tuh-nom′-ik): independent or self-regulating

autonomic nervous system (aw″-tuh-nom′-ik nur′-vus sis′-tum): collection of nerves, ganglia, and plexuses through which visceral organs, heart, blood vessels, glands, and smooth (involuntary) muscles receive their innervation

autosome (aw′-to-sohm): non-sex determining chromosome

axial muscle group (ack′-see-ul mus′-ul groop): muscles of the head, face, neck, and trunk

axial skeleton (ak′-see-ul skel′-e-tun): skeleton of head and trunk

axilla (ak-sil′-uh): armpit

axis (ack′-sis): (1) imaginary line passing through center of the body, (2) second cervical vertebra

axon (ack′s-on): nerve-cell structure which carries impulses away from cell body to dendrites

B

bactericidal (back-teer″-i-sigh′-dul): bacterial destruction

base (bays): (1) lowest part of a body, (2) main ingredient of a substance, (3) chemical compound yielding hydroxyl ions (OH^-) in an aqueous solution which will react with acid to form a salt and water

basophil (bay′-suh-fil): (1) cell, substance, or tissue that shows an attraction for basic dyes, (2) one of two cell types found in the anterior lobe of the pituitary gland. Basophils secrete thyroid-stimulating hormone (TSH), adenocorticotrophic hormone (ACTH), follicle-stimulating hormone (FSH), luteinizing hormone (LH), and interstitial cell-stimulating hormone (ICSH)

benign (be-nine′): non-malignant

bicarbonate ion (by-kahr′-buh-nate eye′-on): salt of carbonic acid characterized by ion HCO_3-

biceps (bye′-seps): large flexor muscle of upper arm or leg

bicuspid (bye-kus′-pid): having two cusps

bicuspid or mitral valve (bye-kus′-pid [my′-trul] valv): atrioventricular valve of left side of heart

bifurcation (bye″-fur-kay′-shun): division into two branches

bilateral symmetry (bye-lat′-ur-ul sim′-e-tree): relating to both sides of body

bilirubin (bil″-ee-roo′-bin): one of two pigments that determines the color of bile. Bilirubin is reddish in color

biliverdin (bil″-ee-vur′-din): one of two pigments that determine the color of bile. Biliverdin is greenish in color

biospy (bye′-op-see): excision of a piece of tissue from a living body for diagnostic study

bipedal (bye-ped′-ul): having two feet

bolus (bo′-lus): rounded mass; food prepared by mouth for swallowing

bowel (bow′-ul): intestine

brachial (bray′-kee-ul): pertaining to the upper arm

brachiocephalic artery (bray′-kee-o-se-fal′-ik ahr′-tur-ee): artery rising from right side of aortic arch; it divides into right subclavian and right common carotid arteries

bradycardia (brad″-ee-kahr′-dee-uh): abnormally slow heartbeat, less than 60 beats per minute

brainstem (brayn′-stem): portion of brain other than cerebral hemispheres and cerebellum

bronchiole (bronk′-ee-ole): one of small subdivisions of a bronchus (1 mm or less)

bronchiolectasis (bronk″-ee-o-lek′-tuh-sis): condition in which the bronchi are dilated

bronchus (bronk′-us): one of two primary branches of trachea

buccal (buck′-ul): pertaining to the cheek or mouth

buccal cavity (buck′-ul kav′-i-tee): mouth cavity bounded by the inner surface of the cheek

bulbourethral glands (bul″-bo-you-ree′-thrul glans): two tubular glands in the male urogenital system, located in front of the prostate gland

bunion (bun′-yun): swelling of bursa of foot

bursa (bur′-suh): small sac interposed between parts that move on one another

bursitis (bur-sigh′-tis): inflammation of a bursa

C

calcaneus (kal-kay′-nee-us): heel bone

calciferol (kal-sif′-ur-ol): vitamin D_2

calcify (kal′-si-fie): to deposit mineral salts

calcitonin (kal″-si-to′-nin): hormone secreted by thyroid gland that controls calcium ion concentration in body by preventing excessive calcium build-up in blood

calculus (kal′-kew-lus): stone-like formation in any part of the body, usually composed of mineral salts

callus (kal′-us): area of hardened and thickened skin

calyx (kay′-liks): cup-shaped part of the renal pelvis

canine (kay′-nine): sharp teeth of mammals, between incisors and premolars

capillary (kap′-i-lair-ee): microscopic blood vessel which connects arterioles with venules

carboxyhemoglobin (kahr-bock″-see-hee′-mo-glo-bin): compound of carbon monoxide and hemoglobin formed when carbon monoxide is present in blood

carboxypolypeptidase (kahr-bock″-see-pol″-ee-pep′-ti-dace): one of the three protein-digesting enzymes which breaks down polypeptides into their component amino acids; secreted by the pancreas

carcinoma (kahr″-si-no′-muh): a malignant tumor

cardiac (kahr′-dee-ack): relating to the heart

cardiac arrest (kahr′-dee-ack uh-rest′): syndrome resulting from failure of heart as a pump

cardiac arrhythmia (kahr′-dee-ack a-rith′-mee-uh): any change or abnormality in the normal heart rhythm or beat

cardiac muscle (kahr′-dee-ack mus′-ul): muscle of the heart

cardiac sphincter (kahr′-dee-ack sfink′-tur): circular muscle fibers around cardiac end of esophagus

cardiopulmonary resuscitation (kahr″-dee-o-puhl′-muh-nair-ee ree-sus″-i-tay′-shun): prevention of asphyxial death by artificial respiration

caries (kair′-eez): decay of tooth or bone

carotid (ka-rot′-id): an artery which supplies blood to the neck and head

carpal (kahr′-pul): bones of the wrist

cartilage (kahr′-ti-lidj): white, semi-opaque, nonvascular connective tissue

casein (kay′-see-in): protein obtained from milk

catalyst (kat′-uh-list): chemical substance which alters a chemical process but does not enter into the process

cataract (kat′-uh-rakt): condition in which the eye lens becomes opaque

cecum (see′-kum): pouch at the proximal end of the large intestine

cells of Leydig (sels-of-lay′-dig): another name for the interstitial cells in the male reproductive system. These cells are named after Franz von Leydig, a German histologist (1821–1908)

centrioles (sen′-tree-oles): two cylindrical organelles found near the muscles in a tiny-body called the centrosome. They are perpendicular to each other

centromere (sen′-tro-meer): a small body that joins two chromatid strands

centrosome (sen′-tro-sohm): tiny area near the nucleus of an animal cell; it contains two cylindrical structures called centrioles

cerebellar peduncle (serr″-e-bel′ur pe-dunk-′ul): the cerebellum communicates with the rest of the central nervous system by three pairs of tracts called the inferior, middle, and superior cerebellar peduncles

cerumen (see-roo′-men): ear wax

cervix (sur′-vicks): neck; usually refers to the rounded, conical protrusion of the uterus into the vagina

"Charley horse" (char′-lee horse): an injury, common among athletes, in which a muscle is torn or bruised; it is accompanied by severe pain and cramps

chemotaxis (kem″-o-tack′-sis): chemotaxis is a response of an organism or a cell to a chemical stimulus by either moving towards or away from the chemical stimulus. Moving towards a chemical stimulus is classified as positive chemotaxis and away as negative chemotaxis

cholecystectomy (kol″-e-sis-tek′-tuh-mee): removal of the gallbladder

cholecystokinin (ko″-lih-sis″-tih-kigh′-nen): hormone secreted by the duodenum and jejunum which stimulates pancreatic juice secretion.

cholesterol (ko-les′-tur-ol): a sterol normally synthesized in the liver and also ingested in egg yolks, animal fats and tissues

chromatid (kro′-muh-tid): each strand of a replicable chromosome

chromosomal mutation (kro″-muh-so″-mul mew-tay′-shun): a mutation that involves change in the number of chromosomes in the organism's nucleus or a change in the structure of a whole chromosome

chromosome (kro′-muh-sohm): nuclear material which determines hereditary characteristics

chyme (kime): food which has undergone gastric digestion

chymotrypsin (kigh″-mo-trip′-sen): enzyme that digests proteins or incompletely digested proteins turning them into peptides, proteases, polypeptides, peptides, and finally into amino acids

chymotrypsinogen (kigh″-mo-trip-sen′-o-jen): compound that is an inactive form of chymotrypsin

cilia (sil-ee-uh): tiny lashlike processes of protoplasm

coagulum (ko-ag′-you-lum): clot; a coagulated mass; a curd

cochlea (kock′-lee-uh): spiral cavity of the internal ear containing the organ of Corti

cochlear duct (kock′-lee-ur dukt): an endolymph-filled triangular canal containing the spiral organ of Corti

complete proteins (kum-pleet′ pro′-teens): proteins that contain all the essential amino acids; they enable an animal to grow and carry on fundamental life activities

congenital (kun-jen′-i-tul): present at birth

consolidation (kun-sol″-i-day′-shun): the process of becoming firm or solid, as a lung in pneumonia

coronary (kor′-o-nair″-ee): referring to the blood vessels of the heart

corpus (kor′-pus): body

cortex (kor′tecks): outer part of an internal organ

costal (kos′-tul): pertaining to the ribs

cretinism (kree′-tin-ism): congenital and chronic condition due to the lack of thyroid hormone

cryptorchidism (krip-tor′-kih-dizm): failure of testes to descend into the scrotal sac

cutaneous (kew-tay′-nee-us): pertaining to the skin

cyanosis (si″-uh-no′-sis): bluish color of the skin due to insufficient oxygen in the blood

cytokinesis (sigh″-to-kih-nee′-sis): the process of dividing one cell into two new daughter cells

cytoplasm (sigh′-to-plazm): protoplasm of the cell body, excluding the nucleus

D

deciduous teeth (de-sid′-you-us teeth): temporary teeth usually lost by six years of age

defecation (def″-e-kay′-shun): elimination of waste material from the rectum

deglutition (dee″-gloo-tish′-un): act of swallowing

deltoid (del′-toyd): triangular-shaped muscle which covers the shoulder prominence; used for intramuscular injections in adults

dendrite (den′-drīte): nerve cell process that carries nervous impulses toward the cell body

dentin (den′-tin): main part of the tooth located under the enamel

dentition (den-tish′-un): number, shape, and arrangement of teeth

deoxygenate (dee-ock″-si-je-nate): process of removing oxygen from a compound

dermis (dur′-mis): true skin; lying immediately beneath the epidermis

dextrin (decks′-trin): yellow or white powder produced by the incomplete digestion of starch; used as an emulsifying, protective, and thickening agent

dextrose (decks′-troce): glucose, a monosaccharide which may accumulate in the urine

diapedesis (dye″-uh-pe′dee′sis): passage of blood cells through unruptured vessel walls into tissues diaphragm (dye'-uh-fram): muscular partition between the thorax and the abdomen

diastole (dye-as'-tuh-lee): dilation state of the heart; the rest between systoles

digestion (di-jes'-chun): change of foods into compounds that can be assimilated

diploid number of chromosomes (dip'-loyd num'-bur of cro'-muh-sohms): number of chromosomes found in the normal human somatic cell nucleus. In humans the diploid number of chromosomes is 46, symbolized by 2n

dislocation (dis"-lo-kay'-shun): displacement of one or more bones of a joint or of any organ from original position

distal (dis'-tul): farthest from point of origin of a structure; opposite of proximal

dorsal (dor'-sul): pertaining to the back

dropsy (drop'-see): accumulation of serous fluid in a body cavity; edema

ductus deferens or vas deferens (duck'-tus def'-uh-renz or vas def'-uh-renz): the part of the excretory duct system of the testes which runs from the epididymus to the ejaculatory duct

duodenum (dew"-o-dee'-num): first part of small intestine, beginning at pylorus

dura mater (dew'-ruh may'-tur): fibrous membrane forming outermost covering of brain and spinal cord

dysmenorrhea (dis-men"-o-ree'-uh): difficult or painful menstruation

dyspareunia (dis"-puh-roo'-nee-uh): difficult or painful sexual intercourse

dyspnea (disp-nee'-uh): labored breathing or difficult breathing

E

ectopic (eck-top'-ick): in an abnormal position; said of an extrauterine pregnancy or cardiac beats

ectoplasm (eck'-to-plazm): outer dense layer of cytoplasm of cell or unicellular organism

edema (eh-dee'-muh): excessive fluid in tissues

ejaculatory ducts (e-jack'-you-luh-tor"-ee ducks): short and narrow ducts that begin where the ductus deferens and the seminal duct join. The ejaculatory ducts then descend into the prostate gland to join with the urethra

elastic (e-las'-tick): capable of returning to original form after being compressed or stretched

elastin (e-las'-tin): protein base of yellow elastic tissue

electrolytes (e-leck'-tro-lights): electrically-charged particles which help determine fluid and acid-base balance

embolism (em'-bo-lizm): obstruction of a blood vessel by a circulating blood clot, fat globule, air bubble, or piece of tissue

embryo (em'-bree-o): the human young up to the first three months after conception; the young of any organism in early development stage

emesis (em'-e-sis): vomitus

emphysema (em'-fi-see'-muh): lung disorder in which inspired air becomes trapped and is difficult to expire

empyema (em"-pye-ee'-muh): pus in a cavity

emulsify (e-mul"-si-fye): to make into an *emulsion,* a product consisting of small globules of one liquid intermixed throughout the body of a second liquid

endocardium (en"-do-kahr'-dee-um): membrane lining interior of heart

endocrine (en'-do-krin): pertaining to a gland which secretes into the blood or tissue fluid instead of into a duct

endometrium (en"-do-mee'-tree-um): mucous membrane lining uterus

endoplasm (en'-do-plazm): inner cytoplasm of cell of unicellular organism

endothelium (en"-do-theel'-ee-um): epithelial cells lining the blood vessels, heart, and lymph vessels or any closed cavity in the body

enterokinase (en"-tur-o-kigh'-nace): enzyme secreted by glands lining the small intestine; it changes inactive trypsinogen into active trypsin

enzyme (en'-zime): organic catalyst that initiates and accelerates a chemical reaction

eosinophil (ee"-o-sin'-uh-fil): white blood cell or bone marrow whose granules stain red with eosin or other acid dyes

epidermis (ep"-i-dur-'-mis): outermost layer of skin

epididymitis (ep"-i-did"-i-mi'-tis): inflammation of epididymis

epididymus (ep"-i-did'-i-mis): portion of the seminal duct lying posterior to the testes; connected by the efferent ductulis of each testis

epiglottis (ep"-i-glot'is): elastic cartilage covered by mucous membrane forming upper part of larynx; guards glottis during swallowing

epinephrine (ep"-i-nef'-rin): adrenalin; secretion of the adrenal medulla, which prepares the body for energetic action

erythrocyte (e-rith'-ro-sight): red blood cell

erythropoiesis (e-rith"-ro-poy-ee'-sis): formation or development of red blood cells

essential amino acids (e-sen'-chul a'mee'-no as'-ids): amino acids that are necessary for normal growth and development and are not made in the human body. They are argnine (Arg)*, histidine (His),* isoleucine (Ileu), leucine (Leu), lysine (Lys), methionine (Met), phenylalanine (Phe), threonine (Thr), tryptophane (Try), valine (Val)

eupnea (yoop-nee'-uh): normal or easy breathing with usual quiet inhalations and exhalations

exophthalmos (eck"-sof-thal'-mus): abnormal protrusion of the eyes

expiration (eck"-spi-ray'-shun): act of breathing forth or expelling air from lungs

extensor (eck-sten'-sur): muscle which extends or stretches a limb or part

F

fallopian tube (fa-lo'-pee-un tewb): uterine tube or oviduct which carries egg from ovary to uterus

fascia (fash'uh): band or sheet of fibrous membranes covering or binding and supporting muscles

femur (fee'-mur): thighbone

fetus (fee'-tus): the human young from birth until the third month of the intrauterine period

fibrin (fī'-brin): an insoluble protein necessary for the clotting of blood

fibrinogen (fī-brin'-o-jen): a protein which is converted into fibrin by the action of thrombin

fibroblast (figh'-bro-blast): large, flat branching cells that help to form the flexible skin collagen fibers

fibroma (figh-bro'-muh): benign tumor made up mainly of fibrous connective tissue

fibula (fib'-yoo-luh): slender bone at outer edge of lower leg

follicle stage (fol'-i-kul stayj): first stage of the female menstrual cycle during which follicle-stimulating hormone (FSH) secreted from the anterior lobe of the pituitary gland is circulated to an ovary via the bloodstream. When FSH reaches an ovary, it stimulates several follicles; however, only one matures. As the one follicle grows in size, an egg cell begins to grow inside the follicle

*Essential only in growing children

follicle-stimulating hormone (FSH) (fol'-i-kul stim'-yoo-lay-ting hor'-mone): an adenohypophyseal hormone which stimulates follicular growth in the ovary

fontanel (fon"-tuh-nel'): unossified areas in the infant skull; soft spot

foramen (fo-ray'-men): an opening in a bone

fracture (frack'-chur): a break in a bone

fundus (fun'-dus): part farthest from opening of an organ

G

ganglion (gang'-glee-un): a mass of nerve cell bodies outside the central nervous system

gangrene (gang'-green): necrosis of a part due to failure of blood supply

gastric (gas'-trick): pertaining to the stomach

gastric glands (gas'-trick glans): glands lining stomach

gene (jeen): part of the chromosome that transmits a specific hereditary trait

genetics (je-net'-icks): the branch of biology that studies the science of heredity and the difference and similarities between parents and offspring

genitals (jen'-i-tuls): reproductive organs, also called genitalia

gestation (jes-tay'-shun): development period of the human young from conception to birth

glenoid fossa (glee'-noid fos'-uh): articular surface on scapula for articulation with head of humerus

glomerulus (glom-err'-you-lus): compact cluster of capillaries in the nephron of the kidney

glucose (gloo'-koce): a monosaccharide or simple sugar; the principal blood sugar

gluteal (gloo-tee'-ul): pertaining to the area near the buttocks

glycerin or glycerol (glis'-ur-in or glis'-ur-ole): product of fat digestion

glycogen (glye'-kuh-jin): polysaccharide formed and stored largely in the liver; can be converted into glucose when needed

gonads (go'nads): sex glands (ovaries or testes)

graafian follicle (graf'-ee-un fol'-i-kul): mature ovarian follicle

graft (graft): portion of tissue, such as bone, periosteum, skin, or sometimes an entire organ, used to replace a defective body part

granulation (gran"-you-lay'-shun): tiny red granules that are visible in the base of a healing wound; consists of newly formed capillaries and fibroblasts

greenstick fracture (green-stick frack'-chur): incomplete fracture of long bone; seen in children; bone is bent but splintered only on convex side

H

hematoma (hee"-muh-toe'-muh): a localized clotted mass of blood formed in an organ, tissue, or space. It is caused by an injury, like a blow, that can cause blood vessels to rupture

hemiplegia (hem"-i-plee'-jee-uh): paralysis of one side of the body

hemocytoblast (hee"-mo-sigh'-toe-blast): cell considered by some to be primitive stem cell, giving rise to all blood cells

hemoglobin (hee'-muh-glo"-bin): oxygen-carrying pigment of the blood

hemophilia (hee"-mo-fill'-ee-uh): sex-linked, hereditary bleeding disorder occurring only in males but transmitted by females; characterized by a prolonged clotting time and abnormal bleeding

hemorrhoids (hem'-uh-roydz): enlarged an varicose condition of the veins in the lower part of the anus or rectum and the tissues of the anus

heparin (hep'-uh-rin): substance obtained from the liver, which slows blood clotting

hepatic vein (he-pat'-ick vain): vein which drains blood from liver into inferior vena cava

hereditary (he-red'-i-terr-ee): of or pertaining to inheritance; inborn; inherited

hernia (hur'-nee-uh): protrusion of a loop of an organ through abnormal opening

histocompatibility (his"-to-kum-pat"-i-bil'-i-tee): state in which the chemistry of tissues from a donor are acceptable to a recipient

histology (his-tol'-uh-jee): microscopic study of living tissues

hormone (hor'-mone): chemical secretion, usually from an endocrine gland

humerus (hew'-mur-us): upper arm bone

hyoid bone (high'-oyd bone): bone between root of the tongue and larynx, supporting tongue and giving attachment to several muscles

hypernea (high"-pur-nee'-uh): increase in the depth and rate of breathing accompanied by abnormal exaggeration of respiratory movements

hyperopia (high"-pur-o'-pee-uh): farsightedness

hypertension (high"-pur-ten'-shun): abnormally high blood pressure

hypertrophy (high-pur'-truh-fee): enlargement of a part due to increase in size of its already existing cells

hypotension (high"-po-ten'-shun): reduced or abnormally low tension, synonymous with low blood pressure

hysterectomy (his"-tur-eck'-tuh-mee): partial or total surgical removal of the uterus

I

ileum (il'-ee-um): the lower part of the small intestine, extending from the jejunum to the large intestine

ilium (il'-ee-um): upper broad portion of the hipbone

immunosuppressant (im'-you-no-suh-press'-unt): an agent, such as a drug, chemical, or X-ray used to suppress the immune system of a patient. Generally, it is used to enhance acceptance of a foreign skin, tissue graft or organ implant

incisor (in-sigh'-zur): cutting tooth; one of four front teeth of either jaw

incomplete proteins (in"-kum-pleet' pro'-teens): proteins that lack some or most of the essential amino acids

incus (ing'-kus): the middle ear bone, also called the anvil

inflammation (in"fluh-may'-shun): occurs when tissues are subjected to chemical or physical trauma (cut or heat); invasion by pathogenic microorganisms like bacteria, fungi, protozoa, and viruses also can cause inflammation. Characteristic symptoms are redness, local heat, swelling and pain; due to (1) irritation by bacterial toxins, (2) increased blood flow, (3) congestion of blood vessels, and (4) collection of blood plasma in the surrounding tissues

infundibulum (in"-fun-dib'-you-lum): the stalk that connects the pituitary gland to the hypothalamus

ingestion (in-jes'-chun): act of taking substances, especially food, into body

inguinal (ing'-gwi-nul): pertaining to the groin

inhalation (in"-huh-lay'-shun): taking air into the lungs

innominate bone (i-nom'-i-nut bone): hipbone

inspiration (in"-spi-ray'-shun): drawing in of air; inhalation

insulin (in'-suh-lin): hormone secreted by the pancreas; regulates the rate of carbohydrate usage

integument (in-teg'-you-munt): covering, especially the skin

intercostal muscles (in"-tur-kos'-tul mus'-ul): muscles found between adjacent ribs interstitial tissue (in″-tur-stish′ul tish′-ue): intercellular connective tissue

intramuscular (in″-truh-mus′-kew-lur): into the muscle

intravenously (in′-truh-vee′-nus-ly): within, or into, the veins

irradiation (ir-ay′-dee-ay′-shun): exposure to radiation such as infrared, gamma, roentgen, and ultraviolet rays

involuntary (in-vol′-un-terr-ee): opposite of voluntary, not within the control of will

involution (in″-vo-lew′-shun): return of an organ to its normal size after enlargement; also the regressive changes due to aging

ion (eye′-on): an electrically charged atom

(eye′-ris): colored, circular smooth muscle surrounding the pupil and controlling the diameter of pupil

irritability (irr″-i-tuh-bil′-i-tee): ability to react to a stimulus; excitability

ischium (is′-kee-um): lower part of hipbone

isotonic (eye″-so-ton-ick): the same tension or pressure

K

karyokinesis (kare″-ee-o-ki-nee′-sis): division of the nucleus during mitosis

keratectomy (kerr″-uh-teck′-tuh-mee): excision of part of the cornea

keratin (kerr′-uh-tin): chemical belonging to albuminoid or scleroprotein group found in horny tissue, hair, nails, feathers; insoluble in protein solvents, and contains a high percentage of sulfur

kilogram (kil′-uh-gram): 1000 grams or approximately 2.2 pounds

kinesthesia (kin″-es-thee′-shuh): ability to perceive the direction or weight of muscular movement

kinetic (ki-ne′-tick): pertaining to motion

L

labia (lay′-bee-uh): lips

lacrimal (lack′-ri-mul): pertaining to tears

lactation (lack′-tay′-shun): secretion of milk from the breasts

lactose (lack′-toce): milk sugar; a disaccharide used in infant formulas

larynx (lar′-inks): voicebox, found between trachea and base of tongue; contain the vocal cords

lateral (lat′-ur-ul): toward the side

laxative (lack′-suh-tiv): chemical substance that relieves constipation; a mild purgative

lens (lenz): crystal or glass for refraction of light rays

leukocyte (lew′-ko-sight): white blood cell

leukocytosis (lew″-ko-sigh-toe′-sis): an increase in the white blood cell count, above 10,000 cells per cubic millimeter (mm^3)

leukocytosis-inducing factor (LIF) (lew″-ko-sigh-toe′-sis in-dewce′-ing fac′-tur): chemical produced in cases of severe infection; stimulates the production and release of neutrophils into the bloodstream causing an increase in the white blood cell count

leukopenia (lew″-ko-pee′-nee-uh): a decrease in the normal number of white blood cells (leukocytes)

leukorrhea (lew″-ko-ree′-uh): whitish, mucopurulent discharge from vagina

ligament (lig′-uh-munt): a band of fibrous tissue connecting bones or supporting organs

lipid (lip′-id): fatty compound

lobule (lob′-yool): small lobe or a small section of a lobe

locomotion (lo″-kuh-mo′-shun): act of moving from place to place

lordosis (lor-do′-sis): forward curvature of lumbar region of spine

lumbago (lum-bay′-go): backache occurring in the lower lumbar or lumbosacral area of the spinal column

lumbar (lum′-bahr): pertaining to the loins; region between the posterior thorax and sacrum

lumbar vertebrae (lum′-bahr vur′-te-bree): five vertebrae associated with lower part of back

lumen (lew′-min): passageway or opening to a tubular structure such as a blood vessel

lymph (limf): watery fluid in the lymphatic vessels

lymphatic (lim-fat′-ick): vessel carrying lymph

lymphatic system (lim-fat′-ick sis′-tum): system of vessels and nodes supplemental to blood circulatory system, carrying lymph

lymphocyte (lim′-fo-sight): a type of white blood cell

lysosome (lye″-so-sohm): cytoplasmic organelle present in many kinds of cells, especially in liver and kidney cells containing digestive enzymes

M

malleus (mal′-ee-us): largest of three middle ear bones; also called the hammer

maltose (mawl'-tose): disaccharide formed by the hydrolysis of starch

mammary (mam'-ur-ree): pertaining to the breast

mandible (man'di-bul): lower jawbone

manubrium (ma-new'-bree-um): (1) handle-like process; (2) upper part of the sternum (breastbone)

mastectomy (mas-teck'-tuh-mee): amputation of breast

mastication (mas''-ti-kay'-shun): process of chewing

maturation (match''-oo-ray'-shun): process of coming to full development

meatus (mee-ay'-tus): passageway or opening

medial (mee'dee-ul): toward midline of body

mediastinum (mee''-dee-as-tih'-num): intrapleural space separating the sternum in front and the vertebral column behind

medulla (ma-dul'-uh): inner portion of an organ

melanism (mel'-uh-nizm): abnormal deposition of dark pigment (melanin) in organs, in tissues, or in skin

membrane (mem'-brane): a thin layer of tissue which covers a surface or divides an organ

menarche (me-nahr'-kee): time when menstruation begins

menopause (men'-o-pawz): physiologic termination of menstruation, generally between forty-fifth and fiftieth years

menstrual cycle (men'-stroo-ul sigh'-kul): recurring series of changes that take place in the ovaries, uterus, and accessory sexual structures during menstruation

menstruation (men''-stroo-ay'-shun): stage that occurs during the menstrual cycle. During menstruation bloody fluid is periodically discharged from the uterus. The fluid is composed of the unfertilized egg, the lining of the uterus, and a small quantity of blood which comes from capillaries that break as the endometrial lining peels away from the uterus. This fluid is discharged from the female's body through the vagina

metabolism (me-tab'-o-lizm): sum total of processes of digestion, absorption, and the resulting release of energy

metacarpus (met''-uh-kahr'-pus): part of the hand between the wrist and the fingers

metastasis (me-tas'-tuh-sis): transfer of disease from an original site to a distant one by the transmittal of causative agents or cells through the circulatory system or lymph vessels

metatarsus (met''-uh-tahr'-sus): part of the foot between the tarsal bones and the toes

microbe (migh'-krobe): microscopic organisms, especially bacterium

microcephalus (migh''-kro-sef'-uh-lus): individual with an unusually small head

microgram (migh-kro-gram): one one-thousandth of a milligram, abbreviated as mcg and symbolized as μg

microtubules (migh'-kro-tew''-bewls): long, thin microscopic tubes that play a role in cytoplasmic membrane function and cell shape as well as help form the spindle fibers in the mitotic spindle-fiber apparatus. Microtubules also move various substances and organelles within the cell

micturition (mich''-tew-rish'-un): voiding, or urinating

miotic (mi-ot'-ick): causing contraction of pupil

milligram (mil'-i-gram): one one-thousandth of a gram, abbreviated as mg

mineral (min'ur-ul): an inorganic, solid chemical compound found in nature

mitosis (migh-toe'-sis): cell division which is divided into two distinct processes:

(1) mitosis–the exact duplication of the nucleus to form two identical nuclei. DNA hereditary material is doubled followed by nuclear division

(2) cytoplasmic division–after nuclear division, the cytoplasm is divided into two approximately equal parts

mixed nerve (mikst nurv): nerve composed of both afferent (sensory) fibers and efferent (motor) fibers

monocyte (mon'-o-sight): large mononuclear leukocyte with deeply indented nucleus, slate-gray cytoplasm, and fine bluish granulations

monorchidism (mon-or'-kid-izm): presence of only one testis

monosaccharide (mon''-o-sack'-uh-ride): simple sugar; glucose

mucilaginous (mew''-si-ladj'-i-nus): gumlike consistency

mucin (mew'-sin): mixture of glycoproteins forming basis of mucus

mucosa (mew-ko'-suh): mucous membrane

mutagenic agent (mew''-tuh-jen'-ick ay'-junt): any substance causing a genetic mutation

mutate (mew-tate'): to change or alter a characteristic which will make it different from that of the parental type mutation (mew-tay′-shun): the appearance of a new and different organic trait caused by the inheritance of a mutated gene or chromosome

myalgia (migh-al′-juh): muscular pain

myelin (migh′-e-lin): a lipoid substance found in the sheath around nerve fibers

myocarditis (migh″-o-kahr-dye′-tis): inflammation of muscular tissue of heart

myocardium (migh″-o-kahr′-dee-um): muscle of the heart

myoglobin (migh′-o-glo″-bin): form of hemoglobin occurring in muscle fibers

myometrium (migh″-o-mee′-tree-um): uterine muscular structure

myopia (migh-o′-pee-uh): nearsightedness

myositis (migh′-o-sigh′-tis): inflammation of muscle tissue, generally voluntary muscle

myotonia (migh″-o-to′-nee-uh): condition where there is an abnormally slow muscle relaxation after voluntary muscle contraction

N

nares (nair′-eez): pertaining to the nostrils

nasal cavity (nay′-zul kav′-i-tee): one of the pair of cavities between anterior nares and nasopharynx

nasal septum (nay′-zul sep′-tum): partition between the two nasal cavities

negative feedback (neg′-uh-tiv feed′-back): the return of part of the output to the source or beginning; this leads to an adjustment in the system. Negative feedback may occur in hormonal or nervous control systems

neoplasm (nee′-o-plazm): applies to various types of tumors

nephron (nef′-ron): unit of structure and function of kidney, consisting of glomerular capsule, glomerulus, and attached kidney tubules

neurohypophysis (new″-ro-high-pof′-i-sis): posterior lobe of the pituitary gland; it does not produce any hormones. However, it helps store two hormones produced by the hypothalamus: antidiuretic hormone and oxytocin

neuron (new′-ron): nerve cell, including its processes

nongravid (non″-grav′-id): not pregnant

nonpathogenic (non″-path″-o-jen′-ick): incapable of producing disease

nucleoalbumin (new″-klee-o-al-bew′-min): protein secreted from mucous membranes that line the bile ducts and gallbladder; this secretion is added to bile

nucleolus (new-klee′-uh-lus): small spherical structure within cell nucleus

nucleoplasm (new′-klee-o-plazm): protoplasm of the nucleus, also called *nuclear sap* or *karyolymph*

nucleus (new′-klee-us): core or center of a cell containing large quantities of DNA

nutrient (new′-tree-unt): affording nutrition

O

obesity (o-bee′-si-tee): increase of body weight due to fat accumulation of 10 to 20% above normal range for the specific age, height, and sex

occiput (ock′-si-put): pertaining to the back of the head

olecranon process (o-leck′-ruh-non pro′-sess): large projection at upper extremity of ulna

olfactory (ol-fack′-tur-ee): pertaining to the sense of smell

oogenesis (o″-o-jen′-e-sis): process of origin, growth, and formation of ovum in ovary during preparation for fertilization

ophthalmic (off-thal′-mick): referring to the eyes

orchitis (or-ki′-tis): inflammation of testis

organelle (or-guh-nel′): microscopic specialized structure, or part of cell having a special function or capacity

oropharynx (or″-o-far′-inks): oral pharynx, found below level of lower border of soft palate and above larynx

orthopnea (or″-thup-nee′-uh): difficult or labored breathing when the body is in horizontal position; usually corrected by taking a sitting or standing position

osmoreceptor (oz″-mo-re-sep′tur): structures found in the hypothalamus; sensitive to changes in the osmotic blood pressure and control the release of the antidiuretic hormone (ADH)

osmosis (oz-mo′-sis): passage of fluid through a membrane

osmotic pressure (oz-mot′-ick presh′-ur): pressure developed when two solutions of different concentrations of the solute are separated by a membrane permeable only to the solvent

ossa carpi (os-sa kahr′-pye): the eight bones of the wrist

osseous (os′-ee-us): bony; composed of or resembling bone

ossicle (os′-i-kul): a small bone; usually refers to the three small bones of the middle ear

osteitis (os″-tee-eye′-tis): inflammation of bone tissue. In osteitis deformans (Paget's disease), loss of calcium and bone softening occurs, followed by calcium deposition which causes bony thickening and abnormalities

osteoarthritis (os″-tee-o-ahr-thry′-tis): degenerative joint disease

osteoblast (os′-tee-o-blast): cells involved in formation of bony tissue

osteoclast (os′-tee-o-klast): cells involved in resorption of bony tissue

osteoma (os″-tee-o′-muh): benign bony tumor found in the membrane bones of the skull. Osteomas have a tendency to extend into the orbit (eye) or nasal sinuses (cavities)

osteomalacia (os″-tee-o-muh-lay′-shee-uh): softening of bones due to lack of vitamin D in the diet or not enough exposure to sunlight. Mineral content of bone is lowered, due to inadequate absorption of calcium and phosphorus from the intestine; also called *adult rickets*

otosclerosis (o″-to-skle-ro′-sis): chronic, progressive ear disorder in which the bone in the region of the oval window first becomes spongy and then hardened, causing the stirrup or stapes to become fixed or immobile. Otosclerosis is a common cause of deafness in young adults. It can be alleviated by an operation called *stapes mobilization,* the stirrup is fixed and hearing is often restored. Another procedure removes the stapes, replacing them by tissue graft

ovulation stage (o″-vyoo-lay′-shun staydj): second stage of the menstrual cycle, when a ripe egg cell is released from an ovarian follicle cell

oxygenate (ock′-si-ji′-nate): to saturate a substance with oxygen, either by chemical combination or by mixture

oxyhemoglobin (ock″-si-hee′-muh-glo″-bin): hemoglobin combined with oxygen

P

palate (pal′-ut): roof of the mouth

Pap or Papanicolaou (pah″-eh-nick′-o-low) **smear:** cytological, diagnostic cancer technique that studies exfoliated cells, especially those from the vagina

papilla (pa-pil′-uh): small, nipple-shaped elevations

paralysis (puh-ral′-i-sis): loss of power of motion or sensation

parathyroid gland (par″-uh-thi′-royd gland): one of several (usually four) small endocrine glands embedded in the thyroid gland; secrete a hormone which regulates blood calcium levels (parathormone)

paresthesia (par″-es-theezh′-uh): perverted sensation of tingling, crawling, or burning of skin

parotid gland (pa-rot′-id): largest of the salivary glands

patella (pa-tel-uh): kneecap

pathogenic (path″-uh-jen′-ick): disease-causing

pectoral (peck′-tuh-rul): pertaining to the chest

pelvis (pel′-vis): any basin-shaped structure or cavity

pericardium (perr″-i-kahr′-dee-um): closed membranous sac surrounding heart

peripheral (pe-rif′-e-rul): outside surface, or the area away from the center

peristalsis (perr″-i-stal′-sis): progressive wave of contraction in tubular structures provided with longitudinal and transverse muscular fibers, as in esophagus, stomach, small and large intestines

pH: hydrogen ion concentration of solution or air mixture; potential of hydrogen

phagocyte (fag′-o-sight): cell having property of engulfing and digesting foreign particles or cells harmful to body

phagocytosis (fag″-o′-si-to′-sis): ingestion of foreign or other particles by certain cells

phalanges (fa-lan′-jeez): bones of fingers and toes

pharynx (fair′-inks): musculomembranous tube located behind nose, mouth, and larynx, extending from base of skull to point opposite sixth cervical vertebra

phase (faze): (1) condition or stage of a disease or a biological, chemical, physiological, and psychological function at a given time, (2) a solid, liquid, or gas which is similar throughout and physically separated from another phase by a clear boundary

phenylketonuria (PKU) (fen″-il-kee″-to-new′-ree-uh): a human metabolic disorder. The body cannot make an enzyme needed for normal metabolism or breakdown of the amino acid *phenylalanine* so it builds up in the body. Excess phenylalanine will disrupt the normal development of neurons in the brain. As a result people who suffer from untreated phenylketonuria are mentally retarded

phlebitis (fle-bye′-tis): inflammation of a vein, with or without infection and thrombus formation

phlegmasia alba dolens ("milk leg") (fleg-may'-zhuh al'-buh do'-lenz): painful swelling of the leg generally seen after childbirth; due to femoral vein thrombophlebitis or lymphatic blockage

physiology (fiz"-ee-ol'-uh-jee): science that studies functions of living organisms and their parts

physiotherapy (fiz"-ee-o-therr'-uh-pee): physical medicine

pia mater (pee'uh may-tur): innermost vascular covering of brain and spinal cord

pigment (pig'-munt): (1) dye or coloring matter, (2) organic coloring matter of body

plasma (plaz'-muh): liquid part of blood containing corpuscles

pleura (ploor'-uh): serous membrane enclosing lung and lining internal surface of thoracic cavity

pleurisy (ploor'i-see): inflammation of pleura

pleurodynia (ploor"-o-din'-ee-uh): chest pain, specifically in the intercoastal area

plexus (pleck'-sus): network of interlacing nerves, blood vessels, or lymphatics

polypnea (pol"-ip-nee'-uh): very rapid respiration or panting due to increased muscular activity or from emotional trauma

polysaccharide (pol"-ee-sack'-uh-ride): a complex sugar

popliteal (pop-lit'-ee-ul): area behind knee

pores (pores): (1) very small openings on a surface, (2) opening ducts of a sweat gland

posterior (pos-teer'-ee-ur): located behind or at the back; opposite to anterior

presbyopia (prez"-bee-o'-pee-uh): farsightedness of advanced age due to loss of elasticity in lens of eye

progesterone (pro-jes'-tur-ohn): steroid hormone secreted by ovary from corpus luteum to help maintain pregnancy

prolapsed uterus (pro-lapst' you'-tur-us): normal supportive structures around the uterus weaken and allow the uterus to fall from its normal position

pronation (pro-nay'-shun): (1) condition of being prone, (2) turning of palm of hand downward

prostate gland (pros'-tate gland): gland located just under the urinary bladder; it surrounds the opening of the bladder leading into the urethra. The gland is covered by a dense fibrous capsule and contains glandular tissue surrounded by fibromuscular tissue that contracts during ejaculation; secretes a thin, milky alkaline fluid that enhances sperm motility

prostatectomy (pros"-tuh-teck'-tuh-mee): surgical removal of all or part of prostate

prostatic urethra (pros'-ta-tick yoo-ree'-thruh): area at the beginning of the urethra, surrounded by the prostate gland

protoplasm (pro'-tuh-plazm): living colloid material of the cell; contains proteins, lipids, inorganic salts and carbohydrates

proximal (prock'-si-mul): located nearest the center of the body; point of attachment of a structure

psychic (sigh'-kick): (1) pertaining to psyche, which is the mind or self as a functional unit, helping a person adjust to the changes, demands, or needs of the environment, (2) sensitive to nonphysical forces, (3) mental

puberty (pew'-bur-tee): age when reproductive organs become functional

pubis (pew'-bis): pubic bone, portion of hipbone forming front of pelvis

pulmones (pul'-mones): plural of lung (pulmo)

pupil (pew'-pil): opening in iris of eye for passage of light

pus (pus): a product of inflammation; a cream-colored liquid that is a combination of dead tissue, dead and living bacteria, dead white blood cells, and blood plasma

pylorus (pye-lo'-rus): circular opening of stomach into duodenum

pyrexia (pye-reck'-see-uh): fever

pyrogen (pye'-ra-jen): any fever-producing agent

Q

quadripedal (kwah'-dri-pe-dul): four-footed stance

R

receptor (re-sep'-tur): sensory nerve that receives a stimulus and transmits it to the CNS

red muscle (red mus'ul): muscle that appears red in fresh state due to presence of muscle hemoglobin

reflex (ree'-flecks): involuntary action; automatic response

reflex arc (ree'-flecks ahrk): pathway travelled by an impulse during reflex action, going from receptor to effector

reflux (ree'-flucks): return flow

renal (ree'-nul): pertaining to the kidney

rennin (ren'-in): milk-coagulating enzyme found in gastric juice of ruminating animals, not present in the human stomach

replication (rep″-li-kay′-shun): occurs when an exact copy of each nuclear chromosome is made during the early part of the first stage of mitosis (early interphase)

respiratory distress syndrome (res′-peh-ruh-tor-ee distress′ sin′-drome): condition that generally affects premature babies; characterized by the formation of a hyaline-like false membrane within the alveoli which causes the alveoli to collapse. Abbreviated as RDS

rete testis (ree′-tee tes′-tis): intermeshing of the seminiferous tubules to form a small mesh-like network of tubules. The rete testis unite to form the epididymis

retroperitoneal (ret″-ro-perr″-i-to-nee′-ul): located behind the peritoneum

rhinorrhea (rye″-no-ree′-uh): discharge of thin, watery fluid from the nose

ribosome (rye′-bo-sohm): submicroscopic particle attached to endoplasmic reticulum, site of protein synthesis in cytoplasm of cell

rugae (roo′-jee): wrinkles or folds

S

sacroiliac joint (say″-kro-il′-ee-ack joint): joint between sacrum and ilium

sagittal (sadj′-i-tul): longitudinal; shaped like an arrow

sarcoplasm (sahr′-ko-plazm): the hyaline or finely granular interfibrillar material of muscle tissue

sartorius (sahr-to′-ree-us): thigh muscle

scapula (skap′-you-luh): large, flat, triangular bone forming back of shoulder

sclera (skleer′-uh): tough, white covering, part of external coat of eye

scoliosis (sko″-lee-o′-sis): lateral curvature of the spine

scrotum (skro′-tum): pouch that contains the testicles

sebaceous gland (se-bay′-shus gland): gland that secretes sebum, a fatty material

sebum (see′-bum): secretion of sebaceous glands that lubricate the skin

secretin (se-kree′-tin): hormone secreted by the epithelial cells that line the duodenum; stimulated by the acidic gastric juice and the partially digested proteins from the stomach. Secretin is circulated to the pancreas via the bloodstream. Where a large quantity of fluid rich in pancreatic digestive enzymes is secreted

sella turcica (sel′-uh tur′-si-kuh): saddle-shaped depression in sphenoid bone

semen (see′-mun): male reproductive fluid containing sperm

semilunar (sem″-ih-lew′-nur): half-moon shaped valve of aorta and pulmonary artery

seminal vesicles (sem′-i-nul ves′-i-kuls): two highly convoluted membranous tubes. A duct leads away from each seminal vesicle which joins the ductus deferens to form the ejaculatory duct on either side. Seminal vesicles produce secretions that contain amino acids, fructose, mucus, prostaglandins, and a small quantity of ascorbic acid–substances found in the seminal fluid to help nourish and protect sperm on its journey up the female reproductive system

senescence (se-nes′-unce): old age; senility

septum (sep′-tum): partition; dividing wall between two spaces or cavities, such as the septum between left and right side of heart

serous fluid (seer′-us floo′-id): (1) normal lymph fluid, (2) thin, watery body fluid

Sertoli cells (sur′-toe-lee sels): specialized cells that line seminiferous tubules and help in sperm formation

serum (seer′-um): clear, pale yellow fluid that separates from a clot of blood; plasma that contains no fibrinogen

sickle-cell anemia (sick′-ul sel uh-nee′-mee-uh): blood disorder common in individuals of African descent. It is caused by a gene mutation, the formation of an abnormal hemoglobin molecule in a red blood cell. This in turn changes the shape of the red blood cell from biconcave to a sickle shape. The sickle shape makes the red blood cells clump together, thus clogging up small blood vessels and capillaries. A sickle-shaped red blood cell also carries less oxygen to the body cells; therefore, the individuals has less energy, has constant fatigue, and experiences pain

sigmoid (sig′-moid): shaped like the letter S; distal, S-shaped part of colon

sinoatrial node (sigh″-no-ay′-tree-ul node): dense network of Purkinje fibers of conduction system at junction of superior vena cava and right atrium

sinus (sigh′-nus): recessed cavity or hollow space

skeletal muscle (skel′-e-tul mus′-ul): muscle attached to a bone or bones of skeleton and concerned in body movements; also known as voluntary or striated muscle

solute (sol′-yoot): dissolved substance in a solution

somatic cell (so-mat′-ick sel): all of the body cells except for sex cells (egg and sperm)

somatic cell mutation (so-mat'-ick sel mew-tay'-shun): mutations that occur in individual body cells

spermatic cord (spur-mat'-ick kord): the cord that extends from the testis to the deep inguinal ring; contains the ductus deferens, the blood vessels and nerves of the testis and epididymis, and the surrounding connective tissue

sphincter (sfink'-tur): circular muscle, such as the anus

spina bifida (spye'-nuh bye'-fi-duh): congenital defect in closure of spinal canal with hernial protrusion of meninges of spinal cord

spindle fibers (spin'-dul fi'-burs): during the second stage of mitosis (prophase), two centrioles start to separate towards the opposite ends (poles) of the cell. As the two centrioles migrate, cytoplasmic microtubules form between them–these are the spindle fibers

spindle fibers apparatus (spin'-dul fi'-burz ap''-uh-ray'-tus): structure formed during cell division to help distribute chromosomes to opposite ends of the dividing cell; comprised of the astral rays, centrioles, and the spindle fibers in animal cell mitosis

spondylitis (spon''-di-lye'-tis): inflammation of the vertebrae

spondylolisthesis (spon''-di-lo-lis-thees'-is): forward displacement of one vertebra upon the one below it; commonly occurs between the fifth lumbar vertebra and the sacrum, or the fourth lumbar over the fifth lumbar vertebra

sprain (sprain): wrenching of a joint, producing a stretching or laceration of ligaments

stapes (stay'-peez): stirrup-shaped bone in middle ear

steapsin (stee-ap'-sin): pancreatic lipase

sternum (stur'-num): flat, narrow bone in median line in front of chest, composed of three parts: manubrium, body, and xiphoid process

stethoscope (steth'-uh-skope): instrument used for detection and study of sounds arising within body

subluxation (sub''-luck-say'-shun): incomplete dislocation

sudoriferous (sue''-dur-if'-ur-us): producing perspiration

superior (sue-peer'-ee-ur): in anatomy, higher; denoting upper of two parts, toward vertex

supination (sue''-pih-nay'-shun): turning of palm of hand upward, condition of being supine (lying on back)

surfactant (sur-fack'-tunt): surface-active agent

suture (sue'-chur): (1) in osteology, a line of connection or closure between bones, as in a cranial suture. (2) in surgery, a fine thread–like catgut or silk–used to repair or close a wound

synapse (sin'-aps): space between adjacent neurons through which an impulse is transmitted

syncytium (sin-sish'-ee-um): mass of cytoplasm with numerous nuclei

synovia (si-no'-vee-uh): viscid fluid present in joint cavities

synthesis (sinth'-e-sis): in chemistry, processes and operations necessary to build up a compound; in general, a reaction, or series of reactions, in which a complex compound is obtained from elements or simple compounds

systole (sis'-tuh-lee): contraction of ventricles, forcing blood into aorta and pulmonary artery

T

tachycardia (tack''-i-kahr'-dee-uh): abnormally rapid heartbeat

tachypnea (tack''-i-nee'-uh): abnormally rapid rate of breathing

talus (tay'-lus): ankle bone that articulates with bones of leg

tarsus (tahr'-sus): instep

Tay-Sachs disease (tay-saks'): genetic mutation caused by lack of a particular enzyme (hexosaminidase) needed for the breakdown of lipid molecules in the brain. Without the enzyme, lipids accumulate in the brain cells and destroy them, resulting in mental and motor deterioration. Tay-Sachs disorder is found most frequently among Jewish people of Central European ancestry. It appears before one year of age. Death occurs within several years

tendon (ten'-dun): cord of fibrous connective tissue that attaches a muscle to a bone or other structure

tetanus (tet'-uh-nus): infectious disease, usually fatal, characterized by spasm of voluntary muscles and convulsions caused by toxin from tetanus bacillus (clostridium tetani)

thoracocentesis (thor''-ruh-ko-sen-tee'-sis): aspiration of chest cavity for removal of fluid, usually for empyema

thorax (tho'-racks): chest; portion of trunk above diaphragm and below neck

thrombin (throm'-bin): enzyme found in blood; produced from an inactive precursor, prothrombin, inducing clotting by converting fibrinogen to fibrin

thrombosis (throm-bo'-sis): formation of a clot in a blood vessel

thyroxine (thigh-rock'-seen): hormone secreted by thyroid gland or prepared synthetically; contains about 64% iodine

tibia (tib'-ee-uh): larger, inner bone of the leg, below the knee

tinnitis (tin-i'-tus): ringing sensation in one or both ears

trait (trate'): any characteristic, feature, quality, or property of an organism

transmit (tranz'-mit): to pass on to another person, place, or thing

transverse (trans-vurce'): crosswise; at right angles to longitudinal axis of body

triceps (trye'-seps): (1) three-headed, (2) muscle having three heads, as triceps brachii

trypsin (trip'-sin): one of four protein-digesting enzymes found in pancreatic juice

trypsinogen (trip-sin'-uh-jen): the inactive form of trypsin. In the small intestine, trypsinogen is converted to trypsin by the influence of enterokinase, an intestinal enzyme that is secreted by glands lining the small intestine

tunica albuginea (tew'-ni-kuh al-bew-jin'-ee-uh): fibrous tissue covering the testes

turbinate (tur'-bin-ut): shaped like a spiral; the three bones situated on the lateral side of the nasal cavity

tympanic membrane (tim-pan'-ick mem'-brane): membrane that separates the external ear from the middle ear; consists of three layers: an outer skin layer, a fibrous layer, and an inner mucous layer

tympanum (tim'-puh-num): drum; middle ear closed externally by the ear drum

U

ulcer (ul'-sur): an inflammation that occurs on the mucosal skin surface

ulna (ul'-nuh): bone on inner forearm

umbilicus (um-bil'-i-kus): navel

unicellular (you"-ni-sel'-yoo-lur): composed of one cell

unilateral (you"-ni-lat'-ur-ul): pertaining to, or affecting, one side

universal recipient (you"-ni-vur'-sul re-sip'-ee-unt): individual belonging to AB blood group

urethra (you-ree'-thruh): passageway through which urine moves out of the body; extends from the neck of the urinary bladder to the external urethral opening

uvula (you'-vew-luh): projection hanging from soft palate, in back of throat

V

vacuole (vack'-yoo-ole): (1) clear space in cell, (2) cavity bound by a single membrane; usually a storage area for fat, glycogen, secretions, liquid, or debris

vagina (va-jie'-nuh): sheathlike structure; tube in females, extending from the uterus to the vulva

vaginismus (vadj"-i-niz'-mus): painful spasm of the vagina

vaginitis (vadj"-i-nigh'-tis): inflammation of the vagina

valve (valv): structure which permits flow of a fluid in only one direction

varicose veins (var'-i-koce vains): veins that have become abnormally dilated and tortuous, due to interference with venous drainage or weakness of their walls

vasopressin (vay"-zo-pres'-in): hormone secreted by the posterior pituitary gland; has an antidiuretic effect. Also called antidiuretic hormone (ADH)

vein (vane): vessel which carries blood toward the heart

ventral (ven'-trul): front or anterior; opposite of posterior or dorsal

ventricle (ven'-trik-ul): small cavity or chamber, as in heart or brain

venule (ven'-yool): small vein

vermiform appendix (vur'-mi-form a-pen'-dicks): small, blind gut projecting from cecum

vermis (vur'-mis): lobe in the middle part of the brain; connects the two cerebellar hemispheres

vesiculitis (ve-sick"-you-lye'-tis): inflammation of the seminal vesicles

villi (vil'-eye): hairlike projections, as in intestinal mucous membrane

viscera (vis'-er-a): internal organs

vitamin (vye'-tuh-min): any of a group of organic compounds found in very small amounts in natural food; needed for the normal growth and maintenance of an organism

vitreous humor (vit'-ree-us hew'-mur): transparent, gelatin-like substance filling greater part of eyeball

voluntary (vol'-un-terr"-ee): under control of the will

W

white muscle (white mus'-ul): skeletal muscle that appears paler in fresh state than red muscle

whooping cough (hoop'-ing kof): infectious disease characterized by repeated coughing attacks that end in a "whooping" sound; caused by the Bordet Gengou bacillus. Whooping cough is often fatal to very young infants. Also called pertussis

wisdom tooth (wiz'-dum tooth): third molar tooth in adult mouth

Z

zona pellucida (so'-nuh pe-lew'-si-duh): thick, solid, elastic envelope of ovum

zygote (zye'-gote): organism produced by union of two gametes

Index